Performing Time

Performing Time

Synchrony and Temporal Flow in Music and Dance

Edited by
CLEMENS WÖLLNER AND JUSTIN LONDON

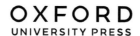

OXFORD
UNIVERSITY PRESS

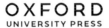

OXFORD
UNIVERSITY PRESS

Great Clarendon Street, Oxford, OX2 6DP,
United Kingdom

Oxford University Press is a department of the University of Oxford.
It furthers the University's objective of excellence in research, scholarship,
and education by publishing worldwide. Oxford is a registered trade mark of
Oxford University Press in the UK and in certain other countries

Published in the United States of America by Oxford University Press
198 Madison Avenue, New York, NY 10016, United States of America

British Library Cataloguing in Publication Data

Data available

Library of Congress Control Number: 2022945553

ISBN 978–0–19–289625–4

DOI: 10.1093/oso/9780192896254.001.0001

Printed and bound by
CPI Group (UK) Ltd, Croydon, CR0 4YY

Oxford University Press makes no representation, express or implied, that the
drug dosages in this book are correct. Readers must therefore always check
the product information and clinical procedures with the most up-to-date
published product information and data sheets provided by the manufacturers
and the most recent codes of conduct and safety regulations. The authors and
the publishers do not accept responsibility or legal liability for any errors in the
text or for the misuse or misapplication of material in this work. Except where
otherwise stated, drug dosages and recommendations are for the non-pregnant
adult who is not breast-feeding

Links to third party websites are provided by Oxford in good faith and
for information only. Oxford disclaims any responsibility for the materials
contained in any third party website referenced in this work.

Acknowledgements

We are grateful to Edith Van Dyck, Jane Ginsborg, Roger Mathew Grant, Devin McAuley (external reviewers), Isabelle Gabolde (assistant to Kent Nagano), Martin Baum and Jade Dixon at Oxford University Press, Geoffrey McDonald, and Kai Siedenburg for suggestions and their time in the preparation of this book.

Contents

SECTION 4. PERFORMANCE TIME EXPERIENCED: ATTENTION, EXPECTATION, AND GROOVE

Abbreviations

AM	apparent motion
BPM	beats per minute
BPS	beat perception and synchronization
DAT	Dynamic Attending Theory
EEG	electroencephalography
ERAN	early right anterior negativity
ESM	experience sampling methodology
GIG	Group Improvisation Game
IDyoM	Information Dynamics of Music
IOI	inter-onset interval
IOS	Inclusion of Other in the Self
ISC	intersubject correlation
MG	mirror game
MRI	magnetic resonance imaging
PoT	passage of time
PPT	preferred perceptual tempo
QoM	quantity of motion
SET	subjective experience of time
SMH	somatic marker hypothesis
SMT	spontaneous motor tempo
TAE	tempo anchoring effect

Contributors

Luc Arnal
Institut Pasteur, France

Richard Ashley
Northwestern University, USA

Asaf Bachrach
EUR ArTec Paris and UMR 7023 CNRS/
Paris, France

Laura Bishop
University of Oslo, Norway

Bettina Bläsing
Technical University Dortmund, Germany

Tanor Bonin
McGill University, Canada

Birgitta Burger
University of Hamburg, Germany

Renee M. Conroy
Purdue University Northwest, USA

Stewart A. Copeland

Simone Dalla Bella
BRAMS, University of Montreal, Canada

Henry Daniel
Simon Fraser University, Canada

Anne Danielsen
University of Oslo, Norway

Roger Dean
Western Sydney University, Australia

Keith Doelling
Institut Pasteur, France

Sylvie Droit-Volet
Université Clermont Auvergne, CNRS
6024, France

Werner Goebl
University of Music and Performing Arts
Vienna, Austria

David Hammerschmidt
University of Hamburg, Germany

Russell Hartenberger
University of Toronto, Canada

Mari Romarheim Haugen
University of Oslo, Norway

Molly J. Henry
Max Planck Institute for Empirical Aesthetics,
Germany

Sophie Herbst
Université Paris-Sud and Université Paris-
Saclay, France

Tommi Himberg
Aalto University, Finland

Michael J. Hove
Fitchburg State University, USA

Alexander Refsum Jensenius
University of Oslo, Norway

Coline Joufflineau
Paris 1 Panthéon-Sorbonne, France

Kristina L. Knowles
Arizona State University, USA

Sonja A. Kotz
Maastricht University, The Netherlands

Mariusz Kozak
Columbia University, USA

Julien Laroche
EUR ArTec Paris, France, and Instituto
Italiano di Tecnologia, Ferrara, Italy

Marc Leman
Ghent University, Belgium

Daniel J. Levitin
McGill University, Canada

Justin London
Carleton College, USA

Psyche Loui
Northeastern University, USA

Guy Madison
Umea University, Sweden

Pieter-Jan Maes
Ghent University, Belgium

Natalia Martinelli
Université Clermont Auvergne, CNRS
6024, France

Stephen McAdams
McGill University, Canada

Kent Nagano
Hamburg State Opera, Germany

Jason Noble
Université de Montréal, Canada

Anna Pakes
University of Roehampton, UK

Jan Stupacher
Aarhus University and The Royal Academy of
Music Aarhus/Aalborg, Denmark

Petri Toiviainen
University of Jyväskylä, Finland

Virginie van Wassenhove
Université Paris-Sud and Université Paris-
Saclay, France

Peter Vuust
Aarhus University and The Royal Academy of
Music Aarhus/Aalborg, Denmark

Marc Wittmann
Institute for Frontier Areas of Psychology and
Mental Health Freiburg, Germany

Clemens Wöllner
University of Hamburg, Germany

Matthew H. Woolhouse
McMaster University, Canada

Introduction to *Performing Time*

Clemens Wöllner and Justin London

For millennia, people have thought and written about time: its fundamental nature, how we perceive and experience it, and how we organize our lives in temporal contexts ranging from minutes to days to lifetimes. For the most part, our experience of time seems natural, as it relates to the rhythms of both our planet and our bodies, so that individuals not only share roughly comparable day–night cycles of sleep and wakefulness, and of the coming of the seasons, but on a more local timescale we naturally gravitate towards preferred speeds for walking, clapping, dancing, or singing.

Recent advances in psychology, neuroscience, and philosophy have elucidated the factors that shape our dynamic, lived experiences of time. The performing arts, and music and dance in particular, provide rich contexts for the study of time, as they foreground our awareness of time and have been empirically shown to change our sense of time. Both dance and music rely on synchronization with auditory events and with other people. They both involve memory and anticipation in audiences and performers, and both facilitate moments of flow and pleasure. Time is at the heart of music and dance, and in this volume we present some of the conceptual and methodological tools currently being used to investigate time in these performing arts.

I.1 Chasing Gibson's Ghosts

James J. Gibson famously stated that 'events are perceivable, but time is not' (Gibson, 1975), a claim that we have no direct perception of time. This was the temporal analogue to his claim regarding visual perception, namely, that we do not have a direct perception of space, although we often talk as if we do. Rather, the visual field presents to our sensory system a set of surfaces, and we come to understand the layout of the world from the information contained in the light we perceive that is reflected from those surfaces. As Gibson (1975) pithily summed it up:

> There is no such thing as the perception of time, but only the perception of events and locomotions. These events and locomotions, moreover, do not occur in space but in the medium of an environment that is rigid and permanent. Abstract space is a sort of ghost of the surfaces of the world, and abstract time is a ghost of the events of the world. (p. 295)

Clemens Wöllner and Justin London, *Introduction to* Performing Time In: *Performing Time*. Edited by: Clemens Wöllner and Justin London, Oxford University Press. © Oxford University Press 2023. DOI: 10.1093/oso/9780192896254.003.0001

Music and dance involve sonic events and bodily locomotion, and in both music and dance we are seemingly aware of space and time as conveyed by the steps of the dancers, the physical actions of the musicians, and the temporally bound sounds they create. In our ordinary, everyday experiences of the world we interact with its surfaces, in terms of our reach and grasp, and sense of near and far. We also interact with events in the world, in terms of our sense of things happening successively or simultaneously, or taking a long time or a short time. Yet when we dance or sing, or go to a ballet or a jazz club, dance and music give us a strong sense of what space and time themselves may be like, even if we cannot perceive them directly. To extend Gibson's metaphor, music and dance animate the ghosts of time and space.

Often the spatial and temporal animations of music and dance correspond to our experience of movements and sounds in everyday contexts; for example, a dancer's steps may be akin to walking, or the repeated chords of a pianist akin to the blows of a carpenter's hammer. Sometimes, however, dance and music can make us acutely aware of space and especially time. In the context of dance, there is the agonizing slowness of movement in Butoh, or the time-stretching choreography of Myriam Gourfink. In music, such slowness has its analogues in the durational extremes of the long-sustained chords of Morton Feldman's *Triadic Memories* for solo piano, Leif Inge's time-stretched version of Beethoven's Ninth Symphony, which lasts 24 hr, and in the most extreme case, John Cage's *Organ²/ASLAP (As Slow as Possible)* for organ, the performance of which began in a church in Halberstadt, Germany, in 2001, and will conclude in the year 2640.

Other pieces of music and dance can involve extreme amounts of repetition, a hallmark of minimalist music of the sort composed by Philip Glass and Steve Reich. Reich's *Violin Phase* involves not only repetition but also problems of simultaneity, as a musical figure constantly slips in and out of sync with itself over the course of the piece. It was choreographed by Anne Teresa de Keersmaeker, whose dance embodies the repetition and phasing of the musical figure that moves in place (see Kozak, 2021, for a discussion of time in de Keersmaeker's performance and choreography). An example of a repetitive piece of music predating those of Glass and Reich is the notorious Vexations by Erik Satie, from his *Pages Mystiques* (1893). This consists of four 8-bar phrases repeated 840 times; a complete performance takes approximately 18 hr. The music theorist and composer Jonathan Kramer reported on his experience of the piece:

> When I first entered the concert, I listened linearly [i.e. hearing one note following from and leading to another]. But I soon exhausted the information content of the work. It became totally redundant. For a brief period I found myself getting bored, becoming imprisoned by a hopelessly repetitious piece. Time was getting slower and slower, threatening to stop. But then I found myself moving into a different listening mode . . . was no longer bored, and I was no longer frustrated, because I had given up expecting . . . After what seemed like forty minutes, I left. My watch told me I had listened for three hours. (Kramer, 1988, p. 379)

I.2 Chasing Gibson's Ghosts in the Laboratory

Understanding how we comprehend the timing of events in the world has preoccupied scientists as well as musicians and dancers. From the earliest days of modern psychology, researchers have sought to document and test the human capacity for the perception of order, synchrony, duration, and continuity, for it is from our perception of these things that we are able to make inferences regarding the nature of time, and articulate our experience of it. These studies—from the first psychophysical experiments of Wundt and Stumpf to more recent neuroscientific studies of temporal processing in the brain—have repeatedly shown that our perception of sound, motion, and time is not always veridical, and various temporal illusions are often due to interactions among our sensory modalities, memories, and cognitive processing.

Many of these illusions and misperceptions involve the coordination of actions with sounds, one of the fundamental activities in both music and dance. Studies of sensorimotor synchronization have shown that the simple task of tapping along with a metronome typically gives rise to a 'negative mean asynchrony' such that, on average, we tend to tap ahead of the metronome click even if we think we are perfectly synchronized (Repp & Su, 2013). Studies in audiovisual perception have shown we have a tolerance for and can adapt to asynchronies in putatively simultaneous events perceived in audition versus vision, for example, when the sound and image tracks of a film are slightly misaligned (Cohen, 2013; Dixon & Spitz, 1980). Other auditory-visual temporal illusions are well documented. These include the oddball effect (a different stimulus in a series of otherwise identical stimuli seems to last longer), the flash-lag illusion (whereby two stimuli presented at the same time, one moving and the other stationary, appear to occur non-simultaneously, the stationary flash lagging behind that of the moving stimulus), and the tau and kappa effects, where larger visual distances and longer temporal durations are confounded, to name but a few (see Arstilla et al., 2019, for an overview and discussion).

Thus, even if we cannot perceive time directly, *pace* Gibson, more than a century of psychological research has probed our sensitivities and abilities with respect to our perception of the order, synchrony, duration, and continuity among events in the world. This research has shown that our perception of these aspects of temporality is fallible and therefore subject to misapprehension, such that music and dance might be called the arts that shape and manipulate our sense of time.

I.3 The Background and Organization of This Volume

A conference entitled 'Time Changes in Experiences of Music and Dance' was hosted in November 2019 by the Institute for Systematic Musicology at the University of

Hamburg, bringing together researchers in dance, musicology, psychology, and neuroscience to discuss and explore the intersections between time in music and dance. The current volume *Performing Time* was conceived as a way of continuing the dialogue between these disciplines.

The book is organized in five sections that aim to capture the many facets of time in dance and music, both performed and perceived. 'Anchor' chapters in each section provide an overview of research, discuss current developments, and suggest potential future studies, while shorter 'focus' chapters present case studies or highlight specifically defined areas of recent research. Section 1 lays the foundations of the book by providing an overview of the state of the art in time research from the perspectives of dance science, musicology, neuroscience, and psychology. Section 2 addresses tempo as one of the main components of perceived time, as well as duration and pacing in music and dance genres. Here, the many parallels between music and dance become particularly evident. Section 3 contains chapters tackling the vast amount of research into synchrony, from entrainment and joint dance improvisations to the levels of social cohesion that can be reached through interactions involving music and dance. Section 4 focuses on experiential qualities in the temporal domain, including a range of topics from experiences of groove and time dilations to what constitutes a 'boring dance'. Finally, Section 5 includes chapters by scientists as well as renowned musicians and a dancer/choreographer, reflecting on how the art and practice of music and dance can inform research into the nature of time and time perception, and vice versa.

In Section 1, Chapter 1 examines dance from an embodied perspective. Bettina Bläsing (Dortmund, Germany) provides an overview of empirical research into the interdependencies of time, rhythmic structures, and the temporal dynamics of the performers' bodies that shape the perception of and memory for dance, for both dancers and spectators. The temporalities of music are discussed in Chapter 2 by Mariusz Kozak (New York, USA). Drawing on psychological and philosophical accounts, he argues that subjective time and lived time do not necessarily align with objective time, and that these differences are reflected in our musical experiences. Chapter 3 by Keith Doelling, Sophie Herbst, Luc Arnal, and Virginie van Wassenhove (Paris, France) presents the neuroscientific and psychological foundations of time perception, focusing on how the processing of temporal structures and, more specifically, rhythm, is organized in the brain. They show how in our performance and perception of music and dance, exogenous rhythms are coupled with both internally and endogenously driven temporal processes, leading to distinct brain rhythms with consequences for synchronized behaviour between individual performers as well as audience members. In Chapter 4, Sylvie Droit-Volet and Natalia Martinelli (Clermont-Ferrand, France) provide an overview of recent psychological research on temporal experience and judgement, with an emphasis on how we feel the passage of time, from past years to present durations. Their work shows that we typically feel time passing faster when engaging in activities such as listening to music and watching dance.

Section 2 starts with the first of three anchor chapters, Chapter 5 by Justin London (Northfield, USA) on musical tempo. On the basis of energistic and embodied accounts, he argues that tempo is a distillation of multiple perceptual cues rooted in memory and bodily affordances, which has consequences for both music and dance. In Chapter 6, Renee Conroy (Hammond, USA) discusses visual, physical, and artistic pacing in dance from the perspectives of audiences, dancers, and choreographers. She presents examples of major contemporary dance works that illustrate aesthetically meaningful discontinuities in time, which she calls 'temporal disconnect' and 'temporal dissonance'. The third anchor chapter, Chapter 7, by Molly Henry (Frankfurt, Germany) and Sonja Kotz (Maastricht, The Netherlands), scrutinizes the topics of temporal flow and one's individual sense of time. They review behavioural and neuroscientific studies, with a particular focus on preferred rate and coupling processes that shape joint behaviours in artistic contexts and beyond.

The four focus chapters in Section 2 offer insights into recent case studies and research projects in tempo and pacing. In Chapter 8, Coline Joufflineau (Paris, France) contributes a case study of very slow dance works by the French choreographer Myriam Gourfink, while in Chapter 9, Alexander Refsum Jensenius (Oslo, Norway) describes experiences of 'standstill' (literally, standing as still as possible for 10 minor more) and the measurement of micromotion in a year-long artistic research project. David Hammerschmidt (Hamburg, Germany) focuses on spontaneous motor tempo in Chapter 10 and presents a large international study and a longitudinal study, and the final focus chapter, Chapter 11 by Mari Romarheim Haugen (Oslo, Norway), explores embodied interdependencies between music and dance, relating body motion to the complex rhythmic periodicities found in one particular genre of Norwegian folk music and dance.

Section 3, on synchrony in music and dance, also comprises three anchor and four focus chapters. In Chapter 12, Guy Madison (Umea, Sweden) scrutinizes the phenomena of entrainment and sensorimotor synchronization that are based on the perception of hierarchically organized regularities in time. Humans share basic neural structures with other species for entrainment, yet human prediction and adaptation are more complex temporal processes that are required for the temporally coordinated actions in music and dance. The second anchor chapter, Chapter 13, by Werner Goebl (Vienna, Austria) and Laura Bishop (Oslo, Norway), extends this research in describing the psychological underpinnings of musical ensemble performance. Adapting to a musical partner may lead to more prototypical performances in terms of microtiming. At the same time, synchronization with each other by means of auditory and visual communication channels may afford feelings of togetherness that are socially rewarding. Synchronization in dance ensembles is tackled in the third anchor chapter, Chapter 14, by Julien Laroche (Paris, France), Tommi Himberg (Helsinki, Finland), and Asaf Bachrach (Paris, France). They explore the multiple timescales that underlie temporally organized behaviours. Rather than referring to some objective clock-time, they argue that joint experiences of time are created together through bodily actions. Collective, rule-based dance improvisations are provided as an example for such temporally organized social interactions.

The focus chapters in Section 3 describe synchronization in music and dance, including Chapter 15 by Birgitta Burger (Hamburg, Germany) and Petri Toiviainen (Jyväskylä, Finland), who used motion capture methods for studying the shape and timing of dance movements in relation to the sound qualities of the music, and Chapter 16 by Simone Dalla Bella (Montreal, Canada), who focuses on individual differences in synchronization abilities and their possible neurodevelopmental bases. Chapter 17 by Anne Danielsen (Oslo, Norway) sheds light on the temporal windows for perceived beats in electronic music genres and the implications of these 'beat bins' for groove perception and synchronization more generally, while Matthew Woolhouse (Hamilton, Canada) in Chapter 18 investigates social bonding through temporally aligned versus non-aligned dancing, and the roles of both auditory and visual cues in social dance contexts.

Section 4 addresses experiential dimensions of time and begins with an anchor chapter by Clemens Wöllner (Freiburg, Germany), who in Chapter 19 discusses the implications of temporal thresholds for perceiving auditory events, from microseconds to larger structures in music, in relation to event detection, memory, and synchronization. He also summarizes recent empirical research into the factors leading to time dilations in music, such as arousal, tempo, and complexity. The second anchor chapter, Chapter 20, was written by Pieter-Jan Maes and Marc Leman (Ghent, Belgium) and discusses expressive timing in music and dance from an embodied perspective. Drawing on research into perception-action coupling, they investigate multiple timescales for temporal experiences, from beat-to-beat sensorimotor synchronization to the larger-scale narrative of expressive timing that is crucial for intentional, goal-directed social interactions. In Chapter 21, Psyche Loui (Boston, USA) takes a closer look at temporal aspects of expectation and its role in musical improvisation. While perception–action coupling is also at the core of her expectancy model, she includes computational, neuroscientific, and psychological perspectives with the goal of bringing together time-based research into the study of improvisation.

The four focus chapters in Section 4 describe studies of different experiences of time in music and dance. In Chapter 22, Anna Pakes (London, UK) discusses why some dance performances may be experienced as boring, and emphasizes the role of time in such perceptions. Jason Noble, Tanor Bonin (both Montreal, Canada), Roger Dean (Sydney, Australia), and Stephen McAdams (Montreal, Canada) conducted empirical case studies of time experiences when listening to Grisey's *Vortex Temporum* (Chapter 23) while Kristina Knowles (Tempe, USA) and Richard Ashley (Evanston, USA) employed a continuous-response method to study the effects of time seeming to pass faster or slower when listening to several other 20th-century compositions (Chapter 24). In Chapter 25, Jan Stupacher (Aarhus, Denmark), Michael Hove (Fitchburg, USA), and Peter Vuust (Aarhus, Denmark) investigate groove, flow, and pleasure, and show that temporally surprising elements may increase groove experiences.

The final section of the book includes reflections on time in music and dance from a distinguished group of artists and scientists: neuroscientists and time researchers (Marc Wittmann and Daniel Levitin), a choreographer (Henry Daniel), a conductor (Kent Nagano), and two percussionists (Russell Hartenberger and Stewart Copeland). The contributors to Section 5 read a selection of chapters from the book, which served as a springboard for their comments and observations in their own chapters or conversations. In Chapter 26, Marc Wittmann (Freiburg, Germany) discusses 'What the psychology and neuroscience of time can learn from the performing arts' and argues that dance and music do not only provide valid stimuli for experiments but are also prime examples of how time is processed in an embodied, dynamic way. Defining temporal processing from micro to macro levels, he claims that the study of both audiences' and performers' lived experiences in music or dance may be a window into consciousness. In Chapter 27, Russell Hartenberger (Toronto, Canada) draws on his vast experience of performing music in Western and non-Western genres, including playing with Sharda Sahai and Steve Reich, and his insights into psychology and music theory, to answer the question of what constitutes musical time. In particular, he focuses on learning to play in time, and on time perspectives in different cultures. Henry Daniel (Burnaby, Canada; in conversation with Justin London), in Chapter 28, reflects on how concepts of time and temporal experience from physics and psychology have influenced his thinking as both a dancer and a choreographer. In Chapter 29, Kent Nagano (Hamburg, Germany; in conversation with Clemens Wöllner) emphasizes the special moment in time when a performance unfolds in an ensemble, and reflects on his vast experiences preparing orchestras to perform. Finally, in Chapter 30, Steward Copeland (Los Angeles, USA) and Daniel Levitin (San Francisco, USA) discuss temporal processes, movement, rhythm, and timing based on their performance experiences and on neuropsychological research, and describe what it means for humans to be together on the beat.

1.4 Conclusion: Time in Music, Time in Dance, and Time in Music and Dance

In dancing or playing a piece of music, issues of order, synchrony, duration, and continuity are inevitable and constant. Music and dance require that certain sounds, steps, and gestures occur at the same time (or not at the same time), that they should take a certain amount of time, and should be more or less connected. Expert musicians and dancers, then, represent some of the most highly skilled examples of human timing behaviour and sensitivity; musicians and dancers could be termed experts in time. Music and dance are therefore a natural laboratory for the study of timing, time perception, and temporal awareness.

Similarly, audiences take note of musicians' and dancers' temporal acuity. Our aesthetic appreciation of these arts and the skills of those who perform them is grounded in our appreciation of the precision with which they coordinate their actions and control the succession of events. Investigating not just what musicians and dancers can do, but also how audiences apprehend and respond to what they do is an important context for the study of timing and time perception. Furthermore, actively dancing and making music even at non-expert levels may change one's experience of time, and can give rise to a sense of flow, defined by Csíkszentmihályi (1990) as losing one's sense of time by being completely absorbed in a task.

But why study time in music and dance *together*, as we do in this volume? The answer is simple, and obvious: dance often involves music, and much music is directly or indirectly written for dancing, or derived from dance-based genres. Indeed, in many contexts we should not refer to works and genres as music or dance, but as music–dance works and genres (see Haugen, this volume). Even music that seems not directly related to dance has a connection through its basic pulse and metre, as almost any piece of music with a beat could be used for dancing. We are studying them together because, in practice, they are together. Indeed, pulling them apart is a distortion of our normative experience of music, dance, and time. The chapters in this volume shed light on the complexities of time research, by placing it in valid contexts that facilitate aesthetic, emotional, and association-rich experiences, and they raise a number of crucial questions for further enquiry.

References

Arstilla, V., Bardon, A., Power, S. E., & Vatakis, A. (Eds.) (2019). *The illusions of time: Philosophical and psychological essays on timing and time perception.* Springer/Palgrave-MacMillan.

Cohen, A. J. (2013). Congruence-Association Model of music and multimedia: Origin and evolution. In S.-L. Tan, A. J. Cohen, S. D. Lipscomb, & R. A. Kendall (Eds.), *The psychology of music in multimedia* (pp. 17–47). Oxford University Press.

Csíkszentmihályi, M. (1990). *Flow: The psychology of optimal experience.* Harper & Row.

Dixon, N. F., & Spitz, L. (1980). The detection of auditory visual desynchrony. *Perception, 9*(6), 719–721. https://doi.org/10.1068/p090719

Gibson, J. J. (1975). Events are perceivable, but time is not. In J. T. Fraser & N. Lawrence (Eds.), *The study of time II* (pp. 295–301). Springer-Verlag.

Kozak, M. (2021). Anne Teresa De Keersmaeker's *Violin Phase* and the experience of time, or why does process music work? *Music Theory Online, 27*(2). https://doi.org/10.30535/mto.27.2.11

Kramer, J. (1988). *The time of music.* Schirmer.

Repp, B. H., & Su, Y.-H. (2013). Sensorimotor synchronization: A review of recent research (2006–2012). *Psychonomic Bulletin & Review, 20*(3), 403–452. https://doi.org/10.3758/s13423-012-0371-2

SECTION 1

FOUNDATIONS

The Flow of Time in Music and Dance

Anchor Chapters

1

Time Experiences in Dance

Bettina Bläsing

1.1 Introduction

Dance, as a fully embodied art form, is deeply anchored in space and time on many levels. Álvarez (2009) describes dance as 'the impermanent art par excellence', stating that dance performance is at a constant vanishing point for creators, performers, and spectators. She identifies four interacting layers of time relevant to dance performance (Álvarez, 2009): *real time* is the measured clock time that coincides with the natural duration of a dance performance; it is chronological and linear, the temporal domain of the dancers' bodies moving in space. *Fictional time* can occur as a deliberate manipulation of real time that is reorganized, compressed, or expanded to serve the presentation of a narrative (e.g. in *ballet d'action* like *The Nutcracker*). *Artificial time* is created intentionally by artistic means; it can be non-linear, non-metric, take other shapes and forms, or even appear as timelessness. *Psychological time* is subjectively experienced time, or the sense of time passing while engaging in an activity like dancing or watching a dance performance; it relates perceived information to memories. Even though psychological time is the main focus of this chapter, all four layers are closely connected and depend on each other for dancers, dance creators, and spectators alike.

Dance and music share common roots in human evolution. Both are ephemeral rhythmic behaviours involving temporal sequences of movement and pitch (Fink et al., 2021; Wang, 2015) with an inherent periodic component based on prediction (Jadoul et al., 2016). Although dance does not have to be accompanied by music, it remains 'musical in nature', a rhythmic behaviour that is based on musicality (Fink et al., 2021; Marcus, 2012). Time experiences related to music per se are the main topic of other parts of this book and will, therefore, not be addressed in this chapter. Yet, in dance, the relation of human motor action to a musical or rhythmic signal remains just as fundamental. Temporal structure in dance primarily arises from the interaction of two factors: the dynamics of the dancers' bodies and musical cues. In addition to body and movement perception, emotion has been identified as a fundamental factor in dance (Christensen & Calvo-Merino, 2013), and effects of emotion on time perception have also been systematically investigated (Droit-Volet & Meck, 2007). Therefore, from a psychological perspective, the human body in motion,

Bettina Bläsing, *Time Experiences in Dance* In: *Performing Time*. Edited by: Clemens Wöllner and Justin London, Oxford University Press. © Oxford University Press 2023. DOI: 10.1093/oso/9780192896254.003.0002 music, and emotion are all but inseparable from each other as factors influencing time experiences in dance (see Van Dyck et al., 2017).

Furthermore, there are two different perspectives to consider: that of the dancer, and that of the dance spectator. Dance has been described as communicative process in which the human body in motion conveys a message with emotional (and other) content that is then decoded by the spectator (Orgs et al., 2016). Dance provides a multimodal experience (Bläsing & Zimmermann, 2021), but vision remains the primary modality of this act of communication between dance artists as sender and the audience as receiver. For the exploration of time experiences in dance, both perspectives have to be taken into account. Information about the dancer's perspective often derives from personal reports. Factors influencing dancers' time perception while dancing include movement dynamics and their level of automatization; attention towards and interaction with partners; episodic memories and emotions; and rhythmic structures in music and movement (Bresnahan, 2017; Waterhouse et al., 2014). A recent line of research explores (non-dancer) participants' experiences while moving together with others in synchrony or rhythmic coordination, focusing on individual emotional and cultural effects arising from social dance scenarios (Himberg et al., 2018; Tarr et al., 2015, 2016).

With regard to the question of how dancers' movement affects spectators' perception of time, insights come from research investigating effects of moving stimuli on observers' perception of duration and passage of time. A complementary line of research has revealed that the perception of human bodies differs significantly from that of other moving objects, on both neurocognitive and behavioural levels (e.g. Blake & Shiffrar, 2007). Networks in the human brain have been identified that specifically process information about the actions or bodily expression of others, facilitating the prediction of others' intentions and the preparation of adequate reactions in social contexts (e.g. Grèzes et al., 2013; Vangeneugden et al., 2014). The aesthetic evaluation of the perceived movement is influenced by the observer's perceptual and motor experience, their background knowledge (Kirsch et al., 2015), the variability and predictability of the movement (Orlandi et al., 2020), the temporal coordination between dancers (Vicary et al., 2017), and by interactions between movement and music (Christensen et al., 2014; Orgs & Howlin, 2022).

This chapter will provide insights into time experiences while watching dance (Section 1.2) and while dancing (Section 1.3). It will consider different lines of empirical research in psychology and related disciplines, as well as dance artists' and scholars' perspectives. It does not claim to present a full account of how time is perceived in the context of dance; this topic is vast, given the central role time plays for dance as an art form, social activity, and form of communication. The aspects raised in this chapter may rather stimulate ideas, fostering further research and creative engagement with time experiences related to dance as it is presented throughout this book.

1.2 Time Experiences While Watching Dance

In recent decades, factors influencing spectators' perception of dance and processes underlying these effects have become a major topic of research (Bläsing et al., 2012; Sevdalis & Keller, 2011), and most of the identified factors and skills can be directly or indirectly linked to temporal processing. This section will take a closer look at (a) which characteristics of (dance-related) stimuli influence observers' judgement of duration under laboratory conditions; (b) how dancer's speed of movement affects spectators' time perception in live performance; (c) how slowness or arbitrariness of movement, as choreographic means of expression, challenges audiences' perception of time and self; and (d) real-time processes in perception that link the spontaneous segmentation of dance movement to long-term memory.

1.2.1 Time Effects of Real and Implied Motion

The extent to which different characteristics of a stimulus representing human body movement influence an observer's time perception has been studied extensively. A variety of factors have been identified, including stimulus type, intervals between static images presented sequentially, and participants' response tasks; however, the reported effects were often contradictory (see Sgouramani et al., 2019). Nather and colleagues (2011) presented images of Degas' ballerinas in body postures implying either considerable or no movement and asked participants to judge whether the presentation duration resembled a short or a long standard reference duration. Participants overestimated presentation durations for images implying considerable compared to no movement, in particular for shorter presentation durations. The authors attributed this finding to a transient short-term arousal effect elicited by the perceived movement intensity speeding up the internal clock system. In a complementary study, overestimation effects were observed for longer presentations (36 s) of images depicting dancers performing dynamic movements; this finding was interpreted with reference to change models, according to which duration judgements depend on the number of changes contained in the stimulus (Nather & Bueno, 2011). Orgs and colleagues (2011) presented static images of human body postures in an apparent motion task. Variations in sequence suggesting longer or shorter movement paths resulted in participants perceiving faster or slower movements, respectively. Duration estimations for the presentation of an additional frame stimulus were biased by the perceived speed of the apparent motion. The same applied when interstimulus intervals were varied in addition to apparent path length (Orgs et al., 2013), suggesting that the involvement of higher-order visual and motor areas produce a temporal bias.

Further studies in this field have compared implied and real motion stimuli. Sgouramani and colleagues (2019) presented video clips of a dancer performing ballet steps varying in movement intensity and static images of dynamic peak moments taken from the same video material. They hypothesized that video and static image stimuli would not differ with regard to observers' duration estimations, given their identical origin and the resulting equal number of (implied) changes. They also expected that movements of higher intensity would lead to more overestimation in both conditions. Unexpectedly, presentation duration was overestimated for the real compared to the implied motion stimuli, and time overestimation was linked to movement intensity only for the real motion stimuli. These results question the correspondence between real and implied motion of human bodies in the timing domain and point to a differentiation of movement and posture processing in visual working memory (Vicary et al., 2014; Vicary & Stevens, 2014). Sgouramani and Vatakis (2014) examined effects of movement speed and expertise on duration judgements. Dancer and non-dancer participants were asked to estimate the duration of ballet steps naturally performed at slow or fast speed, and presented at different time intervals, to control for stimulus changes. The authors expected to find a stronger overestimation of time for faster movement in a reproduction task and the reverse pattern in a production task, but, surprisingly, results showed the opposite pattern. It was concluded that attention must also be considered as a relevant factor, with higher stimulus speed being more attentionally demanding than lower speed. In a study by Allingham and colleagues (2020), participants were recorded moving at different speeds and later watched point-light displays of their own and others' movements. The effects of movement type and speed on duration estimation were stronger for others' than for own movements, supporting the theory that motor familiarity also influences the temporal processing of observed movement.

Taken together, in studies carried out under laboratory conditions, duration estimation was modified by perceived movement speed and intensity, mode of stimulus presentation, response task, attentional processes, and observers' expertise. Duration overestimation effects were stronger for real than implied movement and for higher compared to lower movement intensity, and overestimation was counteracted by stimulus familiarity. Effects, however, were too diverse to be explained by single models, suggesting that the perception of stimuli representing human motion involves a rather complex interaction of factors.

1.2.2 Speed of Movement in Live Dance Performance

While the findings discussed in the previous section contribute to the understanding of internal timing mechanisms of the perception of human motor action, their experimental scenarios nevertheless bear little resemblance to situations in which dance is typically presented. Among the factors influencing dance spectators' experience of time under real-world conditions are rich multimodal perception, the audiovisual spatial perspective, the presence of human bodies, and the social context of live performance. Together, these result in an immersive, fully embodied experience that facilitates empathy (Boucher, 2004; Reason & Reynolds, 2010). A small yet increasing number of empirical studies have used live performance scenarios with dancers presenting choreographed 'stimulus' material on stage.

In a study by Deinzer and colleagues (2017), participants watched live performances in which a dancer performed two short pieces that differed in speed of movement. After the performance, spectators completed questionnaires asking about their attentional focus, emotional reactions, and sense of self, space, and time during the performance. It was expected that time would be perceived as passing more quickly during the faster of two dance performances (see Wittmann, 2015). On average, participants preferred the faster dance piece and felt more positively aroused while watching it. They also focused more on the dancers' breathing and less on their own bodies during the fast dance. The performance mediated the perceived passage of time, but not the estimated duration of the performance (Deinzer et al., 2017). The contradictory finding that time seemed to pass more quickly during the fast dance performance even when it was estimated to have lasted longer was interpreted with reference to the concept of flow (Csikszentmihalyi, 1990). According to the literature on flow states, immersion in an activity can be coupled with intense enjoyment and an attenuated awareness of time and self, which might have resulted in the impression that 'time had flown by' during the fast dance performance. Hancock and colleagues (2019) point out that, while the perceived transformation of time is an important phenomenological representation of flow, time perception might be affected in different ways for the antecedents, characteristics, and consequences of flow (Csikszentmihalyi & Csikszentmihalyi, 1992), rather than simply representing 'one dimension of flow'.

In the study by Deinzer and colleagues (2017), audiences in the slow dance performance reported enhanced attention towards their own bodily signals, as well as to the passing of time. Attention to their own bodies mediated perceived time intensity and slowed down the perceived passage of time. Because participants also reported lower emotional well-being during the slow performance, the authors attributed these findings to boredom. While the awareness of time was modulated by attention to the bodily self, however, no direct relation was found between these factors and lower enjoyment of the performance. The proposed link between increased awareness of body and time, decreased well-being, and boredom can be called into question; indeed, there are situations in dance training and somatic practice in which an inward focus on bodily signals eliciting changes in time experience are considered desirable. Describing training practice in Butoh dance, Kasai and Parsons (2003) conceptualize social time and body time as two psychological modes that vary in perception. During a typical Butoh training session, a transition from social time to body time is achieved through a deep relaxation phase in which the awareness of bodily signals becomes intensified, enabling the dancers to 'notice authentic impulses, explore their dissonance from a socially conditioned or programmed response, and release the developed urge to suppress the motion' (Kasai & Parsons, 2003, p. 262). In the following section, choreographic approaches are presented that explore similar effects on audiences—applying extreme slowness or arbitrariness of movement.

1.2.3 Choreographing Time

While spectators might feel more positively engaged and aroused by faster movement (Deinzer et al., 2017), somatic states of contemplation in which subjective time is slowed down may also be experienced as meaningful and increase feelings of well-being. Watching slow movement or unexpected stillness can provoke intense somatic reactions and changes in time perception via kinaesthetic empathy (Reason & Reynolds, 2010). Myriam Gourfink has developed a choreographic style that makes use of extensive slowing down of movement to such a degree that the dancers appear almost static:

> Sometimes the dancers are almost immobile, or their movement is imperceptible for the spectator's eye, to the point that they can generate a blindness to change: the spectator is surprised to find out that the configuration of the bodies in space has changed without having perceived the movement itself. (Joufflineau & Bachrach, 2016, p. 96)

For dancers, keeping movement slow over long periods of time is extremely demanding (Burger & Wöllner, 2021). Gourfink's dancers' specific skill is based on regular training in 'energy yoga', a contemplative yoga style with an interoceptive focus of attention. Joufflineau and Bachrach (2016) describe the dancers' facial expression while dancing as not directed at the audience, but rather introversive, pensive, and absorbed in the task. In a series of studies, Joufflineau, Bachrach and colleagues explored audience reactions to live performances of Gourfink's choreographic works using a range of complementary measures, including somatic and emotional responses and aesthetics judgements. They found that spectators' time perception was significantly modified (Joufflineau et al., 2018; see also Joufflineau, this volume). While some spectators felt bored and perceived time as passing slowly, others reported a strong somatosensory experience, with long-lasting enhanced attention towards their own bodily sensations that caused them to experience performance time as passing very quickly. Spectators' increased attention to both their own and the dancers' breathing was associated with breath synchronization; their underestimation of performance duration was correlated with their enjoyment of the piece and engagement with their own breathing, as well as with the dancers' physical activity and muscular tension (Bachrach et al., 2015). The authors summarized the observed effects as the 'expansion of the "specious present" that is related to the slowing of physiological rhythms, and an attentional resonance between spectators and the choreography' (Joufflineau et al., 2018, p. 1).

Not only extreme slowness, but also other time-related anomalies of dancers' movement can elicit spectators' emotional reactions and modify their perception of time and bodily self. Álvarez (2009) describes her reactions to watching Merce Cunningham's choreography *Beach Birds*, in which the dancers move with arbitrary timing, like a flock of birds engaging in individual behaviours in which spectators might infer emergent patterns. Álvarez (2009) describes the time structure in this choreography as artificial, irregular, and unpredictable, eliciting in the audience a 'dynamic tension of movement and stillness' that evokes vaguely familiar moments. As spectator, she experiences a pleasurable attentive contemplation and feels 'actively engaged in a subjective experience inspired by the created temporal layers in the dance work but grounded on my past experiences'. Cunningham's choreography (informed by his partnership with composer John Cage) experimented with temporal structure, for example, by applying chance procedures in service of 'making the connection between the dance and the music one of individual autonomy connected at structural points' (Cunningham, 1952/ 1998, p. 39).

The previous two sections have focused on effects of dancers' timing and movement speed on spectators' sense of time, body, and self during live dance performance. As illustrated, these effects arise from choreographers' skills in creating fictional and artificial time, and their ability to integrate the dancers' actions with the spectators' memories (Álvarez, 2009). The following section will investigate more deeply the processes that connect real-time processing in watching dance with long-term memory.

1.2.4 Parsing and Encoding Dance

While watching dance, perception of time is modulated, not only by the dancers' movement speed and timing, but also by attention and memory-based processes that link the dancers' movements and the context in which these are presented to the observers' experience and knowledge. Temporal structure of complex movement material plays a crucial role in pedagogy and choreography; it determines how dance phrases are built up from basic elements, communicated to dancers, and perceived by spectators (deLahunta & Bernhard, 2005). Stevens (2017) summarizes: 'contextual and intellectual meaning enables movement material to be sequenced and chunked. Meaning, then, in connecting movement phrases and ideas, serves as a kind of cognitive glue. Meaningful material is remembered' (p. 50).

Insights into the interactions of real-time parsing and memory in dance perception can be gained from studies based on *Event Segmentation Theory* (Zacks et al., 2007). This line of research provides evidence that observers parse perceived scenarios into segments in real time, and that this spontaneous segmentation of the perceived stream of information is fundamental for the encoding and recall of the scenario (e.g. Sargent et al., 2013; Zacks et al., 2009). Crucial to Event Segmentation Theory is the idea that perception links sensory cues to knowledge structures in long-term memory. These serve action understanding, prediction of upcoming information, preparation for appropriate reactions, and learning. Boundaries between segments occur whenever the prediction of upcoming information is vague and anticipation errors become more frequent; at these instances, event models in working memory are updated based on incoming information, and learning takes place. Coarse- and fine-grained segmentation layers refer to levels of action organization, with coarse-grained segmentation layers mainly reflecting interactions with persons or objects, and fine-grained layers referring to kinematic and dynamic movement characteristics (Sargent et al., 2013; Zacks et al., 2009).

While most studies in this line of research used object-related tasks from everyday contexts, few studies have applied event segmentation paradigms to dance movement (Di Nota et al., 2020; Noble et al., 2014; Pollick et al., 2012). Bläsing (2015) presented a movement sequence from a video-recorded contemporary dance solo to professional dancers, advanced dance amateurs, and non-dancers. Only the dance amateurs participated twice, before and after learning the sequence. All participants marked segment boundaries while repeatedly watching the video clip on a computer screen. Professional dancers defined fewer segment boundaries (i.e. longer segments) than non-dancers, and showed a slight effect of visual familiarity by defining longer segments in earlier trials, whereas no such effect was found in the non-dancers. The difference between the amateurs' and the non-dancers' segment lengths increased from the amateurs' pre-learning to their post-learning condition, suggesting that their parsing became 'more expert' after they had gained motor experience of the movement. The results support the idea that successful action anticipation (due to domain-specific expertise or motor familiarity) reduces the number of segment boundaries perceived (Zacks et al., 2007). Post-experimental questionnaires revealed that segmentation criteria also varied with dance expertise. Only dancers and dance amateurs applied time-related segmentation criteria (speed, dynamics, impulses, accents), whereas non-dancers exclusively applied body-related and spatial criteria (body part, height level, direction). These findings suggest that kinematic information leading to rather fine-grained segmentation might be accessible to all observers, while dynamic information leading to broader segmentation might be accessible only to observers with dance experience, via enhanced motor simulation.

The second section of this chapter has aimed to provide selected findings on spectators' perception of time while watching dance. Laboratory studies using human motion stimuli resulted in diverse findings—corroborating, expanding, or even contradicting comparable studies using non-human stimuli. In live dance performance, even more factors might affect spectators' perception of time, including kinaesthetic empathy, states of arousal or flow, and awareness of own bodily signals, all of which can result in strong emotional reactions. Appealing to these reactions, choreographers can create artificial or fictional time experiences, using speed and the temporal relation of movement to modify audiences' perception.

1.3 Time Experiences While Dancing

While the second section of this chapter has addressed temporal aspects of dance perception from the spectator's perspective, this section is dedicated to dancers' own experiences of time while dancing. Although time perception is fundamental to the creation and execution of choreographic work, there is little empirical research exploring dancers' (as opposed to observers') sense of time. For the dancer, who is confined in real time by the physical body moving in space, psychological time can be shaped by diverse factors: the degree of automatization in movement dynamics, attention (both towards other dancers and relevant cues), episodic memories and emotions, and rhythmic structures (both in music and movement). It is, therefore, not surprising that dancers' perception of time while dancing has been described as multilayered and even, at times, contradictory (e.g. Bresnahan, 2017). Experiences of 'time while dancing' will be addressed in the following, with reference to empirical findings as well as individual artists' and scholars' perspectives, focusing on (a) dancers' sense of time and timing abilities; (b) time perception while dancing together and underlying processes of entrainment; and (c) experiences of synchrony and togetherness in social or club dancing scenarios.

1.3.1 Timing Movement Beyond Thinking in Eights

Adapting one's own movement to counts that refer to a musical rhythm., is a skill learned by dancers from the beginning of their training. Valerie Preston-Dunlop (cf. Álvarez, 2009) points out that dancers can perceive time phenomenally from the inside—feeling and strengthening 'the now'—as well as objectively, organizing it from the outside with counts. Mary Wigman (1963, p. 44) elaborates on the omnipresence of counts in dance, as a means of coordinating the 'two languages' of dance and music: 'The musicians count, and the dancers count. And often one counts past one another. Because the musicians count in the sense of the musical line, while the dancers get to the number from the rhythm of the physical movement.' Dancers are indeed experts in adapting the 'rhythm of the physical movement' to musical cues. Empirical studies corroborate that dancers are, compared to non-dancers, more precise and consistent at synchronizing full body movement or gestures to an external beat, music, or other dancers. Honisch and colleagues (2009) showed that ballet dancers synchronized their movement with greater accuracy to both temporal cues and others' movements than dance novices. Dancers' movement synchronization was better for familiar than for less familiar movements, and more accurate when they aimed to synchronize movement dynamics (peak velocity) than target positions (goal postures). It was concluded that dancers are exceptionally skilled in anticipating and adjusting in real time to changes in the actions of others. Skoe and co-workers (2021) showed that dancers who had continuously trained in their discipline since childhood had an enhanced temporal resolution, and Stevens and colleagues (2009) found evidence that trained dancers have highly attuned internal clock mechanisms. Similarly, effects of domain-specific sensorimotor expertise on the perceptual accuracy and variability have been shown in expert musicians, supporting perceptual resonance in the timing domain (Wöllner & Cañal-Bruland, 2010).

Elaborating on dancers' timing abilities and temporal experiences, Bresnahan (2017) argues that dancers are 'trained to count in sets of eight', and any consciousness arising from dance training is inherently linked to the temporality of the music that typically accompanies the training. Even a skilled dancer's ability to intentionally apply accents or vary movement timing with regard to musical cues is based on this learned and embodied musical temporality. Dancers are thus specifically trained to synchronize or coordinate their movement with temporal, musical, and other parameters, such as other dancers' movements, and to adjust their actions during performances based on anticipating upcoming information. Bresnahan states: 'The expert dancer who is moving in time has both the memory of the past and the imagination of the future. She experiences in consciousness the step she has just taken and anticipates the one she will take next.' She continues:

> [T]hinking-while-dancing takes place in an ever-changing present of which she is aware even while it is constantly changing, even if this is specious rather than the precise dividing line between future and past. This is particularly true during dance improvisations or in improvisational moments of a set dance. (2017, p. 343)

Dancers' sophisticated timing skills are particularly important for coordinating with other dancers in duet or group choreography/improvisation. The processes underlying these skills are fundamental for coordination in many situations, including social interaction and communication, team sports, and musical ensemble performance. The next section will examine processes beyond simply counting that facilitate dancing together, enabling dancers (and musicians) to stay in tune with each other.

1.3.2 Performing Together, Connected

Peter Jarchow, professor of composition and improvisation, accompanied Gret Palucca's dance lessons and performances as pianist for more than two decades. Jarchow describes his perception of time while improvising on the piano together with the dancers as volatile and, at times, confusing: 'then there are several people together fiddling about with time' (2021, personal communication). In this situation, attention is crucial for establishing and maintaining a connection with the dancers:

> While I play, I have to watch the dancers continuously and not miss any detail of their actions. If there are several dancers, I switch between them, but there is no definite leading

and following. The dancers' movement goes from my eyes right into my fingers on the piano. If I lose the dancer only for a moment, the connection is broken. (P. Jarchow, 2021, personal communication)

The connection Jarchow describes is fundamental for musicians playing together (see Goebl & Bishop, this volume), as well as for dancers, as a basis for skilful joint performance. It relies upon processes of entrainment that support the coordination of human activities in social contexts (Sebanz et al., 2006). Knoblich and colleagues (2011) differentiate between emergent coordination (whereby people coordinating their movement unwittingly or without purpose) and planned, deliberate coordination in pursuit of a joint action goal; these authors identify entrainment as one of the processes underlying emergent coordination. Planned coordination has been studied extensively in music (e.g. Goebl & Palmer, 2009; Keller, 2008; Repp & Keller, 2004) and less so in dance (but see Maduell & Wing, 2007; Naveda & Leman, 2010). Especially in dance, where movement often is not goal related in the same sense as in everyday activities (Schachner & Carey, 2013), planned coordination can become an action goal, in itself, rather than the means to an end.

The concept of entrainment goes back to the physicist Christiaan Huygens who used it to describe the phase coupling between mechanical clocks (see Waterhouse, 2018). Human entrainment has been defined as 'spatiotemporal coordination between two or more individuals, often in response to a rhythmic signal' (Phillips-Silver & Keller, 2012; see also Philips-Silver et al., 2010). Waterhouse and colleagues (2014) point out that, although entrainment can be described on a basic level as 'coordination of rhythmic movement', this definition is not sufficient for the context of dance, where entrainment is often intentional, serving higher strategic goals of artistic performance and depending on extensive rehearsal. They describe spatiotemporal entrainment in contemporary dance as 'a form of subjectivity requiring not only the ability to sense and produce rhythm, but also a process of integration that enables an apparent temporary continuity and accumulation of experience' (p. 10). Like entrainment between ensemble musicians (Goebl & Bishop, this volume), it requires the basic skills of adaptive timing, prioritized integrative attending, and anticipatory imagery, as proposed by Phillips-Silver and Keller (2012).

With reference to a case study of William Forsythe's choreography *Duo* (Waterhouse, 2018), Waterhouse and colleagues (2014) propose that entrainment in dance might be partner specific, involving 'conceptual pacts' (Brennan & Clark, 1996), and that it might have subjective dimensions that are accessible exclusively to the entrained agents (Clayton, 2012; Leman, 2012). Modes of entrainment in dance, especially as conceptualized by The Forsythe Company, include levels of unison as well as counterpoint, or complementary movement (Waterhouse et al., 2021). Agreeing with Jarchow, Waterhouse (2010) points out that the concept of connectedness is fundamental to these entrainment modes as a basis for visual and tactile signalling between the dancers. Riley Watts, who has danced *Duo* together with Brigel Gjoka since 2012 (Waterhouse et al., 2021), describes the choreographic structure of the piece as consisting of phrases in which the two dancers move in unison and then separate again, going 'in and out of counterpoint' (Waterhouse et al., 2014). For Watts, dancing together in *Duo* comprises real-time collaboration, 'moving together in its many permutations, performing the art of *elastic temporal integrity*'. Watts and Gjoka thus perform the piece as well-aligned dialogue in which the timing can be adapted spontaneously by the dancers reacting attentively to each other, playfully challenging and relying on each other like musicians in a jazz ensemble (Doffman, 2011). Watts remarks:

> When Brigel surprises me with a musical or spatial anomaly, it is actually for the purpose of introducing a cognitive anomaly from the series of actions in which I am already fluent. Maybe in that way, entrainment is used like the groundwork or pathway for us to communicate through learned cognitive patterns and anomalies in a performance setting. (Waterhouse et al., 2014, p. 8)

Taking a closer look at entrainment in dance reveals how complex the connection between dancers is that facilitates their coordinated interaction in live performance. This is not only true for the online situation of live performance as presented in this section, but also for offline processes involving representations of dance movement in long-term memory (Stevens, 2017). Studies of dancers' long-term memory have shown that in group or duet choreographies, cues and alignments play a significant role in how movement material is recalled and reproduced. Long-term memory for dance combines procedural and shared declarative modes of memory, as dancers integrate labels and cues with dance movement during learning and repetition in rehearsal (Stevens et al., 2011, 2019). Stevens and colleagues (2019) conclude that contemporary dance ensembles that work collaboratively epitomize distributed cognition and collective memory. Dancers, like musicians, develop sophisticated forms of interaction and non-verbal communication that are based on entrainment and shared attention, that are subjectively perceived as interpersonal connection. These processes are not only crucial for the temporal organization of live performance, but also for the recall and reconstruction of choreographies, as cues from other dancers become inherent elements embedded in the temporal structure of action representations in long-term memory.

1.3.3 Chronos Is a DJ: Synchrony and Togetherness in Social and Club Dancing

The previous sections have focused on how entrainment between highly skilled dancers can support sophisticated forms of planned coordination, non-verbal dialogue, and collective memory. Related processes underlie the spontaneous concerted actions of crowds at parties, in clubs, or in sports arenas. Common to these situations are collective, often rhythmic, movements as well as evolving emotional reactions.

Himberg and colleagues (2018) explore the experience of togetherness arising from collective dance improvisation in social or arts contexts. They claim that the experience is accessible to participants and observers of the collective dance activity, and measurable on phenomenological, behavioural, and neurocognitive levels. Based on findings supporting that movement synchronization leads to feelings of connectedness and social closeness, they propose: 'moving together is not merely the quality of similarity or synchronicity of the movements, but intrinsically related to the *feeling of togetherness* that arises in interaction' (p. 2).

In situations of improvised collective dancing in clubs or at parties, music with a high groove factor typically provides a strong rhythmic signal to entrain with (Janata et al., 2012; Madison, 2006), supporting collective positive emotions and feelings of flow. Bernardi and colleagues (2018) showed that flow experience was higher during spontaneous dancing to groovy music compared to just listening to music without moving or performing dance movement without music. Flow was particularly enhanced while participants danced to groovy compared to non-groovy music. Vital or sublime emotions were evoked by listening to music with or without movement, while emotional responses to music were positively correlated to whole-body acceleration profiles. Newson and colleagues (2021) conducted an online survey study with attendees of rave parties and found that extensive dancing in a ritualized social context was rated among the most relevant factors for experiences of awe, personal transformation, and social cohesion, especially for participants scoring high in trait openness.

Synchronizing one's own movement with others', especially in coordination with a musical beat, can have significant emotional and social effects, and even reduce pain perception by activating the endogenous opioid system (Lang et al., 2017; Tarr et al., 2015, 2016). Ellamil and colleagues (2016) recorded accelerometer data from participants dancing in the Carwash disco club (London, UK). They found that synchrony of torso movement was associated with pulsations approximating walking rhythm, and songs that were played with greater frequency facilitated greater group synchrony. The authors suggest that shared intentionality arising from familiarity of music and rhythm promotes movement synchronization within groups. Common performance goals and knowledge of musical structure and co-performers' intentions may thus facilitate the coordination of joint actions. Tarr and colleagues (2016) used a silent disco paradigm with participants listening to music and performing dance moves under different synchrony conditions, according to instructions they received via headphones. Perceived social closeness and pain thresholds were increased in full synchrony conditions, but not in partial synchrony or asynchrony. Von Zimmermann and colleagues (2018) showed that personal affiliations within groups moving in synchrony arise from distributed coordination between individuals moving in synchronized dyads, rather than unitary synchrony of individuals moving in unison to a common rhythm.

Synchrony between dancers is not only a strong social signal for those engaged in joint dancing, but also for observers of it, due to empathy and entrainment, both rhythmic and social (Reason & Reynolds, 2010; Sevdalis & Keller, 2012). Synchrony in group dance can signal coalitional strength and quality of group cohesion, as well as coordinative skill of individual group members (see Fink et al., 2021). Dyads of hip-hop dancers were rated as most attractive when dancers were moving in synchrony with the music and each other, and least attractive when only one dancer was dancing with the music (Tang Poy & Woolhouse, 2020). Coordination between the dancers had a stronger influence on attractiveness ratings than on dancers' coordination with the music. Vicary and colleagues (2017) showed that spectators' aesthetic evaluation of movements is influenced by the synchrony and temporal coordination between the dancers. In their study, a choreography that manipulated synchrony among the dancers in the absence of music was performed live. Performers' acceleration and observers' heart rates were measured using wrist sensors, and enjoyment ratings were collected from audience members throughout the performance. Synchrony among the dancers was found to be a stronger predictor of audience engagement and enjoyment than dancers' motion and acceleration.

To summarize the third section of this chapter, time experiences while dancing underlie partially different processes from those relevant to merely watching dance. Timing movement, organizing its dynamical structure through counts, and adapting it to external cues belong to dancers' basic skills. Trained dancers possess enhanced temporal resolution and internal clock mechanisms, and they outperform non-dancers in synchronizing either to a musical rhythm or to other dancers. Sophisticated processes of entrainment, interaction, and non-verbal communication underlie dancers' skilful coordination in joint performance; they also support interpersonal connection and collective memory. Independent of dance skill and training experience, related processes underlie the experience of togetherness in social or club dancing scenarios. Research in this field suggests that rhythmic synchronized movement can have significant emotional, social, and analgesic effects, and, additionally, act as strong social signals for observers, supporting the claim that dance represents a basic human means of communication. As has been stated at the beginning of this chapter, the topic of time experiences in dance is too vast to be covered here in full length. It is also too closely related to time-related experiences in music (see Kozak, this volume) to be regarded in isolation, given the shared evolutionary roots and underlying neurophysiological processes (see Doelling et al., this volume). The chapters of this book highlight individual findings and perspectives, illustrating how time is experienced in dance and/or music, and hopefully contributing to an enhanced understanding of human experiences of time and the relevance of music and dance for human psychology and culture.

1.4 Conclusion

In dance, temporal structures arise from interactions between musical cues and the dynamics of the dancers' bodies; hence, human bodies in motion, music, and emotion are the main factors influencing time experiences in dance. Dance, like music, is an ephemeral art form that is based on capacities for rhythmic behaviours and musicality. In this chapter, time experiences in dance have been regarded from two different perspectives: that of the dancer, and that of the dance spectator. These two perspectives, however, are not mutually exclusive: dancers often observe dance when learning new movement or choreography; and at parties or in clubs, everyone moves along with the music, sharing a collective dance experience. Hence, the experience of dance is always multimodal, with visual, auditive, kinaesthetic, proprioceptive, interoceptive, vestibular, and haptic perception interacting and contributing to a consistent impression (Boucher, 2004; Reason & Reynolds, 2010).

Perceived time in dance, in its different forms, can be influenced by all somatosensory modalities, as well as by the interactions between them, potentially leading to enhanced or contradictory interpretations and emotional effects. While visual perception of others' movement speed and dynamics might affect duration estimation, time perception in live performance and other real-world dance scenarios is also influenced by other factors, including attention towards (multi-)sensory cues, states of arousal or flow, and emotional reactions to social interactions. Event segmentation processes link real-time perception to long-term memory through the spontaneous parsing of observed actions, supporting anticipation of intentions and social learning (Zacks et al., 2007). Entrainment facilitates temporal coordination on many levels, from alignment in communication to emergent movement synchronization; it does not depend on external rhythmic signals, but rather supports and intrinsically rewards adaptation to perceived rhythmic cues, strengthening group cohesion and emotional bonding.

How the different processes affecting time perception are linked to each other is a worthwhile question for future research, and relevant insights might come from dance research and practice. Temporal processing, in general, seems to be sensitive to training, and effects of dance expertise have been found with regard to many time-related skills, including the perception and representation of rhythms, timing and coordination of movement, entrainment with other dancers, and the encoding and recall of complex movement material.

References

Allingham, E., Hammerschmidt, D., & Wöllner, C. (2020). Time perception in human movement: Effects of speed and agency on duration estimation. *Quarterly Journal of Experimental Psychology, 4*(3), 559–572.

Álvarez, I. (2009). Time as a strand of the dance medium. In *Proceedings of the IV Mediterranean Congress of Aesthetics, Art and Time*, 22–25 Jun 2008, Yarmouk University, Irbid, Jordan. http://oro.open.ac.uk/26381/

Bachrach, A., Fontbonne, Y., Joufflineau, C., & Ulloa, J. L. (2015). Audience entrainment during live contemporary dance performance: Physiological and cognitive measures. *Frontiers in Human Neuroscience, 9*, 179.

Bernardi, N. F., Bellemare-Pepin, A., & Peretz, I. (2018). Dancing to 'groovy' music enhances the experience of flow. *Annals of the New York Academy of Science, 1423*, 415–426.

Blake, R., & Shiffrar, M. (2007). Perception of human motion. *Annual Review of Psychology, 58*, 47–73.

Bläsing, B. (2015). Segmentation of dance movement: Effects of expertise, visual familiarity, motor experience and music. *Frontiers in Psychology, 5*, 1500.

Bläsing, B., Calvo-Merino, B., Cross, E. S., Jola, C., Honisch, J., & Stevens, C. J. (2012). Neurocognitive control in dance perception and performance. *Acta Psychologica, 139*(2), 300–308.

Bläsing, B., & Zimmermann, E. (2021). Dance is more than meets the eye—How can dance performance be made accessible for a non-sighted audience? *Frontiers in Psychology, 16*(12), 643848.

Boucher, M. (2004). Kinetic synesthesia: Experiencing dance in multimedia scenographies. *Contemporary Aesthetics (Journal Archive), 2*(1), 13.

Brennan, S. E., & Clark, H. H. (1996). Conceptual pacts and lexical choice in conversation. *Journal of Experimental Psychology. Learning, Memory, and Cognition, 22*(6), 1482–1493.

Bresnahan, A. W. (2017). Dancing in time. In I. Phillips (Ed.), *The Routledge handbook of philosophy of temporal experience* (pp. 339–348). Routledge.

Burger, B., & Wöllner, C. (2021). The challenge of being slow: Effects of tempo, laterality, and experience on dance movement consistency. *Journal of Motor Behavior*, 1–14. Advance online publication. https://doi.org/10.1080/00222895.2021.1896469

Christensen, J. F., & Calvo-Merino, B. (2013). Dance as a subject for empirical aesthetics. *Psychology of Aesthetics, Creativity, and the Arts, 7*(1), 76–88.

Christensen, J. F., Gaigg, S. B., Gomila, A., Oke, P., & Calvo-Merino, B. (2014). Enhancing emotional experiences to dance through music: The role of valence and arousal in the cross-modal bias. *Frontiers in Human Neuroscience, 8*, 757.

Clayton, M. (2012). What is entrainment? Definition and applications in musical research. *Empirical Musicology Review, 7*, 49–56.

Csikszentmihalyi, M. (1990). *Flow: The psychology of optimal experience*. Harper & Row.

Csikszentmihalyi, M., & Csikszentmihalyi, I. S. (1992). *Optimal experience: Psychological studies of flow in consciousness*. Cambridge University Press.

Cunningham, M. (1998). Space, time and dance. In R. Kostelanetz (Ed.), *Merce Cunningham: Dancing in space and time* (pp. 37–40). Da Capo Press. (Original work published 1952)

Deinzer, V., Clancy, L., & Wittmann, M. (2017). The sense of time while watching a dance performance. *SAGE Open, 7*(4), 2158244017745576.

deLahunta, S., & Barnard, P. J. (2005). What's in a phrase. In J. Birringer and J. Fenger (Eds.), *Tanz im Kopf/Dance and cognition* (pp. 253–266). LIT Verlag.

Di Nota, P. M., Olshansky, M. P., & DeSouza, J. F. (2020). Expert event segmentation of dance is genre-specific and primes verbal memory. *Vision, 4*(3), 35.

Doffman, M. R. (2011). Jammin' an ending: Creativity, knowledge, and conduct among jazz musicians. *Twentieth-Century Music, 8*, 203–225.

Droit-Volet, S., & Meck, W. H. (2007). How emotions colour our perception of time. *Trends in Cognitive Sciences, 11*(12), 504–513.

Ellamil, M., Berson, J., Wong, J., Buckley, L., & Margulies, D. S. (2016). One in the dance: Musical correlates of group synchrony in a real-world club environment. *PLoS One, 11*(10), e0164783.

Fink, B., Bläsing, B., Ravignani, A., & Shackleford, T. (2021). Evolution and functions of human dance. *Evolution and Human Behaviour, 42*(4), 351–360.

Goebl, W., & Palmer, C. (2009). Synchronization of timing and motion among performing musicians. *Music Perception, 26*(5), 427–438.

Grèzes, J., Adenis, M. S., Pouga, L., & Armony, J. L. (2013). Self-relevance modulates brain responses to angry body expressions. *Cortex, 49*(8), 2210–2220.

Hancock, P. A., Kaplan, A. D., Cruit, J. K., Hancock, G. M., MacArthur, K. R., & Szalma, J. L. (2019). A meta-analysis of flow effects and the perception of time. *Acta Psychologica, 198*, 102836.

Himberg, T., Laroche, J., Bigé, R., Buchkowski, M., & Bachrach, A. (2018). Coordinated interpersonal behaviour in collective dance improvisation: The aesthetics of kinaesthetic togetherness. *Behavioral Sciences, 8*(2), 23.

Honisch, J. J., Roach, N., & Wing, A. M. (2009). Movement synchronization to a virtual dancer: How do expert dancers adjust to perceived temporal and spatial changes whilst performing ballet versus abstract dance sequences. In *Proceedings of the ISSP 12th World Congress of Sport Psychology*. International Society of Sport Psychology.

Jadoul, Y., Ravignani, A., Thompson, B., Filippi, P., & De Boer, B. (2016). Seeking temporal predictability in speech: Comparing statistical approaches on 18 world languages. *Frontiers in Human Neuroscience, 10,* 586.

Janata, P., Tomic, S. T., & Haberman, J. M. (2012). Sensorimotor coupling in music and the psychology of the groove. *Journal of Experimental Psychology: General, 141*(1), 54–75.

Joufflineau, C., & Bachrach, A. (2016). Spectating Myriam Gourfink's dances; Transdisciplinary explorations. In Z. Kapoula & M. Vernet (Eds.), *Aesthetics and neuroscience* (pp. 93–116). Springer.

Joufflineau, C., Vincent, C., & Bachrach, A. (2018). Synchronization, attention and transformation: Multidimensional exploration of the aesthetic experience of contemporary dance spectators. *Behavioral Sciences, 8*(2), 24.

Kasai, T., & Parsons, K. (2003). Perception in butoh dance. *Memoirs of Hokkaido Institute of Technology, 31,* 257–264.

Keller, P. E. (2008). Joint action in music performance. In F. Morganti, A. Carassa, & G. Riva (Eds.), *Enacting intersubjectivity: A cognitive and social perspective on the study of interactions* (pp. 205–221). IOS Press.

Kirsch, L. P., Dawson, K., & Cross, E. S. (2015). Dance experience sculpts aesthetic perception and related brain circuits: Dance experience, aesthetics, and the brain. *Annals of the New York Academy of Sciences, 1337,* 130–139.

Knoblich, G., Butterfill, S., & Sebanz, N. (2011). Psychological research on joint action: Theory and data. In B. Ross (Ed.), *The psychology of learning and motivation* (Vol. 54, pp. 59–101). Academic Press.

Lang, M., Bahna, V., Shaver, J. H., Reddish, P., & Xygalatas, D. (2017). Sync to link: Endorphin-mediated synchrony effects on cooperation. *Biological Psychology, 127,* 191–197.

Leman, M. (2012). Musical entrainment subsumes bodily gestures—its definition needs a spatiotemporal dimension. *Empirical Musicology Review, 7*(1–2), 63–67.

Madison, G. (2006). Experiencing groove induced by music: Consistency and phenomenology. *Music Perception, 24*(2), 201–208.

Maduell, M., & Wing, A. M. (2007). The dynamics of ensemble: The case for flamenco. *Psychology of Music, 35*(4), 591–627.

Marcus, G. F. (2012). Musicality: Instinct or acquired skill? *Topics in Cognitive Science, 4*(4), 498–512.

Nather, F. C., & Bueno, J. L. O. (2011). Static images with different induced intensities of human body movements affect subjective time. *Perceptual and Motor Skills, 113*(1), 157–170.

Nather, F. C., Bueno, J. L., Bigand, E., & Droit-Volet, S. (2011). Time changes with the embodiment of another's body posture. *PLoS One, 6*(5), e19818.

Naveda, L. A., & Leman M. (2010). The spatiotemporal representation of dance and music gestures using topological gesture analysis (TGA). *Music Perception, 28*(1), 93–111.

Newson, M., Khurana, R., Cazorla, F., & van Mulukom, V. (2021). 'I get high with a little help from my friends'—How raves can invoke identity fusion and lasting co-operation via transformative experiences. *Frontiers in Psychology, 12,* 719596.

Noble, K., Glowinski, D., Murphy, H., Jola, C., McAleer, P., Darshane, N., Penfield, K., Kalyanasundaram, S., Camurri, A., & Pollick, F. E. (2014). Event segmentation and biological motion perception in watching dance. *Art & Perception, 2*(1–2), 59–74.

Orgs, G., Bestmann, S., Schuur, F., & Haggard, P. (2011). From body form to biological motion: The apparent velocity of human movement biases subjective time. *Psychological Science, 22*(6), 712–717.

Orgs, G., Caspersen, D., & Haggard, P. (2016). You move, I watch, it matters: Aesthetic communication in dance. In S. S. Obhi, & E. S. Cross (Eds.), *Cambridge social neuroscience. Shared representations: Sensorimotor foundations of social life* (pp. 627–653). University Press.

Orgs, G., & Howlin, C. (2022). The audio-visual aesthetics of music and dance. In M. Nadal & O. Vartanian (Eds.), *The Oxford handbook of empirical aesthetics* (pp. 638–659). Oxford University Press.

Orgs, G., Kirsch, L., & Haggard, P. (2013). Time perception during apparent biological motion reflects subjective speed of movement, not objective rate of visual stimulation. *Experimental Brain Research*, *227*(2), 223–229.

Orlandi, A., Cross, E. S., & Orgs, G. (2020). Timing is everything: Dance aesthetics depend on the complexity of movement kinematics. *Cognition*, 205, 104446.

Phillips-Silver, J., Aktipis, C. A., & Bryant, G. A. (2010). The ecology of entrainment: Foundations of coordinated rhythmic movement. *Music Perception*, *28*(1), 3–14.

Phillips-Silver, J., & Keller, P. (2012). Searching for roots of entrainment and joint action in early musical interactions. *Frontiers in Human Neuroscience*, *6*, 26.

Pollick, F., Noble, K., Darshane, N., Murphy, H., Glowinski, D., McAleer, P., Jola, C., Penfield, K., & Camurri, A. (2012). Using a novel motion index to study the neural basis of event segmentation. *i-Perception*, *3*(4), 225–225.

Reason, M., & Reynolds, D. (2010). Kinesthesia, empathy, and related pleasures: An inquiry into audience experiences of watching dance. *Dance Research Journal*, *42*(2), 49–75.

Repp, B. H., & Keller, P. E. (2004). Adaptation to tempo changes in sensorimotor synchronization: Effects of intention, attention, and awareness. *Quarterly Journal of Experimental Psychology. A, Human Experimental Psychology*, *57*(3), 499–521.

Sargent, J. Q., Zacks, J. M., Hambrick, D. Z., Zacks, R. T., Kurby, C. A., Bailey, H. R., Eisenberg, M. L., & Beck, T. M. (2013). Event segmentation ability uniquely predicts event memory. *Cognition*, *129*(2), 241–255.

Schachner, A., & Carey, S. (2013). Reasoning about 'irrational' actions: When intentional movements cannot be explained, the movements themselves are seen as the goal. *Cognition*, *129*(2), 309–327.

Sebanz, N., Bekkering, H., & Knoblich, G. (2006). Joint action: Bodies and minds moving together. *Trends in Cognitive Sciences*, *10*(2), 70–76.

Sevdalis, V., & Keller, P. E. (2011). Captured by motion: Dance, action understanding, and social cognition. *Brain Cognition*, *77*(2), 231–236.

Sevdalis, V., & Keller, P. E. (2012). Perceiving bodies in motion: Expression intensity, empathy, and experience. *Experimental Brain Research*, *222*(4), 447–453.

Sgouramani, H., Moutoussis, K., & Vatakis, A. (2019). Move still: The effects of implied and real motion on the duration estimates of dance steps. *Perception*, *48*(7), 616–628.

Sgouramani, H., & Vatakis, A. (2014). 'Flash' dance: How speed modulates perceived duration in dancers and non-dancers. *Acta Psychologica*, *147*, 17–24.

Skoe, E., Scarpati, E. V., & McVeety, A. (2021). Auditory temporal processing in dancers. *Perceptual and Motor Skills*, *128*(4), 1337–1353.

Stevens, C. J. (2017). Memory and dance: 'Bodies of knowledge' in contemporary dance. In P. Hansen & B. Blasing (Eds.), *Performing the remembered present: The cognition of memory in dance, theatre and music* (pp. 39–68). Bloomsbury.

Stevens, C. J., Ginsborg, J., & Lester, G. (2011). Backwards and forwards in space and time: Recalling dance movement from long-term memory. *Memory Studies*, *4*(2), 234–250.

Stevens, C. J., Schubert, E., Wang, S., Kroos, C., & Halovic, S. (2009). Moving with and without music: Scaling and lapsing in time in the performance of contemporary dance. *Music Perception*, *26*(5), 451–464.

Stevens, C. J., Vincs, K., DeLahunta, S., & Old, E. (2019). Long-term memory for contemporary dance is distributed and collaborative. *Acta Psychologica*, *194*, 17–27.

Tang Poy, C., & Woolhouse, M. H. (2020). The attraction of synchrony: A hip-hop dance study. *Frontiers in Psychology*, *11*, 2991.

Tarr, B., Launay, J., Cohen, E., & Dunbar, R. (2015). Synchrony and exertion during dance independently raise pain threshold and encourage social bonding. *Biology Letters*, *11*(10), 20150767.

Tarr, B., Launay, J., & Dunbar, R. I. (2016). Silent disco: Dancing in synchrony leads to elevated pain thresholds and social closeness. *Evolution and Human Behavior*, *37*(5), 343–349.

Van Dyck, E., Burger, B., & Orlandatou, K. (2017). The communication of emotions in dance. In M. Lesaffre, P-J. Maes, & M. Leman (Eds.), *The Routledge companion to embodied music interaction* (pp. 122–130). Routledge.

Vangeneugden, J., Peelen, M. V., Tadin, D., & Battelli, L. (2014). Distinct neural mechanisms for body form and body motion discriminations. *Journal of Neuroscience, 34*(2), 574–585.

Vicary, S. A., Robbins, R. A., Calvo-Merino, B., & Stevens, C. J. (2014). Recognition of dance-like actions: Memory for static posture or dynamic movement? *Memory & Cognition, 42,* 755–767.

Vicary, S., Sperling, M., Von Zimmermann, J., Richardson, D. C., & Orgs, G. (2017). Joint action aesthetics. *PLoS One, 12*(7), e0180101.

Vicary, S. A., & Stevens, C. J. (2014). Posture-based processing in visual short-term memory for actions. *Quarterly Journal of Experimental Psychology, 67*(12), 2409–2424.

Von Zimmermann, J., Vicary, S., Sperling, M., Orgs, G., & Richardson, D. C. (2018). The choreography of group affiliation. *Topics in Cognitive Science, 10*(1), 80–94.

Wang, T. (2015). A hypothesis on the biological origins and social evolution of music and dance. *Frontiers in Neuroscience, 9,* 30.

Waterhouse, E. (2010). Dancing amidst the Forsythe company: Space, enactment, and identity. In G. Brandstetter & B. Wiens (Eds.), *Theater without vanishing points. The legacy of Adolphe Appia: Scenography and choreography in contemporary theatre* (pp. 153–181). Alexander Verlag.

Waterhouse, E. (2018). In-sync: Entrainment in dance. In B. Bläsing, M. Puttke, & T. Schack (Eds.), *The neurocognition of dance* (pp. 55–75). Routledge.

Waterhouse, E., Jenett, F., Hager, M., & Coniglio, M. (2021). 'I gave that cue.' Integrating dance studies, praxeology, and computational perspectives to model change in the case study of William Forsythe's Duo. *International Journal of Performance Arts and Digital Media, 17*(1), 160–181.

Waterhouse, E., Watts, R., & Bläsing, B. E. (2014). Doing Duo—A case study of entrainment in William Forsythe's choreography 'Duo'. *Frontiers in Human Neuroscience, 8,* 812.

Wigman, M. (1963). *Die Sprache des Tanzes.* Battenberg.

Wittmann, M. (2015). Modulations of the experience of self and time. *Consciousness and Cognition, 38,* 172–181.

Wöllner, C., & Cañal-Bruland, R. (2010). Keeping an eye on the violinist: Motor experts show superior timing consistency in a visual perception task. *Psychological Research, 74*(6), 579–585.

Zacks, J. M., Kumar, S., Abrams, R. A., & Mehta, R. (2009). Using movement and intentions to understand human activity. *Cognition, 112*(2), 201–216.

Zacks, J. M., Speer, N. K., Swallow, K. M., Braver, T. S., & Reynolds, J. R. (2007). Event perception: A mind-brain perspective. *Psychological Bulletin, 133*(2), 273–293.

2

Varieties of Musical Time

Mariusz Kozak

2.1 Introduction

There is an intimate relationship between music and time; notions of musical time mirror notions of time in general. A dramatic shift in thinking about time occurred in the early modern period (Bardon, 2013; Lochhead, 1982). First, Galileo emancipated time from movement, turning it into an independent variable on a par with space. Shortly thereafter, Newton (1726/1972) posited an 'absolute, true, mathematical time' which, uniform and unalterable, was ontologically separate from all other universal forms. This shift—traced assiduously by Roger Grant (2014)—replaced an Aristotelian view that had been the bedrock of temporal epistemology for nearly two millennia, and according to which time was the measure of motion. By contrast, Newton's calculus gave time a conceptual autonomy that allowed it to constitute its own flow. In consequence, time no longer required a unique moment that functioned as the present, an enigmatic point of separation between the past and the future that so troubled St Augustine (2009, Book 11, section 7.9). Instead, all such points became anonymous, unconditional labels like notches on a measuring stick, and as such could be used interchangeably to indicate when, according to an agreed-upon measuring standard, an event takes place.

As evidenced by centuries of debates, Galileo's emancipation and Newton's reconstitution of time hardly settled the matter of its nature (see, e.g. Scherzinger, 2020). If anything, we are now faced with dozens of varieties of time, including musical ones (Almén & Hatten, 2012). In this chapter, I will examine the different ways in which musical time shows up in theoretical and philosophical writings about music. I look at music's temporality through three ontological lenses: (a) objective time, (b) subjective time, and (c) lived time. Each perspective reveals preoccupations with different aspects of music, including its status as an object, its capacity to create narratives and physical/emotional trajectories, its myriad functions in cultural practices, and even its role as a model for dynamical processes that characterize patterns of human behaviour. The variety and richness of musical times is conditioned by specific epistemic commitments regarding musical understanding, some of which may be incompatible with the others. These commitments point to time as a vital

Mariusz Kozak, *Varieties of Musical Time* In: *Performing Time*. Edited by: Clemens Wöllner and Justin London, Oxford University Press. © Oxford University Press 2023. DOI: 10.1093/oso/9780192896254.003.0003 foundation of our musical knowledge, and in what follows I will unpack this relationship by focusing on a small selection of texts taken from the vast pool of writings on time.

2.2 Objective Time

The Newtonian idea that time exists independently of events that occur in it persists in Western cultural consciousness under different guises: objective time, physical time, public time, clock time, and so on. All of these labels indicate a markedly atomized, precisely quantifiable time that is isomorphic with the mathematical properties of serial continuity. This can be captured, for example, with an image of a zero-dimensional point marking a location on an infinite timeline. We regularly take advantage of this isomorphism when we project onto time ideas from our direct knowledge of space, allowing us not only to model phenomena outside of those immediately available to experience, but also to coordinate and regulate the behaviour of a large number of individuals. We do this through our metaphors, when we talk about moments *in* time, movement *through* time, or events as objects coming towards us (Cox, 2017; Lakoff & Johnson, 1980). When using expressions like 'We are coming up on Christmas' or 'Let's move the meeting closer to the deadline', we are turning time into a physically extended entity that can be conceived as a circumscribed, measurable region that functions as a container for events with boundaries marked off by durationless instants.

As Grant (2014) notes, Newton's conceptually emancipated time had a profound impact on music theory, especially as it propagated through the work of Johann Phillip Kirnberger (1771/1968). Now music itself could be regarded as a measurable phenomenon because it could be compared to a neutral unit: literally, the *measure*. What is more, since this measure stands as an objective standard of musical measurement, musical time could be understood without taking into account the perspective of the listener. Such objective musical time functions as the dimension in which music unfolds—it is the medium for musical transmission, an independent flow on which music, like a leaf on a river current, passively glides towards some goal. Indeed, Thomas Mann (1924/1999) beautifully captures this notion when he writes: 'Into a section of mortal time music pours itself, thereby inexpressibly enhancing and ennobling what it fills' (p. 541).

Objective time, its isomorphism with space, and the concomitant spatial metaphors used to describe it manifest themselves in music scholarship concerned with questions of musical structure, of durations and formal proportions, and of relationships between sounds themselves, irrespective of a particular listening situation. For example, the idea of durationless points that create an idealized temporal grid underlying musical flow is explicit in Lerdahl and Jackendoff's metrical theory (1983). In their view, musical beats serve as points of orientation as the listener navigates the musical work and reconstructs its underlying structure, but are not themselves reflective of any individual experience. Music, in its idealized state, is essentially timeless: there is no present, no before and after, only simultaneity. This represents an extreme adherence to the notion of time as an independent entity in which things take place. Events can be altogether extricated from flux as if pulled out of the river-like flow of time; music can be scooped up and later poured back into a container.

The container model is even more vividly present in the work of Richard Cohn (1992), who draws on the isomorphism between objective time and the serial order of numbers, in combination with the cyclical property of musical metre, to conceptualize rhythm in terms of *beat classes* and *beat-class sets*. Beat-class sets denote which beat in a metrical pattern is articulated in any given measure. These sets are formally analogous to pitch-class sets, which allows Cohn to use operations familiar from 12-tone theory, such as transposition and inversion, to make observations about musical processes that are not immediately perceivable, including formal similarities between rhythms that at first sound drastically different (see also Roeder, 2003).

Despite music theorists' widespread reliance on objective time, its reality is by no means a settled matter. As noted by Thomas Clifton (1983) in his phenomenological account of musical experience, 'objective time (or real, or absolute time) is a contradiction in terms' (p. 51). Clifton drew on Husserl's tripartite structure of temporal consciousness (see below) to argue that objective time 'presupposes the existence of a time which exists independently of us, and of a "time sense" whereby a person perceives this time. [. . .] It is useless to measure the sense of time against a clock which is alleged to keep real time' (Clifton, 1983, p. 51; see also Hasty, 1997). Clifton's assessment reflects a century of debates about the nature of time, initiated by a heated exchange between Henri Bergson and Albert Einstein, in which the humanistic and scientific worldviews collided with a force that reverberates to this day (see Canales, 2015).

2.3 Subjective Time

Setting aside philosophical disagreements about the objective nature of time, in the case of music it is often useful to bracket the listener's experience and think about the structure persisting in an architectural, spatial sense. Such a perspective provides a kind of time-map that highlights moments of special interest and suggests paths one might take to reach them. Even as a theoretical construct, drawing on the notion of objective time can guide the attention of listeners and give shape to their experience.

When listening to music, this experience is hardly ever uniform, and, at least relative to an external clock, time occasionally seems to behave in strange ways, now moving slower, now faster (see Wöllner, this volume). Listeners often sense temporal dilation and contraction, and may even select their musical encounters to engender one or the other effect (e.g. while meditating, or while performing a tedious task). The effect has not been lost on composers, who might deliberately try to control it by systematically varying the tempo, texture, or even the density of a piece (see, e.g. Boulez, 1971; Carter, 1977; Stravinsky, 1947). As Stockhausen (1958) claimed, 'If we realize, at the end of a piece of music—quite irrespective of how long it lasted, whether it was played fast or slowly, and whether there were very many or very few notes—that we have "lost all sense of time", then we have in fact been experiencing time most strongly' (p. 65; see also Rofe, 2014).

The individual perception of temporal phenomena is known as *subjective time*. It is predicated on the notion that time itself can be experienced directly. As defined by the editors of *Subjective Time*, the term refers to 'the experience of the temporal properties of events and processes: their order, duration, time of occurrence, context among simultaneous events and events before and after, and more' (Arstila & Lloyd, 2014, p. x). Since it deals with the internal processing of temporal information, the study of subjective time is of interest to cognitive scientists. In the case of music, these scientists are largely preoccupied with judgements of duration and with accuracy in predicting or remembering so-called temporal locations.

Kristina Knowles (2016; see also this volume) explains that the subjective experience of musical time is typically assessed using one of two paradigms: prospective and retrospective. In the prospective paradigm, listeners are informed in advance that they will be asked to compare two time intervals, assuming that findings reflect their real-time experience of durations. By contrast, in the retrospective paradigm, listeners first hear a stimulus and are only told to judge its duration afterwards, which assumes that the task requires the engagement of long-term memory. Studies employing these methods have found that time can be experienced as contracting or dilating depending on the density of events (Ziv & Omer, 2011), their 'complexity' (Bueno et al., 2002; although, as Knowles rightly posits, the term 'complexity' is very imprecise), the context in which these events occur, and even the emotional valence of the stimulus (Droit-Volet et al., 2010). However, Knowles shows that many of these studies offer conflicting explanations for observable behaviour, depending on which paradigm is taken as the lens through which this behaviour is interpreted.

As Mari Riess Jones (2019) points out, what participants are asked to do in prospective and retrospective judgement studies bears little resemblance to situations encountered in the real world. In her groundbreaking work inspired by J. J. Gibson's (1986) ecological approach to perception, Jones has shown that people use temporal information contextually, and rely on both the structure of the phenomenon to which they are attending and their own behaviour. For example, if we hear three clicks at equal time intervals, our attention becomes focused on the temporal location in/at which we expect the fourth click to occur, even to the point of misjudging events that occur outside of this location. Findings like these have led Jones to propose her *Dynamic Attending Theory*, according to which our attention is guided by the temporal structure of the world itself.

Justin London (2012) has enlisted Jones's findings to construct a theory of musical metre based on the concept of *entrainment*, the mechanism by which a listener synchronizes with an auditory signal (see also Clayton et al., 2005; Merker et al.,

2008; Trainor, 2007). According to London, the attention of listeners is guided by regularly recurring sonic events that create a kind of scaffold that shapes auditory perception—comparable to invariant features of the environment that serve as the background for visual perception (Gibson, 1986). As listeners neurally and corporeally entrain to these events, for example, by synchronizing their movements with the auditory signal, they are able to cognitively project a temporal framework that organizes rhythms heard on the musical surface. It is this framework that constitutes musical metre: an embodied schema that organizes patterns of musical sounds in a particular way.

2.4 Musical Times

The objective/subjective duality of time addressed above presents no problem for theories of musical time if one accepts that (a) there exists a well-defined entity that we call *time*, and (b) that this entity is a process that listeners experience according to their own physical and mental dispositions. Since ideas about the independent existence of time have become thoroughly ingrained in the modern consciousness, it is easy to accept the first premise as terra firma on which to build musical understanding: time functions as a medium for the transmission of sonic events, and these events are given specific context by an attentive listener whose individual experience may be at odds with so-called reality. One question that emerges, then, concerns the very nature of this reality: just what *is* musical time?

Barbara Barry (1990) offers a very succinct definition of musical time, which for her is 'the experiential amount of time passing in the course of listening to the performance, either live or recorded, of a musical work—the way that the work is perceived by the listener' (p. 8). This includes the perception of musical rhythms at different temporal scales, from the 'ebb and flow' of tension and resolution, through the intermediate level of pulse, metre, and harmonic rhythm, all the way down to the minute micro-rhythmic nuance responsible for various expressive effects. For Barry, when the listener is fully absorbed in the experience of rhythms at varying timescales, their awareness of the passage of clock time is attenuated. Attending to 'the process of coming-into-being of successive elements in performance' constitutes the subjective experience of the passage of musical time, in contrast to the 'objective evaluation of the musical work in score' (Barry, 1990, p. 8). Musical time is thus the interaction between 'the innate organization of the work' (p. 12) on the one hand, and the listener's ability to respond to this organization by making sense of it, on the other. To perceive musical time, then, is to 'sort out and structure often complex information into coherent patterns' (p. 13) as these patterns unfold during the act of listening to music. Crucially, for Barry the basis of one's temporal experience lies in a time that functions as a neutral medium *in which* events take place (pointing to a container model of time). From this, the listener can take up different 'interpretive viewpoints of events which occur in time' (p. 83), drawing on a matrix of musical time depending on how temporality is considered: analytically, experientially, for-mally, or empirically. In this way, Barry embraces a range of subject positions, in-cluding both static and dynamic conceptions of time, and engaging in both holistic and more atomic modes of listening.

Susanne Langer's (1953) aesthetic theory, inspired by Bergson's concept of dura-tion (Bergson, 1889/1960; see also Hulse, 2008) addresses musical time under the guise of what she calls 'musical duration'. For her, musical time is virtual in the sense that it is a quality drawn out of, but distinct from, the material world. By quality she means that, rather than a measurable chunk of ordinary time, musical time is char-acterized by a fragility that resists symbolic or spatial representation. Langer often refers to it as an 'illusion' created by music: a process of abstracting from the natural world. In music, 'sonorous forms move in relation to each other—always and only to each other, for nothing else exists there' (Langer, 1953, p. 109). There is an obvious reference here to Aristotle's conception of time as the measure of motion, but set in a context of an idealized understanding of music familiar from Eduard Hanslick, who famously wrote that musical elements are constituted by 'sounding forms in motion' (quoted in Langer, 1953, p. 107). Motion, or the sensation thereof, is the condition for the appearance of musical time. Since musical events do not undergo physical displacement, this motion has to be virtual, and it happens in the 'tonal space' of har-monic 'orientations'.

Important here is the fact that Langer's virtual musical time is not the same as our subjective time; it is not meant as an individual experience of objective time. Thus, when she writes that 'music makes time audible, and its form and continuity sen-sible' (Langer, 1953, p. 110) she does not mean that music makes clock time audible. If anything, she advances an extended and pointed critique of clock time, excoriating its one-dimensional continuum and abstraction of pure moments without temporal extension. Clock time for her is composed of 'ideal events indifferent in themselves, but ranged in an infinite "dense" series by the sole relation of succession' (p. 111), making it 'irrelevant' to the experience of musical time, which, by contrast, is vo-luminous and filled with 'tensions—physical, emotional, or intellectual' (p. 112). Langer's musical time is thus linked with the living body: it is 'an image of what might be termed "lived" or "experienced" time—the passage of life that we feel as expecta-tions become "now", and "now" turns into unalterable fact. Such passage is meas-urable only in terms of sensibilities, tensions, and emotions; and it has not merely a different measure, but an altogether different structure from practical or scientific time' (p. 109).

Langer's ideas about musical time continue to appear in summaries and critiques (e.g. Addis, 1999; Alperson, 1980; Guter & Guter, 2021), but perhaps their longest and most substantive extension can be found in Jonathan Kramer's *The Time of Music* (1988). In this tremendously influential monograph, Kramer opens with the already familiar quote from Langer that 'music makes time audible' (p. 1). He fol-lows Langer's lead in conceptualizing musical meaning as arising 'in and through time', or, more precisely, through 'abstract sonorous shapes' that '[move] through yet simultaneously [create] time' (p. 2). However, Kramer departs from Langer when he claims that music does not suspend 'ordinary' or 'absolute' time, but instead ordinary time and 'musical time' interact (p. 3). That said, he does not explicitly define musical time. Rather, he remarks cryptically that 'music unfolds in time' while 'time unfolds in music' (p. 1). The contradiction is possible for him because he concurs with J. T. Fraser (1990) that time is not bound by the 'law of contradiction', or the logical principle that a proposition and its negation cannot be simultaneously true. Kramer (1988) doesn't elaborate on this position, but goes on to note that, as a result, music can exist in time, understood absolutely as 'an external reality . . . apart from the experiences it contains', while also time can exist in music, in which case 'we begin to glimpse *the power of music to create, alter, distort, or even destroy time itself, not simply our experience of it*' (p. 5).

For Kramer, this power manifests itself most fundamentally in two broad categories of temporality: what he calls *linear* time and *non-linear* time. Standing in opposition to each other and hailing from different cultural traditions—the West and the East, respectively—these ontologically distinct times receive different musical representations. Linear time is the time of becoming, the time of process. Musically, linearity is represented most readily in cadence-driven tonal progressions, where 'the determination of some characteristic(s) of music [are made] in accordance with implications that arise from earlier events in the piece' (Kramer, 1988, p. 20). By contrast, non-linear time is the stationary time of being, of 'existence in unchanging continuity' (p. 18), the experience of which Kramer compares to Eastern meditative techniques. In music, non-linear time 'is a concept, a compositional attitude, and a listening strategy that concerns itself with the permanence of music: with aspects of a piece that do not change, and, in extreme cases, with compositions that do not change' (p. 19). Non-linearity—of which the most extreme examples, such as Steve Reich's process music, exhibit what Kramer calls 'vertical time'—concerns 'the determination of some characteristic(s) of music in accordance with implications that arise from principles or tendencies governing an entire piece or section' (p. 20). Linear time in music moves towards a goal; non-linear time stands in permanent stillness.

Arguably, the conceptual ground on which Kramer builds his account is somewhat shaky, not least because we are asked to accept on principle contradictory claims about the basic nature of time. Kramer himself seems to throw in the towel when he asserts, in an echo of St Augustine, that 'time must ultimately be taken as undefinable. We have intuitive knowledge of what time is, but it is impossible to draw up a list of attributes that belong exclusively to time' (Kramer, 1988, p. 6). There is little clarity about either the individual forms time can take, or their ontological status—absolute, musical, personal, daily, sacred, profane, being-time, and becoming-time are just some of the key terms that disappear from the discussion just as soon as they are brought up. Once again, this speaks to the difficulty in giving a comprehensive account of the many forms time takes in human experience.

2.5 Musical Time: Lived, Embodied, and Enacted

Although the distinction between objective and subjective time appears to point to different ontologies, these are really two perspectives on the same entity. In other words, what we call 'subjective time' is the subjective experience of what we call 'objective time'. However, a more fundamental distinction exists between this and what Langer refers to as 'lived time'.

Lived time is time as it shows up in human lives. Although frequently conflated with subjective time because it also concerns first-person experience, lived time is different. First, it is external to the subject, by which I mean that it is physically real and not a mere mental construct. Second, this time is partly constituted by the external world, and partly emergent from the subject's interactions with this world (Kozak, 2020; see also Coorevits et al., 2020; Maes et al., 2015). Think, for example, of the coordination necessary to catch a fly ball, or step off an escalator, or get off a chair lift. All such non-periodic activities require a momentary and temporary coupling of two autonomous systems, and the timing of one's actions is negotiated by the body in relation to the affordances of other bodies and objects in the environment: balls, escalators, chairlifts, and so on. Thus, lived time is not independent of the subject, but is *enacted* insofar as it emerges from the dynamical system that includes embodied subjects situated in the world.

The concept of lived time has its basis in Bergson's metaphysics, but it finds its most elaborate treatment in the existential phenomenology of the French philosopher Maurice Merleau-Ponty (2012). In this view, time consists of what he calls an 'upsurge' that constitutes the present imbued with the context that immediately precedes and follows it. Here Merleau-Ponty elaborates on Husserl's tripartite structure of temporal consciousness (see also Godøy, 2010), which consists of the immediate (primal) impression flanked by gradually receding retentions on one side, and gradually emerging protentions on the other (Figure 2.1). The upsurge is not a durationless point, but a quality of experience with both thickness and breadth, dimensions that come from the embodied, situated nature of our perception. Moreover, the upsurge emerges from our interactions with the entities populating our world, including ephemeral ones like music. We ourselves enact time by turning, through our physical and mental acts, what is implicitly given in our situation (the future) into what is explicit (the present), and what is explicit (the present) into what becomes implicit (the past). Put differently, the present moment is not just what we currently perceive, but implicated in it are things we have just perceived and things we are about to perceive. Importantly, we ourselves are the source of the passage from the future to the present and into the past as we act upon the world that solicits our bodily responses (Kozak, 2020).

This phenomenological perspective considers the world to be in flux, but the flux by itself does not imply the existence of time. Accordingly, there is no future or past 'out there' by itself. An ordering of events requires a particular form of embodied consciousness that humans have come to possess over millennia of social

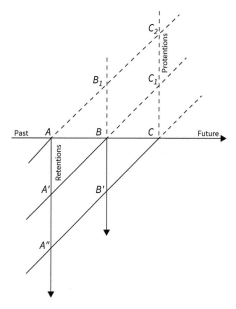

Figure 2.1 Merleau-Ponty's (2012) modifications to Husserl's diagram of the structure of time consciousness. The horizontal line connects a series of successive now-points A, B, and C on a timeline that runs from left (past) to right (future). Diagonal lines connect each 'now' as seen from a later point (e.g. C, B′, A″). Vertical lines show successive retentions of the same 'now' (e.g. A, A′, A″), and protentions (e.g. C, C_1, C_2).

and cultural development. That is, it requires an embodied consciousness that draws on its capacities for memory and anticipation not just to remember and anticipate, but to remember and anticipate in a way that *imbues* events with a sense of pastness (that it had happened) and futurity (that it will happen).

Consider the musical beat, typically defined as a regularly occurring series of sounds that often serve as targets for bodily movements (Zbikowski, 2004). From the perspective of lived time, such a beat does not exist independently of the body that moves in synchrony with the sound. Sound by itself is a fluctuation of air pressure waves, undifferentiated insofar as it has no past and no future: sound just is. Only by doing something in relation to this fluctuation—like tapping our fingers or bobbing our heads—do we turn certain sounds *into* beats. With our bodies we create articulations in ongoing flux. A finger tap perfectly coordinated with a change in some sonic parameter turns this change into a musical event that is folded into the body's temporal framework of retentions, primal impressions, and protentions. A tap orients the body towards the sound, giving it a present, and simultaneously, through memory and anticipation, a past and a future.

Depending on how we move, we are able to enact a variety of musical beats, and with each movement we commit to our experience of sound such that we understand all the other sounds in relation to this feeling of a beat. On the one hand, our commitment involves what I have called our kinaesthetic knowledge of what it is to move to music at a regular pace in coordination with certain sounds (Kozak, 2020). On the other hand, each synchronized gesture expands the body's capacity to affect subsequent sounds, marking those gestures as beats as well (Kozak, 2021b). For instance, a back-and-forth displacement of the body, or change in emphasis from one tap to the next, can create just enough difference to establish a bodily framework that we might call 'metre' (London 2012). In this way, we enact a particular temporal structure for this music, replete with certain kinaesthetic qualities—like 'fleeting', 'rushing', 'dragging', or 'wavering'—that make our lived time flow just so.

Drawing on this perspective, in my own work I have argued that musical time is neither ontologically different from time in general, nor something that exists virtually (Kozak, 2020, 2021a). Instead, music isolates and intensifies those relationships between ourselves and our world that emerge from particular ways of conceptualizing time and temporality. To take musical metre again as an example, it is a culturally situated form of behaviour that draws on concepts of regularity and periodicity (Agawu, 1995; Iyer, 1998). Similarly, music in which metre is attenuated or non-existent draws on concepts like temporal flexibility or even annihilation of time (Kramer, 1988). Musical time more generally is the quality of our experience when we engage in musical behaviour (playing, listening, dancing, establishing affective relationships with others, etc.). That is, it is the quality of our turning of implicit sonic relationships into explicit ones within the norms endemic to our culture and society (norms that include bodily synchronization as well as other temporal relations).

This view grounds time in individual agents who are socially and physically embedded, while simultaneously paving the way for intersubjective time to emerge from the interaction between several agents. Music facilitates this emergence by offering different opportunities for bodily movement, and the perception of these opportunities—what Gibson (1986) called 'affordances'—is culturally transmitted among members of a social group as they participate in the same musical activities. In turn, different forms of musical time are *enacted* when the temporal flux itself is given meaning by being incorporated into the temporality of the body, thus inheriting the body's present (through direct perception), its past (through memory), and its future (through anticipation).

2.6 Conclusion: Why Musical Time?

All existence is temporal in a trivial sense that it requires time to be realized: all events take place *in* time. But to say that music is a uniquely temporal art is to make a stronger claim: musical events not only take place *in* time, but there is a deeper relationship between the two domains. As Zuckerkandl (1956) notes: 'Music is a temporal art not in the barren and empty sense that its tones succeed one another "in time"; it is a temporal art in the concrete sense that it enlists the flux of time as a force to serve its ends' (p. 181). This view is echoed by Stambaugh (1964), who writes that 'music is a temporal structure; it is not a structure in time' (p. 266). Indeed, one could argue that any time we write or talk about music we are implicitly talking about time.

Zbikowski (2016) quips that 'to speak of time, in any substantive way, is to court madness' (p. 3), but the deep relationship between music and time means that we should risk it anyway. This chapter only scratches the surface of the rich scholarship on musical time. Discussions of the nature and significance of music's temporality reflect what Grant (2014) characterizes as 'larger networks of knowledge on time' (p. 4). Time as a concept is itself historical, and Grant's own work shows how the change in its conceptualization in the early modern period had a long-lasting ripple effect on music. Time is also a cultural and social construct (Blum, 2016; Clayton, 2000; Qureshi, 1994), and the perspectives considered above are admittedly ethnocentric. Hence, any purchase we might gain on understanding time will be markedly different depending on which historical or cultural framework we take into account (Scherzinger, 2020). The acknowledgement of this contingency of time—of the conditional nature of temporal concepts that Western society has come to accept as fact—opens up a path towards creating new possibilities for understanding musical time.

References

Addis, L. (1999). *Of mind and music*. Cornell University Press.

Agawu, V. K. (1995). *African rhythm: A Northern Ewe perspective*. Cambridge University Press.

Alperson, P. (1980). 'Musical time' and music as an 'art of time'. *Journal of Aesthetics and Art Criticism*, *38*(4), 407–417.

Almén, B., & Hatten, R. (2012). Narrative engagement in twentieth-century music: Possibilities and limits. In M. L. Klein & N. Reyland (Eds.), *Music and narrative since 1900* (pp. 59–85). Indiana University Press.

Arstila, V., & Lloyd, D. (2014). *Subjective time: The philosophy, psychology, and neuroscience of temporality*. MIT Press.

Augustine of Hippo. (2009). *Confessions* (H. Chadwick, Trans.). Oxford University Press.

Bardon, A. (2013). *A brief history of the philosophy of time*. Oxford University Press.

Barry, B. (1990). *Musical time: The sense of order*. Pendragon Press.

Bergson, H. (1960). *Time and free will* (F. L. Pogson, Trans.). Harper & Row. (Original work published 1889)

Blum, S. (2016). Ethnomusicologists and questions of temporality. In S. Clark & A. Rehding (Eds.), *Music in time: Phenomenology, perception, performance* (pp. 55–70). Harvard University Press.

Boulez, P. (1971). *Boulez on music today* (S. Bradshaw & R. R. Bennett, Trans.). Faber & Faber.

Bueno, J. L. O., Firmino, A. E., & Engelman, A. (2002). Influence of generalized complexity of a musical event on subjective time estimation. *Perceptual and Motor Skills*, *94*(2), 541–547.

Canales, J. (2015). *The physicist and the philosopher: Einstein, Bergson, and the debate that changed our understanding of time*. Princeton University Press.

Carter, E. (1977). Music and the time screen. In E. Stone and K. Stone (Eds.), *The writings of Elliott Carter* (pp. 343–365). Indiana University Press.

Clayton, M. (2000). *Time in Indian music: Rhythm, metre, and form in North Indian rag performance*. Oxford University Press.

Clayton, M., Sader, R., & Will, U. (2005). In time with the music: The concept of entrainment and its significance for ethnomusicology. *European Meetings in Ethnomusicology*, *11*, 3–142.

Clifton, T. (1983). *Music as heard: A study in applied phenomenology*. Yale University Press.

Cohn, R. (1992). Transpositional combination of beat-class sets in Steve Reich's phase-shifting music. *Perspectives of New Music, 30*(2), 146–177.

Coorevits, E., Maes, P. J., Six, J., & Leman, M. (2020). The influence of performing gesture type on interpersonal musical timing, and the role of visual contact and tempo. *Acta Psychologica, 210*, 103166.

Cox, A. (2017). *Music and embodied cognition: Listening, moving, feeling, and thinking.* Indiana University Press.

Droit-Volet, S., Bigand, E., Ramos, D., & Bueno, J. L. O. (2010). Time flies with music whatever its emotional valence. *Acta Psychologica, 135*(2), 226–232.

Fraser, J. T. (1990). *Of time, passion, and knowledge: Reflections on the strategy of existence.* Princeton University Press.

Gibson, J. J. (1986). *The ecological approach to visual perception.* Psychology Press.

Godøy, R. I. (2010). Thinking now-points in music-related movement. In R. Bader, C. Neuhaus, & U. Morgenstern (Eds.), *Concepts, experiments, and fieldwork: Studies in systematic musicology and ethnomusicology* (pp. 241–258). Peter Lang.

Grant, R. (2014). *Beating time and measuring music in the early modern era.* Oxford University Press.

Guter, E., & Guter, I. (2021). Susanne Langer on music and time. *Estetika: The European Journal of Aesthetics, 58/59*(1), 35–56.

Hasty, C. (1997). *Meter as rhythm.* Oxford University Press.

Hulse, B. (2008). On Bergson's concept of the virtual. *Gamut, 1*(1), 1–41.

Iyer, V. (1998). *Microstructures of feel, macrostructures of sound: Embodied cognition in West African and African-American musics* (Publication No. 9922889) [Doctoral dissertation, University of California, Berkeley]. ProQuest Dissertations Publishing.

Jones, M. R. (2019). *Time will tell: A theory of dynamic attending.* Oxford University Press.

Kirnberger, J. P. (1968). *Die Kunst des reinen Satzes in der Musik.* Facsimile edition, Georg Olms. (Original work published 1771–79).

Knowles, K. L. (2016). *The boundaries of meter and the subjective experience of time in post-tonal, unmetered music* (Publication No. 10160530) [Doctoral dissertation, Northwestern University]. ProQuest Dissertations Publishing.

Kozak, M. (2020). *Enacting musical time: The bodily experience of new music.* Oxford University Press.

Kozak, M. (2021a). Anne Teresa De Keersmaeker's Violin Phase and the experience of time, or why does process music work? *Music Theory Online, 27*(2).

Kozak, M. (2021b). Feeling meter: Kinesthetic knowledge and recent progressive metal. *Journal of Music Theory, 65*(2), 185–237.

Kramer, J. D. (1988). *The time of music: New meanings, new temporalities, new listening strategies.* Schirmer Books.

Lakoff, G., & Johnson, M. (1980). *Metaphors we live by.* University of Chicago Press.

Langer, S. (1953). *Feeling and form. A theory of art developed from Philosophy in a new key.* Scribner.

Lerdahl, F., & Jackendoff, R. (1983). *A Generative Theory of Tonal Music.* MIT Press.

Lochhead, J. (1982). *The temporal structure of recent music* [Doctoral dissertation, Stony Brook University].

London, J. (2012). *Hearing in time: Psychological aspects of musical meter* (2nd ed.). Oxford University Press.

Maes, P. J., Giacofci, M., & Leman, M. (2015). Auditory and motor contributions to the timing of melodies under cognitive load. *Journal of Experimental Psychology: Human Perception and Performance, 41*(4), 1336–1352.

Mann, T. (1999). *The magic mountain* (H. T. Lowe-Porter, Trans.). Vintage. (Original work published 1924)

Merker, B., Madison, G., & Eckerdal, P. (2008). On the role and origin of isochrony in human rhythmic entrainment. *Cortex, 45*(1), 4–17.

Merleau-Ponty, M. (2012). *Phenomenology of perception* (D. A. Landes, Trans.). Routledge.

Newton, I. (1972). *Philosophiae naturalis principia mathematica* (A. Koyré, I. B. Cohen, & A. Whitman, Eds.). Harvard University Press. (Original work published 1726)

Qureshi, R. B. (1994). Exploring time cross-culturally: Ideology and performance of time in the Sufi Qawwālī. *Journal of Musicology, 12*(4), 491–528.

Roeder, J. (2003). Beat-class modulation in Steve Reich's music. *Music Theory Spectrum*, *25*(2), 275–304.

Rofe, M. (2014). Dualisms of Time. *Contemporary Music Review*, *33*(4), 341–354.

Scherzinger, M. (2020). Temporalities. In A. Rehding and S. Rings (Eds.), *The Oxford handbook of critical concepts in music theory* (pp. 234–271). Oxford University Press.

Stambaugh, J. (1964). Music as a temporal form. *Journal of Philosophy*, *61*(9), 265–280.

Stockhausen, K. (1958). Structure and experiential time. *Die Reihe*, *1–4*, 64–74.

Stravinsky, I. (1947). *Poetics of music in the form of six lessons* (A. Knodel & I. Dahl, Trans.). Harvard University Press.

Trainor, L. (2007). Do preferred beat rate and entrainment to the beat have a common origin in movement? *Empirical Musicology Review*, *2*(1), 17–20.

Zbikowski, L. M. (2004). Modeling the Groove: Conceptual Structure and Popular Music. *Journal of the Royal Musical Association 129*(2), 272–297.

Zbikowski, L. M. (2016). Musical time, embodied and reflected. In S. Clark and A. Rehding (Eds.), *Music and time: Phenomenology, perception, performance* (pp. 33–54). Harvard University Press.

Ziv, N., & Omer, E. (2011). Music and time: The effect of experimental paradigm, musical structure, and subjective evaluations on time estimations. *Psychology of Music*, *39*(2), 182–195.

Zuckerkandl, V. (1956). *Sound and symbol: Music and the external world*. Routledge.

3
Psychological and Neuroscientific Foundations of Rhythms and Timing

Keith Doelling, Sophie Herbst, Luc Arnal, and Virginie van Wassenhove

3.1 Introduction

Rhythms are everywhere: in the motion of planets that sets the pace of our day/night routines, in the rhymes that humans enjoy reading, and in the music and dance they generate. At each scale of life, from molecules to flocks of birds, rhythms mark time and provide the metrics for information flow. In György Ligeti's *Poème Symphonique* (1962), 100 metronomes, each set to a distinct tempo, are launched as simultaneously as possible, marking time for a few minutes. This symphonic poem could be thought of as an idealized metaphor of brain rhythms: hundreds of neural populations can be rhythmically active at the same time, at the same or at different frequencies, in phase or out of phase with each other. The multiple time metrics, endogenous to brain function, may serve the coding, segmentation, regulation, and transmission of information. This chapter provides a broad neuroscientific view of the psychological and neural constraints of rhythms and rhythmic processing, leaving the subtleties of individual areas of expertise to the other chapters in this book. We first discuss the importance and definition of rhythms in human productions, then turn to the role of neural oscillations, illustrating specific roles of rhythms for prediction, attention, and anticipation—notions that are central to artistic productions. Finally, we highlight a tension inherent to biology and psychology, namely, the interfacing between exogenous temporalities and endogenous bodily rhythms that make individuals' clocks relative.

3.2 Rhythms

In this chapter, rhythms are defined as periodic patterns in signals (e.g. sounds, body movements, or neural dynamics) over a wide range of timescales. Temporal patterns do not have to be strictly isochronous to qualify as rhythm; indeed, these rhythms can be very complex, such as the hierarchically nested structures in music, dance, or speech that humans readily produce. For this chapter, our case study will mostly be a quasi-isochronous single stream of sounds (i.e. notes, syllables, or anything else).

Keith Doelling, Sophie Herbst, Luc Arnal, and Virginie van Wassenhove, *Psychological and Neuroscientific Foundations of Rhythms and Timing* In: *Performing Time*. Edited by: Clemens Wöllner and Justin London, Oxford University Press. © Oxford University Press 2023. DOI: 10.1093/oso/9780192896254.003.0004

The accompanying constructs representing higher-order temporal abstractions such as beat, tempo, and metre are thoroughly described in other chapters (e.g. London, this volume; Henry & Kotz, this volume; Hammerschmidt, this volume). Herein, we focus on the sequence itself, which unfolds chronologically, with the expectation of when the next note or gesture will occur given the preceding temporal context. To keep the scope of this chapter open to a variety of research areas, our focus will remain at this low-level definition of rhythm.

3.2.1 Human Production of Rhythms

Across cultures and eras, human activities and the artefacts generated by them, which we refer to as human productions, have been characterized by time constants that occur and reoccur as we create new works of art or complete menial tasks. For example, handwriting, a behaviour not typically thought of as rhythmic, can be modelled as a coupled oscillator system, as if the pen were being pulled by two pendulums swinging in perpendicular directions (Gangadhar et al., 2007; Hollerbach, 1981). Similar rhythmicity can be found in sweeping, painting, walking, and swimming, and, of course, in speech, dance, and music. These rhythmic sequences of behaviours tend to occur whenever repetition is required. When a single act is not enough to accomplish the task, repeating it allows us to build on past actions, creating more complex structures. In performing similar acts repeatedly, we necessarily create rhythms.

At first inspection, a behaviour might only be considered rhythmic when the same temporal interval, or an exact integer multiple of it, is repeated precisely over a sequence. A metronome might come to mind as a possible example of a prototypical isochronous rhythm being used to dictate the tempo of a musical piece. Most human behaviours would fail by this definition, even ones that we would expect to succeed. Walking, for example, an undeniably rhythmic action, shows fractal variance over time (Hausdorff et al., 1996). Instead, by our definition, rhythms are sequences with temporal structures, whereby each event provides some—but not necessarily exact—information about when the next event will occur: a balance between predictability and complexity.

To illustrate the point further, consider audition, in which rhythmic human production leads to rhythmic sensory stimuli. In speech and music, each unit of action (e.g. articulating a syllable or singing a note) is comparable to each other unit—for example, in the opening and closing of the vocal tract—as they occur within similar temporal constraints. Still, despite their similarity, each unit is intentionally distinguished from one another to form the building blocks of complex concepts for listeners. These differences create variety not only in the actions generated, but also in the time it takes to execute them. These signals are therefore rhythmic, in the sense that they maintain temporal regularities and structures without being isochronous. Furthermore, the timing of speech, dance, or music is not passive; instead, it actively nuances communication. Consider the slowing down of the syllabic rate to indicate the end of a thought (Local et al., 1986), or the expressive timing of a musician to give a performance greater feeling (Clarke, 1989; Todd, 1985). Herein, 'rhythms' refer to repetitive temporal structures that do not precisely match isochrony although they rely on periodic processes. While human productions like speech, music, or dance are sourced from the rhythmic tools provided to us by our biology, we must also appreciate the complexity of our timing, which is added to accommodate the semantic and emotional processes that these signals are intended for.

Evidence for rhythmicity in human productions often comes from corpus studies, which analyse large databases of audio signals to investigate their temporal properties. Using the Fourier transform (Figure 3.1), we can glean whether a signal contains high- or low-frequency content. The presence of rhythmicity depends on finding a peak in the spectrum, noting, for example, that there is a dominance of power in the 5 Hz range, that is, at a periodicity of 200 ms. The width of the spectral peak will vary with how precise or isochronous a rhythm is. For instance, in Ligeti's *Poème Symphonique*, the rhythmic complexity is apparent in the number of spectral peaks that also overlap (Figure 3.1a) or as 'spiderwebs of rhythm emerg[ing] from the cloud of ticks' as Alex Ross put it (2007, p. 508). Ding and colleagues (2017) used this method to investigate a wide array of recordings for speech and music. The languages they analysed showed an average peak frequency of 5 Hz with a variance of about ±1 Hz and the music they analysed, an average peak around 2 Hz (a periodicity of 500 ms) across a wide array of instruments (single or ensemble pieces) and musical styles. The authors suggest that the observed spectral peaks may reflect the beat rate with their metrical subdivisions, such as those typically reported in Western music (London, 2012) and readily tracked by cortical activity (Nozaradan et al., 2011, 2012, discussed below). While the presence of rhythm in music is uncontroversial, how these rhythms compare across cultures is less clear. Recent work (Jacoby & McDermott, 2017; Polak et al., 2018) has taken an innovative, iterative tapping approach to find which rhythmic patterns are endemic to particular cultures. They found that while each culture had a different pattern seemingly typical of their own culture (e.g. Balkan folk music contains 3–3–2, a pattern that was more heavily represented in people from that region), they also reported a universal preference for rhythms with low-integer ratio relationships between them.

The preference for rhythmicity in speech and music (and likely dance) results from temporal constraints of at least two types: the temporal constraints of our body effectors and those of our neural architecture. Regarding the effectors, successful musical performance requires the manipulation of a wide range of articulators to dynamically control the timing and quality of the outcome. For example, playing the piano requires both the fine-grained movement of the fingers as well as more large-scale arm, shoulder, and core movements. The requirement for coordination between our articulators creates temporal constraints on its movement. There are limits to how fast and how slow we can reliably control these movements (see Wöllner, this volume). By contrast, the nature of our neural architecture requires

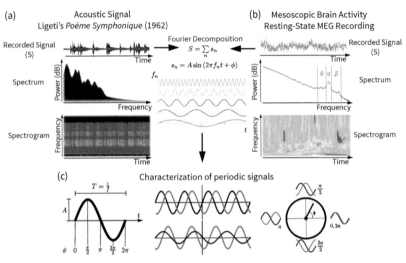

Figure 3.1 Signal processing of time series. (a) Example of an audio recording of Ligeti's *Poème Symphonique* for 100 metronomes (left) and (b) resting-state data acquired with magnetoencephalography (MEG). The *Fourier decomposition* provides a quantitative description of signals as a sum of sinusoids. The power spectral density or spectrum is characterized by a $1/f$ spectrum in all physical systems so that the lower frequencies display a higher power than higher frequencies. Peaks in the spectrum indicate the most prominent periodicities. In Ligeti's spectrum, each peak is a metronome. In the brain's spectrum, alpha (α) band (8–12 Hz) is a spontaneous neural oscillation seen during the resting state. We also see peaks of activity at 4–7 Hz in the theta (θ) band, and 20–30 Hz in the beta (β) band. Time-frequency analyses result in spectrograms preserving the temporal dimension of spectral fluctuations, which a spectral representation dismisses. The extreme regularities of Ligeti's symphonic poem become evident (bottom left panel; yellow pattern) in contrast to the abrupt increases in a specific part of the spectrum in brain activity (bottom right panel, red). (c) The outcome of Fourier decomposition helps characterizing the periodic components of signals by their frequencies (f), period (T), amplitudes (A), and relative phases (ϕ) (left panel). The middle panel illustrates two sinusoids with the same frequency but different phases (top) or with different frequencies and amplitudes (bottom). The full range of phase differences between two signals sharing the same frequency or period is illustrated on the unit circle (right panel). The in-phase and out-of-phase relations of the two sinusoids (0 and π, respectively) illustrate that sharing the same frequency does not equate synchrony or shared temporal alignment.

time for processing as well. An artificially highly sped-up melody will create the perception of blurred individual notes and groupings not present at the intended tempo. To borrow an example from language, while both speech and sign languages are produced by vastly different effectors, their units of information move at nearly the same speed (Wilbur & Nolen, 1986). That such remarkably different effectors have similar time constants suggests these actions are constrained by a third component, the neural time constraints of the listener.

As members of the same species, humans share similar neural and effector constraints. Our ability to enjoy and generate music that others can contribute to depends on creating a stimulus that behaves in a manner that is coherent with these shared constraints. It is possible then that these shared temporal properties can help explain the universal features of rhythmicity at the cultural level; still, why do humans exhibit a universal tendency to synchronize and embody auditory rhythms, as they do, for example, in dance?

3.2.2 Embodied Time in a Predictive Brain

Rhythmicity yields the capacity to predict the timing of future events, which in turn has the potential to enhance perception and facilitate action. Internalizing and forming abstract representations of external temporal regularities (music or seeing others dancing), confers considerable evolutionary advantages by enabling adaptive and proactive behaviours. The temporal scales of spontaneous human productions range from tens to hundreds of milliseconds (see Hammerschmidt, this volume). Many phenomena related to perception and action occur at this scale, which likely accounts for the human propensity to synchronize movements to rhythms (Patel & Iversen, 2014).

At these timescales, the motor system is often recruited during the processing of rhythmic sequences, and it aligns its ongoing activity to anticipated and unattended events (Arnal & Giraud, 2012; Fujioka et al., 2009, 2012). This predictive alignment increases with sensorimotor expertise (Doelling & Poeppel, 2015) and improves with periodic motor priming (vocally) or auditory motor training (Cason et al., 2015). The relationship between the motor system and the perceptual processing of rhythmic sequences supports behavioural findings that temporal prediction in perception and action might rely on similar systems (Wöllner & Cañal-Bruland, 2010), and computational/neurophysiological mechanisms (Schubotz, 2007).

Whether the recruitment of the motor system is necessary for perception or merely useful in noisy or unfavourable listening or viewing conditions remains a matter of debate (Stokes et al., 2019). Many cerebral regions, for instance, the cerebellum (Bareš et al., 2019), can internalize implicit or explicit knowledge about the timing of sensory environments. This can arguably contribute to the anticipation of upcoming sensorimotor events, as well as control temporal predictions and expectations in sensory regions. It is also noteworthy that sensorimotor feedback loops create rhythmic behaviours even in the absence of external signals: postural control is generally viewed as a feedback loop in which the alternation between the sensory detection of the body's current position (proprioception) and its stabilization by motor correction creates perceptible cyclic behaviours (Massion, 1994).

In fact, the motor system can exploit a rich repertoire of actions (e.g. head nodding, tapping with the feet, and dancing) in which the associated temporal trajectories of effectors can be internally emulated in the temporal dynamics of brain activity to predict the sensory consequences of actions. In doing so, the motor system uses top-down signals (i.e. volition) to tune the ongoing activity (and, specifically, the phase of ongoing oscillations) in sensory regions. This top-down control of the motor system over sensory activity enables the fine-tuning and temporal calibration of sensory regions to the impending sensory consequences. Owing to its expertise in exerting motor trajectories with sensorimotor control at the millisecond time-scale, the motor system is particularly well suited for time-related anticipatory computations, including the estimation of one's timing errors (Kononowicz et al., 2019). In this sense, the performance of dance (the realization of these motor trajectories) may serve as a physical instantiation of our own internal anticipation of time.

The experimental evidence showing that the motor system automatically synchronizes with external temporal patterns (periodic or aperiodic) suggests that top-down signals proactively track temporal patterns to facilitate their processing. In this view, temporal predictions in the auditory domain correspond to a covert form of active inference (Adams et al., 2013) in which top-down signals that are generated to dynamically control the production of audible actions are also generated during the perception of predictable auditory streams. By comparing simulated and real sensory outcomes, prediction errors can be computed, and used to learn, correct, and improve temporal predictions in the system.

Anticipation in time is essential to theories of brain function which propose that the brain generates internal models of the sensory world to predict the future (Bar, 2011). Brain theories like *predictive coding* or *active inference* provide a unified perspective on perception and action (Adams et al., 2013; Brown et al., 2011; Friston, 2005, 2018). Internal models use the same computational strategies to predict external events and the sensory consequences of our own actions, suggesting that the brain exploits all available sources of internal knowledge to reduce external and internal noise. The predictive and anticipatory exploration of the environment often requires several repetitions of basic movements (visual saccades, sniffing) to accumulate sufficient evidence and capture the full picture of a scene or of a scent. This sensory exploration, or *active sensing* (Schroeder et al., 2010), does not only occur in modalities that possess moveable motor effectors; it is also seen in audition and in somatosensation. Although humans cannot move their ears, exploring an acoustic scene is not a passive, continuous process, but a discrete and repetitive one involving multiple looks in time (Viemeister & Wakefield, 1991). Empirical support for active sensing and the sampling of sensory evidence in the brain can be found in rhythmic patterns of neural activity, often referred to as neural oscillations.

3.2.3 Brain Rhythms in Perception, Action, and Cognition

Neural oscillations and oscillatory dynamics are a prominent feature of neural activity (Buzsáki, 2006; Wang, 2010). In the last decades, the field of neuroscience has shifted its opinion on the utility of neural oscillations: from epiphenomenal 'fumes of computation' to functional implementation of binding, predicting, and orchestrating neural information, both locally and globally, in the networks (e.g. the 'communication through coherence' hypothesis; Engel et al., 2001).

The origins of rhythmic and oscillatory neural activity depend on the scale of observation (Wang, 2010). Microscopic membrane fluctuations and the intrinsic properties of single neurons display resonant properties so that neuronal spikes are elicited at a preferred frequency (Llinás, 1988; Whittingstall & Logothetis, 2009). At the mesoscopic scale, neural oscillations reflect the mean activity of local neural assemblies; at the macroscopic scale, rhythmic fluctuations capture interareal synchronizations over time and space (Varela et al., 2001; Wang, 2010). Brain rhythms reflect the tendency of single neurons (and groups of neurons) to act as self-sustained oscillators, resonating in restricted frequency ranges. Neural oscillations display specific temporal periodicities (Figure 3.1b): delta (δ) occurs at 1–3 Hz, theta (θ) at 4–7 Hz (i.e. periodicity of about 250 ms), and the most prominent alpha (α) at 7–12 Hz (i.e. periodicity of about 100 ms). Strikingly, these characteristic temporal scales or frequencies are preserved across species—independent, even, of brain sizes (Buzsáki et al., 2013). Therefore, these temporal scales reflect biophysically relevant timescales for behaviours across species, which may provide universal constants for cognition.

Neural oscillations can be identified in the spectral domain through a peak amplitude emerging at a restricted frequency (Donoghue et al., 2020). The identification often uses the Fourier transform (Figure 3.1), which assumes a sinusoidal shape of the underlying neural signals. This is a strictly signal processing approach, one that can be readily applied to any time-varying signals (e.g. Ligeti's symphonic poem (Figure 3.1a) or an individual's brain activity in quiet wakefulness (Figure 3.1b)). The 'Fourier fallacy' (Jasper, 1948) oversimplifies the characterizations of neural rhythms by neglecting their morphology (Cole & Voytek, 2017). This concern has prompted novel approaches to assess oscillatory activity more accurately, for instance, by trying to preserve the dynamic spectral properties of the signals (Cole & Voytek, 2019) or using a statistical modelling approach (Dupré la Tour et al., 2017). Rhythmic activity depicted as a sinusoid is largely acknowledged as an oversimplification, although it is useful for conveying basic ideas.

Neural oscillations provide the temporal dimensions of how the mind works (Jones, 1976; Pöppel, 1971; Varela, 1999) and rely on a parsimonious account of brain functions. Neural oscillations and recurrent neural activity provide natural temporal structures with which information can be sampled in (perception) and out (action), likely forming a structural basis of cognition in the time domain. In the context of the predictive brain theories discussed above, neural oscillations embody the temporal metrics of predictions. In her early theoretical formalization of attentional processes, Jones (1976) described attention as a hierarchy of temporal metrics (rhythms) so that the loci of attention in time could occur at multiple timescales. The *Dynamic Attending Theory* (DAT; Jones, 1976) was proposed to be implemented through neural oscillations, to account for sampling and the postulated 'attentional pulses' (Large & Jones, 1999; Figure 3.2a). The DAT postulates that the temporal

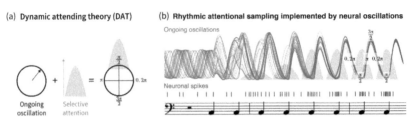

Figure 3.2 Rhythmic sampling. (a) Dynamic attending theory (DAT) (adapted from Large & Jones, 1999). Selective attention (depicted by the grey cone) is aligned to a particular phase of an ongoing oscillation represented here by the phase cycle. The frequency of the oscillation defines the sampling rate, the phase aligns with the moment at which attention is highest. (b) Simulating an implementation of rhythmic attention by oscillatory dynamics. Bottom, a rhythmic sequence of notes that stimulates oscillatory activity. Top, examples of ongoing oscillations as simulated by a Wilson–Cowan model (Wilson & Cowan, 1972). Before the notes begin, oscillatory activity is at a random phase (rest period). The rhythmic stimulation elicits a series of phase shifts, which yields convergence to a specific phase over time, allowing for attention to unfold at the optimal phase. Middle, neuronal spikes biased by the excitability of the oscillation. Spikes are initially random but become locked to an optimal phase when the oscillation is synchronized.

structure of sensory inputs is internalized by endogenous rhythms, to improve the sensory analysis and facilitate reaction times at rhythmically expected timepoints (Rimmele et al., 2018). In agreement with the rhythmic attentional regulation proposed in the DAT, behavioural performance has been shown to fluctuate in discrete, rhythmic sampling patterns, rather than according to a continuous attentional spotlight (Fiebelkorn et al., 2013; Ho et al., 2017; Landau & Fries, 2012).

The facilitation of processing rhythmically predicted inputs is rendered possible by neurophysiology: neuronal spiking activity tends to occur at preferred moments (or phases of oscillatory activity) so that attentional or sensorimotor alignment of ongoing oscillations in time regulate the encoding of sensory information. This mechanism consists mainly of low-frequency neural oscillations (up to about 14 Hz) which synchronize to phasically defining windows of opportunity for neuronal spiking (Buzsáki, 2006; Panzeri et al., 2010; Wang, 2010; Figure 3.2b). In Section 3.3, we will discuss more thoroughly how the phase alignment of neural oscillations to external stimulation optimizes the encoding of sensory information (Lakatos et al., 2008; Panzeri et al., 2010; Schroeder et al., 2010; Whittingstall & Logothetis, 2009).

3.3 Prediction, Attention, and Anticipation in Time

Temporal predictions can be conveyed by (quasi-) isochronous rhythms (e.g. a musical beat occurring every 0.5 seconds), or isolated time intervals that tend to recur (e.g. the time from pushing the start button on your computer to opening your inbox). In the context of periodic sequences, the dynamics of cortical oscillations at a low sensory level represent a powerful means to extract and exploit temporal regularities. By modulating the allocation of processing resources in time, intrinsic oscillators play a functional role in temporal predictions and act as hard-wired temporal priors, periodically aligning neural excitability with the occurrence of repetitive sensorimotor inputs. The DAT proposes that attention allocates limited resources efficiently to the most critical moments in time, selectively enhancing the processing of relevant events (Figure 3.2): the interplay between isochronous sensory inputs and attentional allocation in time may be aligned such that the attended moment (attention driven) and the moment of temporal predictions (temporal statistics) are fully congruent, or in phase.

Prediction (prior knowledge) and attention (selective relevance) are theoretically distinct processes (Summerfield & Egner, 2009; Wyart et al., 2012), but their dissociation must be clarified for the temporal domain, where, depending on task context, expectations might reflect both attentional orienting and sensory prediction (Doherty et al., 2005; Todorovic et al., 2015). In the case of rhythms, the two concepts are related but refer to different aspects of the temporal process (de Lange et al., 2018; Press et al., 2020): attention increases the gain of neural responses for relevant timepoints, and prediction exploits prior event times to assess when those timepoints might be, reducing the costs of processing incoming inputs (Arnal et al., 2015; Arnal & Giraud, 2012; Cravo et al., 2011).

As an illustration, both aspects are necessary when a conductor incrementally changes tempo. The orchestra and the corps de ballet must both predictively entrain their movements to the new rhythm and attend to the critical timepoints, beats, to optimize their perception. Section 3.3.1 discusses this specific scenario. Section 3.3.2 will then introduce the more complex consequences of the coexistence between periodic and aperiodic temporal predictions.

3.3.1 Entrainment: Temporal Predictions and Attention in Time in Unison

Neural entrainment refers to a mechanism by which periodic sensory inputs induce an adaptation of the period, and the alignment of the phase of ongoing neural oscillations. In Figure 3.2b, the sequence of musical notes serves as a rhythmic input entraining ongoing neuronal oscillations; a simulated oscillator thereby develops synchrony and, in turn, regulates neuronal excitability to align to the rhythmic stimulus. Oscillatory entrainment has been proposed to be instrumental in temporal processing and sensory selection (Lakatos et al., 2008, 2019; Obleser & Kayser, 2019) by maintaining a temporal reference frame between sensory stimuli and neural responses (Herrmann et al., 2013).

Many studies have emphasized that the intrinsic auditory brain rhythms (notably, δ and θ; Figure 3.1b) match, to a remarkable degree, those found in speech or music; and there is ample experimental evidence that music and speech induce neural entrainment (Arnal & Giraud, 2012; Doelling et al., 2019; Luo & Poeppel, 2007). We have briefly mentioned the importance of sensorimotor alignment in action (see Section 3.2.2) but neural entrainment also facilitates the processing of sensory inputs, both within and across sensory modalities (Besle et al., 2011; Busch & VanRullen, 2010; Henry & Obleser, 2012; Kösem et al., 2014; Stefanics et al., 2010). For instance, the behavioural detection of short silences while listening to sound fluctuates in phase with the external rhythm and with the measured neural oscillations at that same frequency range (Henry & Obleser, 2012). Visual sensitivity is also modulated in phase with rhythmic inputs (Cravo et al., 2013).

When rhythmic inputs are provided in a different sensory modality, both speed and behavioural performance in experimental tasks can improve. For instance, in a visual conjunction search paradigm, where participants had to detect a horizontal or a vertical bar that changed colour rhythmically, the addition of sounds synchronized to the colour change sped up participants' reaction times (Van der Burg et al., 2008). By contrast, sounds synchronized to visual distractors both slowed participants down and decreased their accuracy (Kösem & Van Wassenhove, 2012; see also Miller et al., 2013). These behavioural results were interpreted in the context of the cross-sensory entrainment hypothesis (Lakatos et al., 2008), whereby a stream of events in one sensory modality (e.g. audition) can serve as a temporal structure for the other sensory stream (e.g. vision) so long as they share the same rhythm or frequency.

Following the observation of behavioural benefits of entrainment, an important working hypothesis is that entrainment flexibly synchronizes, and implicitly regulates, neuronal excitability for efficient processing of environmental inputs, be they auditory, visual, speech related, musical, gestural, or multisensory (Arnal & Giraud, 2012; Giraud & Poeppel, 2012; Lakatos et al., 2008; Schroeder & Lakatos, 2009; Schroeder et al., 2010). Note that this working hypothesis entails the a priori existence of latent neural oscillators that have the propensity to oscillate at a particular frequency. Although some oscillations are readily seen in resting state (Figure 3.1b), this is difficult to establish with full certainty, and recent reconsiderations of the criteria for neural entrainment have been discussed both empirically and theoretically (Doelling & Assaneo, 2021; Lakatos et al., 2019; Obleser & Kayser, 2019). This point will be further discussed in Section 3.4. In the next section, we consider temporal predictions outside of a rhythmic context.

3.3.2 Non-Rhythmic Temporal Predictions

Dancers must be sensitive not only to the rhythm when the piece is played but also to isolated temporal intervals throughout a performance, such as the time from when the conductor arrives on stage and when they will give the first cue, or how long a solo musician will hold a fermata. Such predictions are often memory based, developed over the course of rehearsal. Furthermore, many musical styles employ non-periodic metres (Huron, 2008) that can nevertheless be anticipated and embodied in dance (Godøy et al., 2016; Su, 2016).

The notion of temporal predictions is sometimes conflated with that of entrainment to periodic sensory inputs; but, as we have seen, aperiodic temporal predictions can also occur in human productions (Rimmele et al., 2018). Recent work suggests that behavioural performance is equally enhanced for predictable conditions—whether periodic or not—compared to unpredictable ones (Bouwer et al., 2020; Morillon et al., 2016). This could present a challenge for classical entrainment models, which hypothesize that periodicity should maximize neural entrainment and ensuing behaviours. While potentially useful, entrainment is not the sole neural mechanism involved in temporal prediction.

Implicit predictions of temporal intervals have been studied using the *foreperiod paradigm* (Niemi & Näätänen, 1981; Woodrow, 1914): observers learn to predict from a cue stimulus the moment of appearance of a target stimulus, that is, the foreperiod. Depending on the underlying temporal statistics, reaction times decrease at the most probable foreperiods (fixed foreperiod designs), but also for longer foreperiods (variable foreperiod designs) through conditional updating of the temporal prediction. A temporal prediction of the foreperiod must be initiated anew at each presentation of the cue, which itself cannot be predicted in time, such that no isochronous temporal structure emerges. Importantly, human observers and non-human primates can learn and represent several foreperiod distributions concurrently or in succession (Bueti et al., 2010; Herbst et al., 2018; Janssen & Shadlen, 2005; Trillenberg et al., 2000). Interval-based temporal predictions can align neural oscillations to sensory inputs by phase-resetting oscillations whose period matches the interval (Haegens & Zion Golumbic, 2018; Rimmele et al., 2018; Schroeder & Lakatos, 2009). The phase of endogenous oscillations can be modulated by the internal representation of the temporal statistics of events (Breska & Deouell, 2014; Daume et al., 2021; Herbst & Obleser, 2019) and is sensitive to the shape of the implicit foreperiod distribution (Cravo et al., 2011).

The distinction between rhythmic and non-rhythmic temporal predictions has important consequences for the postulated neural mechanisms. While rhythmic temporal motifs are typically salient enough to be extracted in a bottom-up manner, interval-based predictions range on a continuum from strictly implicit, bottom-up modulations of temporal statistics (Bueti et al., 2010; Cravo et al., 2011; Herbst & Obleser, 2017) to cued top-down temporal orientation (Nobre & van Ede, 2018). Whether oscillatory responses observed during rhythmic stimulation truly reflect an endogenous representation of temporal predictions, or reflect the exogenous structure of the inputs is thus an open question.

The difficulties encountered in Section 3.3 highlight the need for empirical explorations that tease out the origins of temporal predictions, as well as their relation to endogenous attention and sensory saliency. These issues are a prelude to Section 3.4, in which we describe the tension between endogenous and exogenous rhythms. The first issue that arises is the very existence of spontaneous neural oscillations (i.e.

in the absence of driving external stimuli), which stems from scepticism about the functional relevance of brain rhythms to cognition. A second issue results from the need to distinguish the elicitation of neural oscillation from the modulation of ongoing oscillations (as posited and questioned by neural entrainment).

3.4 The Tension in Synchronization

While Section 3.3 outlined a complex system that evolved to align predictively with incoming rhythms, here we show that the perceiver may resist such alignment according to its own internal processing. Our brain exerts endogenous control over how it perceives: deciding which beats are most important, imagining other melodies that might go well with a piece, or perceiving different metres where multiple interpretations are possible. At the same time, we must also consider that stimuli are not isolated: they are generated intentionally by producers, with the aim of eliciting mental constructs in the listeners (e.g. emotions or semantic concepts) through manipulations of internal processes. The dynamism in the musical interaction lies not in fully successful synchronization, but in the attempt to control and align to a constantly shifting experience.

3.4.1 Modulation of Endogenous Oscillations: Uncoupled Coupling

If brain rhythms remain under an individual's endogenous and volitional control, a straightforward prediction is that one should be able to elicit a neural oscillation at will. This was verified in the elegant electroencephalographic study of Nozaradan and colleagues (2011): human participants listening to rhythmic auditory stimuli (2.4 Hz periodicity) were asked to imagine a binary metre (1.2 Hz), or a ternary metre (0.8 Hz), aligned to the 2.4 Hz beat, but to refrain from overt motor movements or counting. As predicted by entrainment, electroencephalographic activity showed clear spectral peaks at the beat frequency corresponding to the acoustic inputs. More interestingly, it also showed spectral peaks at the frequencies of the mentally generated metre. These findings are essential in showing that neural entrainment is not solely a bottom-up brain response to exogenous periodicities, it also reflects an endogenous temporal structure that is experienced by the listener. In fact, oscillatory dynamics can be measured in the absence of exogenous stimulation and resonate during and after rhythmic (Cason et al., 2015; Falk et al., 2017; Pesnot Lerousseau et al., 2021) and non-rhythmic (Teng et al., 2018) stimulation. Such intrinsic spontaneous oscillators support the biological and psychological needs for adaptability and stability.

Furthermore, endogenous control of brain responses can regulate sensory entrainment in subtle ways that are essential to psychological timing. Neural oscillations are not pure sinusoids and rather display non-stationarities, like bursting changes or slow changes in phase response. An example of non-stationarity in the oscillatory phase response has been argued to maintain an endogenous internal metric for the representation of conscious timing (Kösem et al., 2014). In this magnetoencephalographic study, desynchronized audiovisual stimuli were rhythmically presented to elicit a peak following response at the entrainment rate of 1 Hz (δ). The presentation of desynchronized audiovisual stimuli yielded a temporal recalibration phenomenon, in which participants' perception of audiovisual simultaneity shifted. As MEG records the mean response of latent neural oscillators, the entrained 1 Hz response should remain constantly in phase and temporally aligned with the rhythmic presentation of the stimuli (Bauer et al., 2020; Thut et al., 2011). Contrary to this prediction, the phase of the auditory response systematically changed in a manner that linearly predicted participants' time perception. These findings suggested that while the brain may stabilize its internal time metric through external entrainment, the need to maintain a unitary perception of the most probable multisensory event may endogenously adjust the phase response. Consistent with this observation, the (partial) independence of endogenous temporal references with exogenous temporal statistics suggests that some properties of entrained oscillations are physiologically independent from the external inputs, and exist beyond the passive tracking of sensory signals (Obleser & Kayser, 2019).

Altogether, these results support the idea that neural oscillations play a mechanistic role in information processing and that the phase of neural oscillations plays a tangible role in timing under endogenous control. In this sense, what fundamentally distinguishes animals from other living matter is their capacity to generate timing in a manner that remains coherent with, but partially independent from, the temporal properties of their environment (van Wassenhove, 2016, 2017).

3.4.2 Synchronizing With Others: Rhythms, Almost

Given the complex predictive apparatus, why can we not perfectly predict rhythmic behaviours of others? Surprising stimuli attract exogenous attention (Theeuwes, 1991): unexpected stimuli, like a sudden clap of thunder or a bright flash, automatically grab our attention in a bottom-up manner. The same occurs in less dramatic scenarios: surprising words in a sentence ('I like my coffee with cream and socks') attract more attention than predictable ones (Itti & Baldi, 2009; Zarcone et al., 2016). The subtle interplay between anticipation and surprise is essential in music (Huron, 2008). Surprisal, formulated as the error between what is predicted and what occurs, is also a mathematical definition of information content. Inputs that differ from our predictions contain new information (Shannon, 1948). A common example of the utility of surprisal in music is when performers in dance or music vary the timing of their expression. Unscripted and expressive shifts in musical timing, commonly referred to as rubato, further engage the listener and often evoke emotional experiences (Clarke, 1989; Todd, 1985). These behaviours, therefore, differ from the ubiquitous biological rhythms in our environment because they explicitly manipulate the perceiver, rendering them maximally receptive to new information.

How this behaviour should relate to neural oscillations remains a matter of debate. Recent proposals suggest that such synchronization can align with imprecise expressive rhythms (Doelling & Assaneo, 2021). In this sense, it may be in the producer's interest to maintain enough of a rhythm that synchronization is meaningful, while also introducing enough complexity to avoid stationarity. Furthermore, a single oscillator is likely too simple a mechanism to support the full complexity of rhythms that we experience in dance and music. Here is where the motor cortex, with its ability to flexibly simulate temporal trajectories at a wide array of timescales, may come into play. The interplay between motor trajectories and oscillatory synchronization may form the basis of this interaction between producer and listener.

From a temporal prediction perspective, a tension arises between the listener (audience) and the producer (expresser): the former thrives on predicting the timing of events; the latter thrives on attention-grabbing surprise. The result is a feedback-loop system, which must constantly progress: listeners improve their internal model of the producers, the improvement in (non-)rhythmic predictions diminishes surprisal, which forces the invention of new surprising techniques. Despite—or perhaps because of—our endogenous biases towards predicting rhythms and patterns, humans tend to avoid perfect predictability. In music, listeners experience the desire to move, and greater pleasure, when the rhythmic complexity is at a medium level (Matthews et al., 2019; Witek et al., 2014): too complex, and the stimulus becomes unpredictable, and difficult to track; too simple, and it becomes overly predictable. While it may appear that the 'goal' of neural synchronization is to become fully aligned with the outside world, human behaviour suggests a different approach. The tension between our internal rhythms and those of our environment is an important feature of our perception, helping us to learn new rhythms and/or to contribute our own creativity to the process.

3.5 Conclusion

Life is about homeostasis, namely the maintenance of an equilibrium in the face of ever-changing environments. For this equilibrium to remain steady, biological rhythms under automatic and voluntary control require efficient and reliable circuits. In the absence of entrainment to external clocks, intrinsic rhythms maintain their course, displaying distinct, endogenously defined periodicities, including neuronal ones (Webb et al., 2009). It is noteworthy that some neuronal circuits, such as central pattern generators, are specialized in producing rhythmic behaviours like walking, swimming, breathing, or chewing *in the absence of rhythmic inputs* (Marder & Bucher, 2001). Life is also unquestionably a matter of rhythms and most bodily rhythms exist independently of externally imposed stimulations: breathing or beating hearts consist in the periodic alternations of physiological inflows and outflows. In many species, synchronization and entrainment are not solely defined by passive universal time constants, they are also driven by social interactions (Aschoff et al., 1971; Bloch, 2010; Eban-Rothschild & Bloch, 2012). While this may be unsurprising for dancers, musicians, and cognitive neuroscientists, that social synchronization may affect basic biological functioning such as clocking mechanisms (even in passive biological clocks) is intriguing and essential. This is the seed for collective behaviours whose complexity can be increased by some of the fundamental mechanisms we have described—active sensing, dynamic attending, entrainment, temporal predictions, and, ultimately, synchronization. All lead to the creativity of human productions.

References

Adams, R. A., Shipp, S., & Friston, K. J. (2013). Predictions not commands: Active inference in the motor system. *Brain Structure & Function*, *218*(3), 611–643. https://doi.org/10.1007/s00429-012-0475-5

Arnal, L. H., Doelling, K. B., & Poeppel, D. (2015). Delta–beta coupled oscillations underlie temporal prediction accuracy. *Cerebral Cortex*, *25*(9), 3077–3085. https://doi.org/10.1093/cercor/bhu103

Arnal, L. H., & Giraud, A.-L. (2012). Cortical oscillations and sensory predictions. *Trends in Cognitive Sciences*, *16*(7), 390–398. https://doi.org/10.1016/j.tics.2012.05.003

Aschoff, J., Fatranská, M., Giedke, H., Doerr, P., Stamm, D., & Wisser, H. (1971). Human circadian rhythms in continuous darkness: Entrainment by social cues. *Science*, *171*(3967), 213–215. https://doi.org/10.1126/science.171.3967.213

Bar, M. (2011). *Predictions in the brain: Using our past to generate a future*. Oxford University Press.

Bareš, M., Apps, R., Avanzino, L., Breska, A., D'Angelo, E., Filip, P., Gerwig, M., Ivry, R. B., Lawrenson, C. L., Louis, E. D., Lusk, N. A., Manto, M., Meck, W. H., Mitoma, H., & Petter, E. A. (2019). Consensus paper: Decoding the contributions of the cerebellum as a time machine. From neurons to clinical applications. *Cerebellum*, *18*(2), 266–286. https://doi.org/10.1007/s12311-018-0979-5

Bauer, A.-K. R., Debener, S., & Nobre, A. C. (2020). Synchronisation of neural oscillations and cross-modal influences. *Trends in Cognitive Sciences*, *24*(6), 481–495. https://doi.org/10.1016/j.tics.2020.03.003

Besle, J., Schevon, C. A., Mehta, A. D., Lakatos, P., Goodman, R. R., McKhann, G. M., Emerson, R. G., & Schroeder, C. E. (2011). Tuning of the human neocortex to the temporal dynamics of attended events. *Journal of Neuroscience*, *31*(9), 3176–3185. https://doi.org/10.1523/JNEUROSCI.4518-10.2011

Bloch, G. (2010). The social clock of the honeybee. *Journal of Biological Rhythms*, *25*(5), 307–317. https://doi.org/10.1177/0748730410380149

Bouwer, F. L., Honing, H., & Slagter, H. A. (2020). Beat-based and memory-based temporal expectations in rhythm: Similar perceptual effects, different underlying mechanisms. *Journal of Cognitive Neuroscience*, *32*(7), 1221–1241. https://doi.org/10.1162/jocn_a_01529

Breska, A., & Deouell, L. Y. (2014). Automatic bias of temporal expectations following temporally regular input independently of high-level temporal expectation. *Journal of Cognitive Neuroscience*, *26*(7), 1555–1571. https://doi.org/10.1162/jocn_a_00564

Brown, H., Friston, K. J., & Bestmann, S. (2011). Active inference, attention, and motor preparation. *Frontiers in Psychology*, *2*, 218. https://doi.org/10.3389/fpsyg.2011.00218

Bueti, D., Bahrami, B., Walsh, V., & Rees, G. (2010). Encoding of temporal probabilities in the human brain. *Journal of Neuroscience*, *30*(12), 4343–4352. https://doi.org/10.1523/JNEUROSCI.2254-09.2010

Busch, N. A., & VanRullen, R. (2010). Spontaneous EEG oscillations reveal periodic sampling of visual attention. *Proceedings of the National Academy of Sciences of the United States of America*, *107*(37), 16048–16053. https://doi.org/10.1073/pnas.1004801107

Buzsáki, G. (2006). *Rhythms of the brain*. Oxford University Press.

Buzsáki, G., Logothetis, N., & Singer, W. (2013). Scaling brain size, keeping timing: Evolutionary preservation of brain rhythms. *Neuron, 80*(3), 751–764. https://doi.org/10.1016/j.neuron.2013.10.002

Cason, N., Astésano, C., & Schön, D. (2015). Bridging music and speech rhythm: Rhythmic priming and audio–motor training affect speech perception. *Acta Psychologica, 155*, 43–50. https://doi.org/10.1016/j.actpsy.2014.12.002

Clarke, E. F. (1989). The perception of expressive timing in music. *Psychological Research, 51*(1), 2–9. https://doi.org/10.1007/BF00309269

Cole, S. R., & Voytek, B. (2017). Brain oscillations and the importance of waveform shape. *Trends in Cognitive Sciences, 21*(2), 137–149. https://doi.org/10.1016/j.tics.2016.12.008

Cole, S. R., & Voytek, B. (2019). Cycle-by-cycle analysis of neural oscillations. *Journal of Neurophysiology, 122*(2), 849–861. https://doi.org/10.1152/jn.00273.2019Cravo, A. M., Rohenkohl, G., Wyart, V., & Nobre, A. C. (2011). Endogenous modulation of low frequency oscillations by temporal expectations. *Journal of Neurophysiology, 106*(6), 2964–2972. https://doi.org/10.1152/jn.00157.2011

Cravo, A. M., Rohenkohl, G., Wyart, V., & Nobre, A. C. (2013). Temporal expectation enhances contrast sensitivity by phase entrainment of low-frequency oscillations in visual cortex. *Journal of Neuroscience, 33*(9), 4002–4010.

Daume, J., Wang, P., Maye, A., Zhang, D., & Engel, A. K. (2021). Non-rhythmic temporal prediction involves phase resets of low-frequency delta oscillations. *NeuroImage, 224*, 117376. https://doi.org/10.1016/j.neuroimage.2020.117376

de Lange, F. P., Heilbron, M., & Kok, P. (2018). How do expectations shape perception? *Trends in Cognitive Sciences, 22*(9), 764–779. https://doi.org/10.1016/j.tics.2018.06.002

Ding, N., Patel, A. D., Chen, L., Butler, H., Luo, C., & Poeppel, D. (2017). Temporal modulations in speech and music. *Neuroscience & Biobehavioral Reviews, 81*, 181–187.

Doelling, K. B., & Assaneo, M. F. (2021). Neural oscillations are a start toward understanding brain activity rather than the end. *PLoS Biology, 19*(5), e3001234. https://doi.org/10.1371/journal.pbio.3001234

Doelling, K. B., Assaneo, M. F., Bevilacqua, D., Pesaran, B., & Poeppel, D. (2019). An oscillator model better predicts cortical entrainment to music. *Proceedings of the National Academy of Sciences of the United States of America, 116*(20), 10113–10121. https://doi.org/10.1073/pnas.1816414116

Doelling, K. B., & Poeppel, D. (2015). Cortical entrainment to music and its modulation by expertise. *Proceedings of the National Academy of Sciences of the United States of America, 112*(45), E6233–E6242. https://doi.org/10.1073/pnas.1508431112

Doherty, J. R., Rao, A., Mesulam, M. M., & Nobre, A. C. (2005). Synergistic effect of combined temporal and spatial expectations on visual attention. *Journal of Neuroscience, 25*(36), 8259–8266. https://doi.org/10.1523/JNEUROSCI.1821-05.2005

Donoghue, T., Haller, M., Peterson, E. J., Varma, P., Sebastian, P., Gao, R., Noto, T., Lara, A. H., Wallis, J. D., Knight, R. T., Shestyuk, A., & Voytek, B. (2020). Parameterizing neural power spectra into periodic and aperiodic components. *Nature Neuroscience, 23*(12), 1655–1665. https://doi.org/10.1038/s41593-020-00744-x

Dupré la Tour, T., Tallot, L., Grabot, L., Doyère, V., van Wassenhove, V., Grenier, Y., & Gramfort, A. (2017). Non-linear auto-regressive models for cross-frequency coupling in neural time series. *PLoS Computational Biology, 13*(12), e1005893. https://doi.org/10.1371/journal.pcbi.1005893

Eban-Rothschild, A., & Bloch, G. (2012). Social influences on circadian rhythms and sleep in insects. *Advances in Genetics, 77*, 1–32. https://doi.org/10.1016/B978-0-12-387687-4.00001-5

Engel, A. K., Fries, P., & Singer, W. (2001). Dynamic predictions: Oscillations and synchrony in top-down processing. *Nature Reviews Neuroscience, 2*(10), 704–716. https://doi.org/10.1038/35094565

Falk, S., Lanzilotti, C., & Schön, D. (2017). Tuning neural phase entrainment to speech. *Journal of Cognitive Neuroscience, 29*(8), 1378–1389. https://doi.org/10.1162/jocn_a_01136

Fiebelkorn, I. C., Saalmann, Y. B., & Kastner, S. (2013). Rhythmic sampling within and between objects despite sustained attention at a cued location. *Current Biology, 23*(24), 2553–2558. https://doi.org/10.1016/j.cub.2013.10.063

Friston, K. (2005). A theory of cortical responses. *Philosophical Transactions of the Royal Society B: Biological Sciences, 360*(1456), 815–836. https://doi.org/10.1098/rstb.2005.1622

Friston, K. (2018). Does predictive coding have a future? *Nature Neuroscience, 21*(8), 1019–1021. https://doi.org/10.1038/s41593-018-0200-7

Fujioka, T., Trainor, L. J., Large, E. W., & Ross, B. (2009). Beta and gamma rhythms in human auditory cortex during musical beat processing. *Annals of the New York Academy of Sciences, 1169*(1), 89–92. https://doi.org/10.1111/j.1749-6632.2009.04779.x

Fujioka, T., Trainor, L. J., Large, E. W., & Ross, B. (2012). Internalized timing of isochronous sounds is represented in neuromagnetic beta oscillations. *Journal of Neuroscience, 32*(5), 1791–1802. https://doi.org/10.1523/JNEUROSCI.4107-11.2012

Gangadhar, G., Joseph, D., & Chakravarthy, V. S. (2007). An oscillatory neuromotor model of handwriting generation. *International Journal of Document Analysis and Recognition (IJDAR), 10*(2), 69–84.

Giraud, A.-L., & Poeppel, D. (2012). Cortical oscillations and speech processing: Emerging computational principles and operations. *Nature Neuroscience, 15*(4), 511–517. https://doi.org/10.1038/nn.3063

Godøy, R. I., Song, M., Nymoen, K., Haugen, M. R., & Jensenius, A. R. (2016). Exploring sound-motion similarity in musical experience. *Journal of New Music Research, 45*(3), 210–222. https://doi.org/10.1080/09298215.2016.1184689

Haegens, S., & Zion Golumbic, E. (2018). Rhythmic facilitation of sensory processing: A critical review. *Neuroscience and Biobehavioral Reviews, 86*, 150–165. https://doi.org/10.1016/j.neubiorev.2017.12.002

Hausdorff, J. M., Purdon, P. L., Peng, C. K., Ladin, Z., Wei, J. Y., & Goldberger, A. L. (1996). Fractal dynamics of human gait: Stability of long-range correlations in stride interval fluctuations. *Journal of Applied Physiology, 80*(5), 1448–1457. https://doi.org/10.1152/jappl.1996.80.5.1448

Henry, M. J., & Obleser, J. (2012). Frequency modulation entrains slow neural oscillations and optimizes human listening behavior. *Proceedings of the National Academy of Sciences of the United States of America, 109*(49), 20095–20100. https://doi.org/10.1073/pnas.1213390109

Herbst, S. K., Fiedler, L., & Obleser, J. (2018). Tracking temporal hazard in the human electroencephalogram using a forward encoding model. *eNeuro, 5*(2), ENEURO.0017-18.2018. https://doi.org/10.1523/ENEURO.0017-18.2018

Herbst, S. K., & Obleser, J. (2017). Implicit variations of temporal predictability: Shaping the neural oscillatory and behavioural response. *Neuropsychologia, 101*, 141–152. https://doi.org/10.1016/j.neuropsychologia.2017.05.019

Herbst, S. K., & Obleser, J. (2019). Implicit temporal predictability enhances pitch discrimination sensitivity and biases the phase of delta oscillations in auditory cortex. *NeuroImage, 203*, 116198. https://doi.org/10.1016/j.neuroimage.2019.116198

Herrmann, B., Henry, M. J., Grigutsch, M., & Obleser, J. (2013). Oscillatory phase dynamics in neural entrainment underpin illusory percepts of time. *Journal of Neuroscience, 33*(40), 15799–15809. https://doi.org/10.1523/JNEUROSCI.1434-13.2013

Ho, H. T., Leung, J., Burr, D. C., Alais, D., & Morrone, M. C. (2017). Auditory sensitivity and decision criteria oscillate at different frequencies separately for the two ears. *Current Biology, 27*(23), 3643–3649. https://doi.org/10.1016/j.cub.2017.10.017

Hollerbach, J. M. (1981). An oscillation theory of handwriting. *Biological Cybernetics, 39*(2), 139–156.

Huron, D. (2008). *Sweet anticipation: Music and the psychology of expectation*. MIT Press.

Itti, L., & Baldi, P. (2009). Bayesian surprise attracts human attention. *Vision Research, 49*(10), 1295–1306. https://doi.org/10.1016/j.visres.2008.09.007

Jacoby, N., & McDermott, J. H. (2017). Integer ratio priors on musical rhythm revealed cross-culturally by iterated reproduction. *Current Biology, 27*(3), 359–370. https://doi.org/10.1016/j.cub.2016.12.031

Janssen, P., & Shadlen, M. N. (2005). A representation of the hazard rate of elapsed time in macaque area LIP. *Nature Neuroscience, 8*(2), 234–241. https://doi.org/10.1038/nn1386

Jasper, H. H. (1948). Charting the sea of brain waves. *Science, 108*(2805), 343–347. https://doi.org/10.1126/science.108.2805.343

Jones, M. R. (1976). Time, our lost dimension: Toward a new theory of perception, attention, and memory. *Psychological Review, 83*(5), 323–355. https://doi.org/10.1037/0033-295X.83.5.323

Kononowicz, T. W., Roger, C., & van Wassenhove, V. (2019). Temporal metacognition as the decoding of self-generated brain dynamics. *Cerebral Cortex*, *29*(10), 4366–4380. https://doi.org/10.1093/cer cor/bhy318

Kösem, A., Gramfort, A., & van Wassenhove, V. (2014). Encoding of event timing in the phase of neural oscillations. *Neuroimage*, *92*, 274–284. https://doi.org/10.1016/j.neuroimage.2014.02.010

Kösem, A., & Van Wassenhove, V. (2012). Temporal structure in audiovisual sensory selection. *PLoS One*, *7*(7), e40936. https://doi.org/10.1371/journal.pone.0040936

Lakatos, P., Gross, J., & Thut, G. (2019). A new unifying account of the roles of neuronal entrainment. *Current Biology*, *29*(18), R890–R905. https://doi.org/10.1016/j.cub.2019.07.075

Lakatos, P., Karmos, G., Mehta, A. D., Ulbert, I., & Schroeder, C. E. (2008). Entrainment of neuronal oscillations as a mechanism of attentional selection. *Science*, *320*(5872), 110–113. https://doi.org/ 10.1126/science.1154735

Landau, A. N., & Fries, P. (2012). Attention samples stimuli rhythmically. *Current Biology*, *22*(11), 1000–1004. https://doi.org/10.1016/j.cub.2012.03.054

Large, E., & Jones, M. (1999). The dynamics of attending: How people track time-varying events. *Psychological Review*, *106*(1), 119–159. https://doi.org/10.1037/0033-295X.106.1.119

Llinás, R. R. (1988). The intrinsic electrophysiological properties of mammalian neurons: Insights into central nervous system function. *Science*, *242*(4886), 1654–1664. https://doi.org/10.1126/scie nce.3059497

Local, J. K., Kelly, J., & Wells, W. H. (1986). Towards a phonology of conversation: Turn-taking in Tyneside English. *Journal of Linguistics*, *22*, 411–437. https://doi.org/10.1017/S0022226700010859

London, J. (2012). *Hearing in time: Psychological aspects of musical meter*. Oxford University Press.

Luo, H., & Poeppel, D. (2007). Phase patterns of neuronal responses reliably discriminate speech in human auditory cortex. *Neuron*, *54*(6), 1001–1010. https://doi.org/10.1016/j.neuron.2007.06.004

Marder, E., & Bucher, D. (2001). Central pattern generators and the control of rhythmic movements. *Current Biology*, *11*(23), R986–R996. https://doi.org/10.1016/S0960-9822(01)00581-4

Massion, J. (1994). Postural control system. *Current Opinion in Neurobiology*, *4*(6), 877–887. https:// doi.org/10.1016/0959-4388(94)90137-6

Matthews, T. E., Witek, M. A. G., Heggli, O. A., Penhune, V. B., & Vuust, P. (2019). The sensation of groove is affected by the interaction of rhythmic and harmonic complexity. *PLoS One*, *14*(1), e0204539. https://doi.org/10.1371/journal.pone.0204539

Miller, J. E., Carlson, L. A., & McAuley, J. D. (2013). When what you hear influences when you see: Listening to an auditory rhythm influences the temporal allocation of visual attention. *Psychological Science*, *24*(1), 11–18. https://doi.org/10.1177/0956797612446707

Morillon, B., Schroeder, C. E., Wyart, V., & Arnal, L. H. (2016). Temporal prediction in lieu of periodic stimulation. *Journal of Neuroscience*, *36*(8), 2342–2347. https://doi.org/10.1523/JNEURO SCI.0836-15.2016

Niemi, P., & Näätänen, R. (1981). Foreperiod and simple reaction time. *Psychological Bulletin*, *89*(1), 133–162. https://doi.org/10.1037/0033-2909.89.1.133

Nobre, A. C., & van Ede, F. (2018). Anticipated moments: Temporal structure in attention. *Nature Reviews Neuroscience*, *19*(1), 34–48. https://doi.org/10.1038/nrn.2017.141

Nozaradan, S., Peretz, I., Missal, M., & Mouraux, A. (2011). Tagging the neuronal entrainment to beat and meter. *Journal of Neuroscience*, *31*(28), 10234–10240. https://doi.org/10.1523/JNEURO SCI.0411-11.2011

Nozaradan, S., Peretz, I., & Mouraux, A. (2012). Selective neuronal entrainment to the beat and meter embedded in a musical rhythm. *Journal of Neuroscience*, *32*(49), 17572–17581. https://doi.org/ 10.1523/JNEUROSCI.3203-12.2012

Obleser, J., & Kayser, C. (2019). Neural entrainment and attentional selection in the listening brain. *Trends in Cognitive Sciences*, *23*(11), 913–926. https://doi.org/10.1016/j.tics.2019.08.004

Panzeri, S., Brunel, N., Logothetis, N. K., & Kayser, C. (2010). Sensory neural codes using multiplexed temporal scales. *Trends in Neurosciences*, *33*(3), 111–120. https://doi.org/10.1016/j.tins.2009.12.001

Patel, A. D., & Iversen, J. R. (2014). The evolutionary neuroscience of musical beat perception: The Action Simulation for Auditory Prediction (ASAP) hypothesis. *Frontiers in Systems Neuroscience*, *8*, 57. https://doi.org/10.3389/fnsys.2014.00057

Pesnot Lerousseau, J., Trébuchon, A., Morillon, B., & Schön, D. (2021). Frequency selectivity of persistent cortical oscillatory responses to auditory rhythmic stimulation. *Journal of Neuroscience*, *41*(38), 7991–8006. https://doi.org/10.1523/JNEUROSCI.0213-21.2021

Polak, R., Jacoby, N., Fischinger, T., Goldberg, D., Holzapfel, A., & London, J. (2018). Rhythmic prototypes across cultures: A comparative study of tapping synchronization. *Music Perception*, *36*(1), 1–23. https://doi.org/10.1525/mp.2018.36.1.1

Pöppel, E. (1971). Oscillations as possible basis for time perception. *Studium Generale (Berlin)*, *24*(1), 85–107.

Press, C., Kok, P., & Yon, D. (2020). The perceptual prediction paradox. *Trends in Cognitive Sciences*, *24*(1), 13–24. https://doi.org/10.1016/j.tics.2019.11.003

Rimmele, J. M., Morillon, B., Poeppel, D., & Arnal, L. H. (2018). Proactive sensing of periodic and aperiodic auditory patterns. *Trends in Cognitive Sciences*, *22*(10), 870–882. https://doi.org/10.1016/j.tics.2018.08.003

Ross, A. (2007). *The rest is noise: Listening to the twentieth century*. Macmillan.

Schroeder, C. E., & Lakatos, P. (2009). Low-frequency neuronal oscillations as instruments of sensory selection. *Trends in Neurosciences*, *32*(1), 9–18. https://doi.org/10.1016/j.tins.2008.09.012

Schroeder, C. E., Wilson, D. A., Radman, T., Scharfman, H., & Lakatos, P. (2010). Dynamics of active sensing and perceptual selection. *Current Opinion in Neurobiology*, *20*(2), 172–176. https://doi.org/10.1016/j.conb.2010.02.010

Schubotz, R. I. (2007). Prediction of external events with our motor system: Towards a new framework. *Trends in Cognitive Sciences*, *11*(5), 211–218. https://doi.org/10.1016/j.tics.2007.02.006

Shannon, C. E. (1948). A mathematical theory of communication. *The Bell System Technical Journal*, *27*(3), 379–423. https://doi.org/10.1002/j.1538-7305.1948.tb01338.x

Stefanics, G., Hangya, B., Hernádi, I., Winkler, I., Lakatos, P., & Ulbert, I. (2010). Phase entrainment of human delta oscillations can mediate the effects of expectation on reaction speed. *Journal of Neuroscience*, *30*(41), 13578–13585. https://doi.org/10.1523/JNEUROSCI.0703-10.2010

Stokes, R. C., Venezia, J. H., & Hickok, G. (2019). The motor system's [modest] contribution to speech perception. *Psychonomic Bulletin & Review*, *26*(4), 1354–1366. https://doi.org/10.3758/s13423-019-01580-2

Su, Y.-H. (2016). Visual tuning and metrical perception of realistic point-light dance movements. *Scientific Reports*, *6*(1), 22774. https://doi.org/10.1038/srep22774

Summerfield, C., & Egner, T. (2009). Expectation (and attention) in visual cognition. *Trends in Cognitive Sciences*, *13*(9), 403–409. https://doi.org/10.1016/j.tics.2009.06.003

Teng, X., Tian, X., Doelling, K., & Poeppel, D. (2018). Theta band oscillations reflect more than entrainment: Behavioral and neural evidence demonstrates an active chunking process. *European Journal of Neuroscience*, *48*(8), 2770–2782. https://doi.org/10.1111/ejn.13742

Theeuwes, J. (1991). Exogenous and endogenous control of attention: The effect of visual onsets and offsets. *Perception & Psychophysics*, *49*(1), 83–90. https://doi.org/10.3758/BF03211619

Thut, G., Schyns, P., & Gross, J. (2011). Entrainment of perceptually relevant brain oscillations by noninvasive rhythmic stimulation of the human brain. *Frontiers in Psychology*, *2*, 170. https://doi.org/10.3389/fpsyg.2011.00170

Todd, N. (1985). A model of expressive timing in tonal music. *Music Perception*, *3*(1), 33–57. https://doi.org/10.2307/40285321

Todorovic, A., Schoffelen, J.-M., Van Ede, F., Maris, E., & De Lange, F. P. (2015). Temporal expectation and attention jointly modulate auditory oscillatory activity in the beta band. *PLoS One*, *10*(3), e0120288. https://doi.org/10.1371/journal.pone.0120288

Trillenberg, P., Verleger, R., Wascher, E., Wauschkuhn, B., & Wessel, K. (2000). CNV and temporal uncertainty with 'ageing' and 'non-ageing' S1–S2 intervals. *Clinical Neurophysiology*, *111*(7), 1216–1226. https://doi.org/10.1016/S1388-2457(00)00274-1

Van der Burg, E., Olivers, C. N., Bronkhorst, A. W., & Theeuwes, J. (2008). Pip and pop: Nonspatial auditory signals improve spatial visual search. *Journal of Experimental Psychology: Human Perception and Performance*, *34*(5), 1053–1065. https://doi.org/10.1037/0096-1523.34.5.1053

Van Wassenhove, V. (2016). Temporal cognition and neural oscillations. *Current Opinion in Behavioral Sciences*, *8*, 124–130.

van Wassenhove, V. (2017). Time consciousness in a computational mind/brain. *Journal of Consciousness Studies*, *24*(3–4), 177–202.

Varela, F. J. (1999). The specious present: A neurophenomenology of time consciousness. In J. Petitot, F. J. Varela, B. Pachoud, & J.-M. Roy (Eds.), *Naturalizing Phenomenology: Issues in Contemporary Phenomenology and Cognitive Science* (pp. 266–329). Stanford University Press.

Varela, F., Lachaux, J. P., Rodriguez, E., & Martinerie, J. (2001). The BrainWeb: Phase synchronization and large-scale integration. *Nature Reviews Neuroscience*, *2*(4), 229–239. https://doi.org/10.1038/35067550

Viemeister, N. F., & Wakefield, G. H. (1991). Temporal integration and multiple looks. *Journal of the Acoustical Society of America*, *90*(2), 858–865. https://doi.org/10.1121/1.401953

Wang, X.-J. (2010). Neurophysiological and computational principles of cortical rhythms in cognition. *Physiological Reviews*, *90*(3), 1195–1268. https://doi.org/10.1152/physrev.00035.2008

Webb, A. B., Angelo, N., Huettner, J. E., & Herzog, E. D. (2009). Intrinsic, nondeterministic circadian rhythm generation in identified mammalian neurons. *Proceedings of the National Academy of Sciences of the United States of America*, *106*(38), 16493–16498. https://doi.org/10.1073/pnas.0902768106

Whittingstall, K., & Logothetis, N. K. (2009). Frequency-band coupling in surface EEG reflects spiking activity in monkey visual cortex. *Neuron*, *64*(2), 281–289. https://doi.org/10.1016/j.neuron.2009.08.016

Wilbur, R. B., & Nolen, S. B. (1986). The duration of syllables in American Sign Language. *Language and Speech*, *29*(3), 263–280. https://doi.org/10.1177/002383098602900306

Wilson, H. R., & Cowan, J. D. (1972). Excitatory and inhibitory interactions in localized populations of model neurons. *Biophysical Journal*, *12*(1), 1–24. https://doi.org/10.1016/S0006-3495(72)86068-5

Witek, M. A. G., Clarke, E. F., Wallentin, M., Kringelbach, M. L., & Vuust, P. (2014). Syncopation, body-movement and pleasure in groove music. *PLoS One*, *9*(4), e94446. https://doi.org/10.1371/journal.pone.0094446

Wöllner, C., & Cañal-Bruland, R. (2010). Keeping an eye on the violinist: Motor experts show superior timing consistency in a visual perception task. *Psychological Research*, *74*(6), 579–585. https://doi.org/10.1007/s00426-010-0280-9

Woodrow, H. (1914). The measurement of attention. *The Psychological Monographs*, *17*(5), i–158. https://doi.org/10.1037/h0093087

Wyart, V., Nobre, A. C., & Summerfield, C. (2012). Dissociable prior influences of signal probability and relevance on visual contrast sensitivity. *Proceedings of the National Academy of Sciences of the United States of America*, *109*(9), 3593–3598. https://doi.org/10.1073/pnas.1120118109

Zarcone, A., van Schijndel, M., Vogels, J., & Demberg, V. (2016). Salience and attention in surprisal-based accounts of language processing. *Frontiers in Psychology*, *7*, 844. https://doi.org/10.3389/fpsyg.2016.00844

4

The Psychological Underpinnings of Feelings of the Passage of Time

Sylvie Droit-Volet and Natalia Martinelli

4.1 Introduction

> O time, suspend your flight and you, propitious hours, suspend your course!
> Let us savor the quick delights. Of the most beautiful of our days!
> > Poem by Alphonse de Lamartine (1820/1921)

The most delightful hours were perhaps those spent in front of a troupe of dancers who would twirl before your eyes, or those spent listening to symphonies in concert halls. However, those hours could no longer be called hours because time would have ceased to exist. It would have left your mind. How can time no longer exist? The logical reasoning is that if we have an experience of the passage of time (PoT), that is because it is an objective feature of reality. Newton spoke of a 'true time' that flows continuously. The problem with this idea is that our judgements are guided by our beliefs: time exists, so much is obvious! With age and education, we learn to distrust our presuppositions and understand that time is a more complex concept than we thought. However, we continue to talk about time in the same way. Why do we feel the psychological need to talk about the PoT, and what do our judgements of the PoT mean? The purpose of this chapter is not to enter the long philosophical debate about the reality of time. It is simply to present recent studies in psychology on the phenomenological aspects of time and discuss the underlying psychological processes. The ultimate goal would be to try to establish the links between judgements of the PoT and perception of durations from the perspective of an integrated theory of different types of time judgement. However, PoT judgement in human consciousness is a particularly complex psychological phenomenon (Gruber et al., 2018; Thönes & Stocker, 2019) which is not yet understood due to a lack of empirical data. We will therefore discuss some aspects of judgements of the PoT in this chapter.

Studies on the PoT judgement have examined the subjective experience of the flow of time, that is, the feeling of time (Wearden, 2015). This is assessed by asking participants a single question, such as 'How fast does time seem to be passing for you?' However, as pointed out by Droit-Volet and colleagues (2021, p. 335), 'it doesn't

Sylvie Droit-Volet and Natalia Martinelli, *The Psychological Underpinnings of Feelings of the Passage of Time*
In: *Performing Time*. Edited by: Clemens Wöllner and Justin London, Oxford University Press. © Oxford University Press 2023.
DOI: 10.1093/oso/9780192896254.003.0005

make sense to ask people this question if we don't give them a time frame'. People can base their answer on their immediate experience of the PoT, or on a comparison between the pace of their daily life and that of a more or less distant time period in the past. For example, an elderly dancer may express the feeling that time passes quickly if they note that they are old and that a lot of time has passed since childhood, and, at the same time, say that time passes slowly when they compare their current life with years spent dancing in front of audiences. In other words, the experience of flow of time reported by individuals changes depending on the spontaneously adopted point of view, that is, the time periods used as reference. Taking the lifetime period as an anchor point, we distinguish two major types of PoT judgements: the retrospective PoT judgement and the present PoT judgement (Figure 4.1).

4.2 The Retrospective Passage of Time Judgement

The retrospective PoT judgement has been the more extensively investigated of the PoT judgements, although studies remain scarce. It is a judgement about a period of time that has elapsed (i.e. in the past). This period can be more or less distant from the present (now) and it can also cover a long or short period in one's life. Typically, the question asked to participants is: 'How fast has time passed for you during the last day/week/month/year/5–10 years?' The question can also refer to a longer period of life, as in the question: 'Do you think that time passes more quickly as you get older?' The participants generally answer on a 7-point Likert scale from 'very slow' to 'very fast'.

The results described below reveal that retrospective PoT judgements are highly unstable and vary according to several factors. Three main factors have been identified: the time period considered, the nature and/or quantity of events retrieved from memory, and the characteristics of the person making this temporal judgement, such as their age, mental health, or well-being.

As regards the judgement for different time periods, individuals can hold contradictory opinions. They can say, on the one hand, that the years flash by and, on the other hand, that the days last forever. This type of attitude has been observed by Droit-Volet and Wearden (2015) in people living in retirement homes and has been referred to as 'the paradox of our grand-mothers' temporalities'. It can also be found in younger people suffering from depression (e.g. Thönes & Oberfeld, 2015; Vogel et al., 2018). This mismatch in judgements of the PoT over different periods (e.g. 1 day vs years) reveals that different processes underlie the PoT judgement depending on the time period considered. It also indicates that a simple, isolated question about the PoT is insufficient to capture the reality of the feeling of the PoT.

Only a few studies have examined the relationship between these PoT judgements for different time periods. A recent study carried out with people living in nursing homes showed that PoT judgements for the day were not correlated with those for longer periods of time (Droit-Volet et al., 2021). They were, instead, associated with

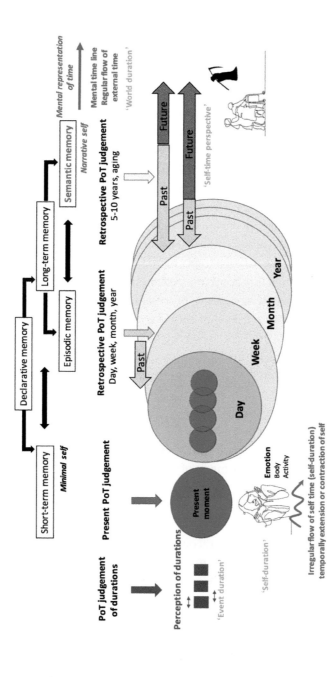

Figure 4.1 Retrospective PoT judgements and present PoT judgement.

the present PoT judgement described below. By contrast, the PoT judgements for the past week, month, and year covaried. When individuals said that time had passed quickly the previous week, they also said the same thing for the month including that week. However, PoT judgements for longer lifetime periods spanning several years were not systematically linked to judgements of these shorter periods. The time judgement for 1 year represented an intermediate stage, being significantly correlated with both the shorter and longer time periods. Therefore, the fact that old participants describe a slowing down of the PoT at the level of the day, week, or month does not mean that they report that time passes slowly with age, or that it has passed more slowly during the past 5 years. Most of them say that time passes more quickly as they get older, or that it has done so during the last 5–10 years. This phe-nomenon is well known in psychology. It has been described in many studies with participants aged 50 years and older (Friedman & Janssen, 2010; Janssen et al., 2013; Lemlich, 1975; Wittmann & Lenhoff, 2005), although some studies have found that this feeling is cross-generational (Droit-Volet & Wearden, 2015; Joubert, 1983).

The difference in the feeling of time for different time periods indicates that dif-ferent processes are used to assess time according to the time periods considered. As suggested by Figure 4.1, the different types of PoT judgement are based on a declara-tive memory system—that is, a conscious, voluntary, and effortful verbal report that requires controlled top-down cognitive processes, and that mobilizes memory be-cause it requires conscious retrieval of episodes and events from long-term storage (Friedman & Janssen, 2010). As explained by Wittmann (2016), the content of long-term memory is crucial for the retrospective PoT judgement. Consequently, the PoT judgement calls on memory mechanisms that are close to those described for the retrospective judgement of time. Retrospective time judgement occurs when participants do not know in advance that they will have to estimate the duration of the stimulus they have seen or the task they have performed, and prospective time judgement occurs when participants do know in advance (Block & Reed, 1978). The latter would depend on the functioning of an internal clock system that provides the raw material for time estimation (units of time) and which is triggered by an atten-tional mechanism (Gibbon, 1991; Gibbon & Church, 1984). When participants are not paying attention to time (i.e. retrospective time judgement), no time unit is re-corded and the duration estimate is reconstructed a posteriori based on the amount of non-temporal information or perceived contextual changes recalled for the tem-poral interval considered (Block, 1992; Block & Reed, 1978; Ornstein, 1969). In the music domain, Wöllner and Hammerschmidt (2021) confirmed that the same mu-sical excerpt (hip-hop music) has a different effect on temporal judgement if subjects are asked to prospectively estimate its duration or to judge the speed of the PoT, with an effect of metrical level for the former and not the latter.

As we will see, retrospective PoT judgements do not simply result from the number of memories retrieved for a time period. In a recent study, Kosak et al. (2019) advocated this long-standing idea with regard to the temporal judgement of the last 5 years. However, in their study, the participants still considered time to have passed quickly during the last 5 years (score >5 on a 7-point scale), regardless of the number of memories recalled in autobiographical memory. Additionally, the small significant variation in the overall feeling that time was passing quickly involved only three and four recalled events—a very small number of memories. Moreover, these memories were autobiographical (e.g. 'When I got married') and not simply a series of episodic events. Finally, without rejecting this interpretation, the authors conclude that 'a number of other factors may play a role' (Kosak et al., 2019, p. 11). The retrospective PoT judgement is thus an even more complex psychological phenomenon than the retrospective duration judgement. Indeed, the same judgement in terms of the speed of the PoT may conceal different types of reasoning and may therefore involve different cognitive processes.

Ever since the seminal chapter published by Endel Tulving (1972), a distinction has been made between semantic and episodic memory. Semantic memory is defined as including general knowledge and/or schematic representations of events or self (self-knowledge) (e.g. 'I was a member of a ballet company'). By contrast, episodic memory refers to experienced events situated in a unique spatial and temporal context, together with their modal (sensorimotor) attributes ('I trembled at the applause when I danced in *Swan Lake*'). As illustrated in Figure 4.1, the components of the declarative long-term memory system underlying the PoT judgement also differ according to the period of time considered. Semantic memory seems to be called on mainly in the PoT judgement of long time periods (5–10 years; as one ages) and episodic memory in that of shorter time periods (last week/month). Obviously, semantic and episodic memory interact extensively with one another and possess similarities at both the cognitive and at the neural level (Renoult et al., 2019). Indeed, semantic knowledge or schemata can emerge from episodic memory or assimilate certain episodic aspects of events or experiences. Conversely, episodic memory can use (or be modified by) abstract knowledge. We can therefore assume that the reactivation of certain episodic memories could also influence the judgement of the speed of the PoT for long life episodes.

As pointed out earlier, PoT judgements for long life periods (as we get older; 5/10 years) seem to derive mainly from semantic memory processes. Semantic memory includes a mental representation of time (mental timeline; conceptualization of time as a regular flow), but also conceptual knowledge related to the self in its temporality. Some authors have spoken of the 'narrative self' (Dennett, 1991; Gallagher, 2000) or the 'self-concept' (Morin, 2006). Both refer to self-awareness, which is made up of a series of personal characteristics and autobiographical knowledge considered in their temporality. Gallagher defined the concept of narrative self as 'a more or less coherent self (or self-image) that is endowed with a past and a future in the various stories that we and others tell about ourselves' (2000, p. 15). The universal feeling of an acceleration of passage of time as one ages would therefore be related to what we call a 'self-time perspective' (Droit-Volet, 2018; Droit-Volet & Dambrun, 2019), that is, this narrative self in the past–present–future perspective (Fuchs, 2001; Zimbardo & Boyd, 1999). People know that their life expectancy is limited; at best, it may exceed 90 or 100 years. They anticipate the future, including the eventuality of their death. When, with age, our past becomes longer and our future shorter, we logically deduce that time is passing quickly (Figure 4.1). Some studies have suggested that other factors contribute to the feeling that time accelerates over the course of one's life, such as an increase in daily routine or a decrease in the frequency of new life experiences (Winkler et al., 2017), or even increasing time pressures (Janssen, 2017; Janssen et al., 2013; Winkler et al., 2017; Wittmann & Lehnhoff, 2005). People who feel that they are under more time pressure will feel that time is currently passing more quickly (Janssen, 2017). However, is it the pressure of everyday life that increases with age or the pressure of life going by that changes the relationship to the present? In sum, the changes in our feeling for time as we get older seem to come mostly from our general knowledge about life—about the self in its temporal perspective; and this temporal reasoning does not correspond to time in real life, that is, in the present (Droit-Volet & Wearden, 2015).

As suggested earlier, the judgement of the course of time for long periods can also change depending on the personal characteristics of the person making this judgement. Some people (very old people, depressed people) feel that time passes more slowly as they grow old or more slowly now than it did 5 years ago (score <4 on the 7-point Likert scale from 'very slow' to 'very fast'). In all these cases, there is a disturbance of lived time that impacts the self-time perspective (Fuchs, 2001; Minkowski, 1968). Indeed, these individuals' mental health, their lack of resilience, and/or their low level of life satisfaction lead to a distortion of the self-time perspective, thereby causing a relative dilation of the present. They find it difficult, even frightening or painful, to project themselves into a future that lacks prospects. By contrast, their present expands as it loses its clarity and is invaded by the past. These patients are indeed focused on their present difficulties, comparing them to a past which they judge to have been better. And as they reflect, 'the past looms in the present in the form of guilt and regret' (Blewett, 1992, p. 195). Their problems in lived time therefore prevent them from reaching a high level of reflection—a positive time perspective—which is necessary if one is to accept that life passes quickly and that we are but small things in the universe. There are nevertheless many therapies, such as mindfulness, that allow individuals to change their time perspective by simply focusing on and appreciating the small moments of the present (Droit-Volet et al., 2019). Depending on the cognitive focus on the self in time, the feeling of the flow of time can thus go slower, faster, or even disappear altogether into timelessness.

Whereas the sense of self in its temporality plays a major role in the retrospective PoT judgement for long periods of life, the emotions felt in daily life are at the source of PoT judgements for shorter periods. In line with this suggestion, Droit-Volet and colleagues (2021) showed that representational abilities are the best predictors of the first type of judgement, while the feeling of happiness best predicts the second. The happier people feel, the faster the last day/week/month is judged to have passed. Conversely, the sadder they feel, the slower time is judged to have passed. Clearly, the emotional colour of everyday life that affects the PoT judgement for these short periods depends on episodic events activated in memory at the moment of the retrospective judgement (Figure 4.1). The question is: what type and volume of episodic events (memorable events) create the emotional colour of the last week or month? These questions about emotional memory have, so far, been handled only by memory experts. It would seem to be important for time experts to work together more closely with memory experts. In our studies in connection with the PoT judgement, we have only observed a difference between the general feeling of happiness as a personality trait ('authentic, durable happiness') and a 'fluctuating happiness' (frequent alternation of pleasure and displeasure) which varies according to daily circumstances (Dambrun et al., 2012). Indeed, PoT judgements for short periods (day/week) depend more on momentary emotions than on personality traits or general mood, although the two may be related (Droit-Volet et al., 2021; Martinelli et al., 2021). Indeed, one can be depressed and still have occasional, fleeting moments of pleasure. In sum, we assume that the judgement of the PoT for short life periods is a valid way to account for feelings of well-being or happiness resulting from experienced events and their characteristics: emotion, activity which captures the attention, and motivation.

4.3 The Present Passage of Time Judgement

The present PoT judgement is the momentary judgement made in the present, that is, the experience of the flow of time here and now. To evaluate the present PoT judgement in daily life, some studies have used the ecological momentary assessment, also named the experience sampling methodology (ESM; Droit-Volet & Wearden, 2015; Larson & von Eye, 2006). In this method, participants are called on their smartphones several times per day over a period of several days and asked to report their current experience of time: 'Right now, what is your feeling about the speed of time?' A series of additional questions are asked to assess the context in which this judgement is made. Droit-Volet and Wearden (2015) asked participants questions about their emotional state (happy, sad), their level of arousal, the attention devoted to their current activity, and the difficulty of this activity. Larson and von Eye (2006) questioned them on their emotional engagement ('How emotionally involved were you in the activity?') and their intellectual engagement ('How intellectually involved in or "into" the activity were you?') (p. 124). Other studies have asked participants to answer a single question: 'How fast does time usually pass for you?' (Winkler et al., 2017). However, it is not clear whether the subjects answered based on their judgement of their experience of time at the point of questioning, on a period of several days or weeks, or simply on life in general.

The few studies on the PoT judgement that have used ESM have clearly shown that the emotional state at the moment of the judgement is the major factor explaining inter-individual differences in the feeling of the flow of time in the present. Indeed, participants experience time as passing more quickly when they feel happier and more aroused. In contrast, time seems to them to slow down when they are sad and calm. These results have been replicated in numerous studies (Droit-Volet, 2019; Droit-Volet et al., 2017; Droit-Volet & Wearden, 2016). The activity undertaken, if it captures attention or is difficult, also affects the present PoT judgement. However, these results are not always replicated across studies, probably due to the diversity of activities performed in daily life. It would be interesting to test the effect of different categories of activities on the judgement of the PoT. For example, the experience of the performing arts examined in this book may have different temporal effects than other activities of daily life, for reasons related to the intensity of emotions and attentional focus. Recent studies have observed a slowing down of PoT during the lockdown imposed by national governments in order to fight against the spread of the COVID-19 pandemic (Cellini et al., 2020; Droit-Volet et al., 2020; Martinelli et al., 2021; Ogden, 2020). These studies confirmed that the slowing down of time was significantly linked to a decrease in the level of happiness, as well as to increased boredom. The association between subjective dilation of time and boredom has been observed in other contexts, such as waiting situations (Witowska et al., 2020; Zakay, 2014). The emotion of boredom is particularly complex because it is intimately linked to both negative emotion and a lack of activity. It has indeed been shown that the relationship between boredom and time is significantly mediated by lack of activity and decrease in happiness (Martinelli et al., 2021). However, the effect of boredom on PoT judgements cannot be reduced to these two factors. Boredom can also be related to a deprivation of meaningful information (van Hooft & van Hooft, 2018). In particular, Avni-Babad and Ritov (2003) found a lengthening of time estimates for a routine activity compared to a non-routine activity. Overall, these results support the dynamic occupation in time model proposed by Larson and von Eye (2006) on the basis of flow theory (Csikszentmihalyi & Csikszentmihalyi, 1988). According to this model, experience of time depends on intellectual and emotional engagement in an activity. In sum, activity-related attention and emotion constitute the two main categories of factors explaining variations in PoT judgement in the present.

Recently, we conducted a laboratory examination of the relationship between the present PoT and these two factors: attention and emotion (Martinelli & Droit-Volet, 2022). In our study, the participants performed a task with three levels of difficulty (easy, medium, and difficult) (Experiment 1), and were presented with emotional stimuli of negative, neutral, and positive valence (Experiment 2). The duration of the task and emotional stimuli were controlled and held constant. The results presented in Figure 4.2 show that the present PoT judgement varied directly with changes in non-temporal information. The feeling that time is passing faster thus increases linearly with the level of task difficulty. Similarly, PoT judgements increased with the valence of the emotional stimuli, such that time was judged to pass faster with the positive than with the neutral or the negative stimuli. These findings were observed for durations in both the seconds and minutes ranges even with the duration of the task and of the emotional stimuli held constant. Overall, these results confirm the

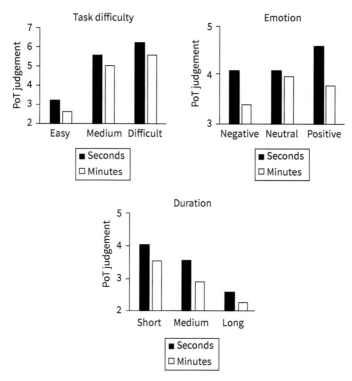

Figure 4.2 Present PoT judgements varying with changes in non-temporal information.

major role of attention and emotion in the momentary judgement of the PoT, but also its extreme intra-individual malleability depending on the context.

As suggested in Figure 4.1, the present PoT judgement would result from intro-spective analysis of oneself as the immediate subject of experience, the so-called 'minimal self' (Gallagher, 2000). Participants would thus translate their phenom-enological experience of changes in their internal state into temporal language. To account for this personal duration, we have adopted the concept of 'self-duration' as introduced by Minkowski (1968), and we contrast this with the 'self-time per-spective' and the 'world duration' mentioned above. This self-duration is elastic and very unstable because it depends on the awareness of temporal extensions or con-tractions of the self in certain contexts. When people are sad, they are aware that they have no more energy and express this by saying that time is dragging, passing slowly—that is, in terms of their own subjective durations. When they become aware that their minds are fully occupied by the task, they say that time is 'flying' or passing quickly. Bodily sensation may also modify this self-duration. However, to be able to say that time is passing faster or slower than usual, participants necessarily have to use a temporal reference scale. This reference scale is the 'external duration' ('world duration'), such as it is conceived of by humans in Western society. It is conceived of as a flow that runs at a constant rate regardless of the events that fill it, like the movement of our watches. Participants therefore experience subjective distortions of self-duration in comparison to objective external time. In sum, given that the self-duration depends on context, different dimensions can be used in the establishment of the present PoT judgement. It will be interesting to try to identify which category of factors prevails over the others, and then to understand why. However, in this contextual self-duration theory of present POT judgements, we assume that it is the emotions that prevail.

4.4 Relationship Between Present Passage of Time Judgements and Perception of Durations

Finally, in our contextual self-duration theory of the present PoT judgement, such judgements are based on the perception of contextual changes (internal or external) in non-temporal information. However, in our recent laboratory study, we also varied task duration while keeping non-temporal information constant (Experiment 3) (Martinelli & Droit-Volet, 2022). In this case, we also found a linear relationship between the present PoT judgement and the stimulus durations in both the seconds and minutes ranges. The PoT was judged to slow down as the duration increased. Furthermore, this decrease in the PoT judgement was proportional to the duration values, in keeping with the scalar properties of the perception of durations. We would not have found this result if PoT judgements were never based on temporal information. This suggests that present PoT judgements can also be based on estimations of duration when the changes in stimulus durations are the most salient information.

It is obvious that we can judge the speed of time for stimulus durations per se, saying, for example, that a short duration passes more quickly than a long duration. Accordingly, in Figure 4.1, we included PoT judgements based on the duration of events. An internal clock system is thought to be involved in the measurement of event duration. There is therefore an additional step in the hierarchical processing of durations in which the encoded duration is represented mentally in terms of the speed of the PoT. However, the way in which one represents and thinks about the flow of time may also (retroactively) influence the judgement of durations. Several studies have already shown how prior verbal instructions or the way we think about time impact the subsequent judgement of stimulus durations (Droit-Volet et al., 2015; Droit-Volet & Rattat, 2007). The prior feeling of the flow of time (verbal context) could thus modify the relationship between the present PoT judgement and perceived event duration.

In our study, the participants were instructed that they had to judge the PoT. We were therefore using a prospective and not a retrospective time judgement paradigm. This explains why the perception of stimulus durations still has an influence on PoT judgements, even though the changes in non-temporal information are the dominant factor in this type of judgement (as observed in the study involving task difficulty and that involving emotional stimuli; see Figure 4.2). However, in the ESM studies that have assessed present PoT in daily life, the present PoT judgement appeared to be unrelated to the judgement of durations. Droit-Volet and Wearden (2016) simultaneously assessed present PoT judgements, verbal estimates, and temporal production of short durations ranging from 350 to 1650 ms and found no significant correlation between these different temporal judgements. They concluded that the feeling of the PoT does not depend on measures of duration provided by an internal clock-like system. This dissociation between the judgement of present PoT and the duration estimation has since been observed with longer durations (from 2 to 33 s) (Droit-Volet et al., 2017). However, a significant correlation appeared when longer durations of several minutes were tested (Droit-Volet et al., 2017). Few studies have investigated the estimation of long durations of several minutes. It is thought that the estimation of very long durations is based on the non-temporal information stored in memory during the interval considered. Similarly, and as explained above, the present PoT judgement is based on non-temporal information (e.g. emotional state). Finally, although the subjects in the ecological studies using ESM were informed that they had to estimate the PoT, the present PoT judgement in daily life is also a retrospective and not a prospective judgement as in Martinelli and Droit-Volet's study (2022, Experiment 3), and concerns the period that has just passed. There are therefore two forms of present PoT judgements, the prospective and the retrospective judgement of PoT, and only the former (called PoT judgement of durations, Figure 4.1) can be linked to the duration perceived when changes in durations are the most salient information.

4.5 Conclusion

The results of studies of PoT judgements differ because of the variety of meanings that this judgement can encompass. Moreover, the PoT judgement is extremely unstable, changing as a function of the situation, the individual, and/or the questions asked. We identified four types of PoT judgement. The first two are retrospective PoT judgements, one for the long periods of life and the other for shorter periods covering the last week or the last month. The other two are the 'present' PoT judgement, made either prospectively (PoT judgement of durations) or retrospectively (present PoT judgement). Only in the prospective condition can the measurement of duration be used in the PoT judgement. In the other condition, the PoT results from the introspective analysis of changes in self-duration related to context (contextual self-duration theory of present PoT judgement). Therefore, the present PoT is elastic and fluctuates with our states, regardless of objectively measured time. But is the PoT really a judgement about time? What is time, after all? Whatever the answer to the deeper philosophical question, when we talk about our subjective experience of the PoT, we must immediately ask ourselves the question of which time it is we are referring to.

References

Avni-Babad, D., & Ritov, I. (2003). Routine and the perception of time. *Journal of Experimental Psychology: General, 132*(4), 543–550.

Blewett, A. E. (1992). Abnormal subjective time experience in depression. *British Journal of Psychiatry, 161*, 195–200.

Block, R. A. (1992). Prospective and retrospective duration judgment: The role of information processing and memory. In M. Macar, V. Pouthas, & W. J. Friedman (Eds.), *Time, action, and cognition: Towards bridging the gap Dordrecht* (pp. 141–152). Kluwer Academic Publishers.

Block, R. A., & Reed, M. A. (1978). Remembered duration: Evidence for a contextual-change hypothesis. *Journal of Experimental Psychology: Human Learning and Memory, 4*(6), 656–665.

Cellini, N., Canale, N., Mioni, G., & Costa, S. (2020). Changes in sleep pattern, sense of time and digital media use during COVID-19 lockdown in Italy. *Journal of Sleep Research, 29*(4), e13074. https://doi.org/10.1111/jsr.13074

Csikszentmihalyi, M., & Csikszentmihalyi, I. S. (1988). *Optimal experience: Psychological studies of flow in consciousness.* Cambridge University Press.

Dambrun, M., Ricard, M., Despr.s, G., Drelon, E., Gibelin, E., Gibelin, M., Loubeyre, M., Py, D., Delpy, A., Garibbo, C., Bray, E., Lac, G., & Michaux, O. (2012). Measuring happiness: From fluctuating happiness to authentic–durable happiness. *Frontiers in Psychology, 3*, 16. https://doi.org/10.3389/fpsyg.2012.00016

Dennett, D. C. (1991). *Consciousness explained.* Little, Brown.

Droit-Volet, S. (2018). Intertwined facets of subjective time. *Current Directions in Psychological Science, 27*(6), 422–428.

Droit-Volet, S. (2019). Time does not fly but slows down in old age. *Time & Society, 28*(1), 60–81.

Droit-Volet, S., Chaulet, M., Dutheil, F., & Dambrun, M. (2019). Mindfulness meditation, time judgment and time experience: Importance of the time scale considered (seconds or minutes). *PLoS One, 14*(10), e0223567. https://doi.org/10.1371/journal.pone.0223567

Droit-Volet, S., & Dambrun, M. (2019). Awareness of the passage of time and self-consciousness: What do meditators report? *PsyCH Journal, 8*(1), 51–65. https://doi.org/10.1002/pchj.270

Droit-Volet, S., Gil, S., Martinelli, N., Andant, N., Clinchamps, M., Parreira, L., Rouffiac, K., Dambrun, M., Huguet, P., Dubuis, B., Pereira, B., COVISTRESS network, Bouillon, J. B., & Dutheil, F. (2020). Time and Covid-19 stress in the lockdown situation: Time free, 'dying' of boredom and sadness. *PLoS One, 15*(8), e0236465. https://doi.org/10.1371/journal.pone.0236465

Droit-Volet, S., Lamotte, M., & Izaute, M. (2015). The conscious awareness of time distortions regulates the effect of emotion on the perception of time. *Consciousness and Cognition, 38*, 155–164. https://doi.org/10.1016/j.concog.2015.02.021

Droit-Volet, S., Martinelli, N., Dambrun, M., Vallet, G. T., & Lorandi, F. (2021). The retrospective and present judgment of the passage of time in the elderly. *Timing & Time Perception, 9*(4), 335–352. https://doi.org/10.1163/22134468-bja10031

Droit-Volet, S., & Rattat, A.C. (2007). A further analysis of temporal bisection behavior in children with and without reference memory: The similarity and the partition task. *Acta Psychologica, 125*(2), 240–256.

Droit-Volet, S., Trahanias, P., & Maniadakis, M. (2017). Passage of time judgments in everyday life are not related to duration judgments except for long durations of several minutes. *Acta Psychologica, 173*, 116–121.

Droit-Volet, S., & Wearden, J. (2015). Experience Sampling Methodology reveals similarities in the experience of passage of time in young and elderly adults. *Acta Psychologica, 156*, 77–82.

Droit-Volet, S., & Wearden, J. (2016). Passage of time judgments are not duration judgments: Evidence from a study using Experience Sampling Methodology. *Frontiers in Psychology, 7*, 176. https://doi.org/10.3389/fpsyg.2016.00176

Friedman, W. J., & Janssen, S. M. (2010). Aging and the speed of time. *Acta Psychologica, 134*, 130–141.

Fuchs, T. (2001). Melancholia as a desynchronization: Towards a psychopathology of interpersonal time. *Psychopathology, 34*, 179–186. https://doi.org/10.1159/000049304

Gallagher, S. (2000). Philosophical conceptions of the self: Implications for cognitive science. *Trends in Cognitive Sciences*, 4(1), 14–21.

Gallagher, S. (2012). Time, emotion, and depression. *Emotion Review*, 4, 127–132. https://doi.org/10.1177/1754073911430142

Gallagher, S. (2013). A pattern theory of self. *Frontiers in Human Neuroscience*, 7, 443. https://doi.org/10.3389/fnhum.2013.00443

Gibbon, J. (1991). Origins of scalar timing. *Learning and Motivation*, 22(1–2), 3–38. https://doi.org/10.1016/0023-9690(91)90015-Z

Gibbon, J., & Church, R. (1984). Sources of variance in an information processing theory of timing. In H. Roitblat, T. Bever, & H. Terrace (Eds.), *Animal cognition* (pp. 465–488). Lawrence Erlbaum Associates.

Gruber, R. P., Smith, R. P., & Block, R. A. (2018). The illusory flow and passage of time within consciousness: A multidisciplinary analysis? *Timing & Time Perception*, 6(6), 125–153. https://doi.org/10.1163/22134468-2018e001

Janssen, S. M. J. (2017). Autobiographical memory and the subjective experience of time. *Timing & Time Perception*, 5(1), 99–122.

Janssen, S. M. J., Naka, M., & Friedman, W. J. (2013). Why does life appear to speed up as people get older? *Time & Society*, 22(2), 274–290.

Joubert, C. E. (1983). Subjective acceleration of time: Death anxiety and sex differences. *Perceptual and Motor Skills*, 57(1), 49–50.

Kosak, F., Kuhbandner, C., & Hilbert, S. (2019). Time passes too fast? Then recall the past! —Evidence for a reminiscence heuristic in passage of time judgments. *Acta Psychologica*, 193, 197–202.

Lamartine, A. (1981). *Les méditations poétiques*. Gallimard (Original work published 1820).

Larson, E., & von Eye, A. (2006). Predicting the perceived flow of time from qualities of activity and depth of engagement. *Ecological Psychology*, 18(2), 113–130. https://doi.org/10.1207/s15326969eco1802_3

Lemlich, R. (1975). Subjective acceleration of time with aging. *Perceptual and Motor Skills*, 41(1), 235–238.

Martinelli, N., & Droit-Volet, S. (2022). What factors underlie our experience of the passage of time? Theoretical consequences. *Psychological Research*, 86(2), 522–530. https://doi.org/10.1007/s00426-021-01486-6

Martinelli, N., Gil, S., Belletier, C., Chevalère, J., Dezecache, G., Huguet, P., & Droit-Volet, S. (2021). Time and emotion during lockdown and the Covid-19 epidemic: Determinants of our experience of time? *Frontiers in Psychology*, 11, 616169. https://doi.org/10.3389/fpsyg.2020.616169

Minkowski, E. (1968). *Le temps vécu: Phénoménologiques et psychopathologiques*. Monfort.

Morin, A. (2006). Levels of consciousness and self-awareness: A comparison and integration of various neurocognitive views. *Consciousness and Cognition*, 15(2), 358371. https://doi.org/10.1016/j.concog.2005.09.006

Ogden, R. S. (2020). The passage of time during the UK Covid-19 lockdown. *PLoS One*, 15(7), e0235871. https://doi.org/10.1371/journal.pone.0235871

Ornstein, R. E. (1969). *On the experience of time*. Penguin Books. https://doi.org/10.1016/0010-0285(77)90012-3

Renoult, L., Irish, M., Moscovitch, M., & Rugg, M. D. (2019). From knowing to remembering: The semantic-episodic distinction. *Trends in Cognitive Sciences*, 23(12), 1041–1057. https://doi.org/10.1016/j.tics.2019.09.008

Thönes, S., & Oberfeld, D. (2015). Time perception in depression: A meta-analysis. *Journal of Affective Disorders*, 175, 359–372. https://doi.org/10.1016/j.jad.2014.12.057

Thönes, S., & Stocker, K. (2019). A standard conceptual framework for the study of subjective time. *Consciousness and Cognition*, 71, 114–122. https://doi.org/10.1016/j.concog.2019.04.004

Tulving, E. (1972). Episodic and semantic memory. In E. Tulving & W. Donaldson (Eds.), *Organization of memory* (pp. 381–403). Academic Press.

van Hooft, E. A. J., & van Hooff, M. L. M. (2018). The state of boredom: Frustrating or depressing? *Motivation and Emotion*, 42(6), 931–946. https://doi.org/10.1007/s11031-018-9710-6

Vogel, D. H. V., Krämer, K., Schoofs, T., Kupke, C., & Vogeley, K. (2018). Disturbed experience of time in depression—Evidence from content analysis. *Frontiers in Human Neuroscience, 12*, 66. https://doi.org/10.3389/fnhum.2018.00066

Wearden, J. H. (2015). Passage of time judgements. *Consciousness and Cognition, 38*, 165–168. https://doi.org/10.1016/j.concog.2015.06.005

Winkler, I., Fischer, K., Kliesow, K, Rudolph, T., Thiel, C., & Sedlmeier, P. (2017). Has it really been that long? Why time seems to speed up with age. *Timing and Time Perception, 5*(2), 168–189. https://doi.org/10.1163/22134468-00002088

Wittmann, M. (2016). *Felt time: The psychology of how we perceive time* (E. Butler, Trans.). MIT Press.

Wittmann, M., & Lehnhoff, S. (2005). Age effects in perception of time. *Psychological Reports, 97*(3), 921–935. https://doi.org/10.2466/pr0.97.3.921-935

Witowska, J., Schmidt, S., & Wittmann, M. (2020). What happens while waiting? How self-regulation affects boredom and subjective time during a real waiting situation. *Acta Psychologica, 205*, 103061.

Wöllner, C., & Hammerschmidt, D. (2021). Tapping to hip-hop: Effects of cognitive load, arousal, and musical meter on time experiences. *Attention, Perception and Psychophysics, 83*(4), 1552–1561. https://doi.org/10.3758/s13414-020-02227-4

Zakay, D. (2014). Psychological time as information: The case of boredom. *Frontiers in Psychology, 5*, 917. https://doi.org/10.3389/fpsyg.2014.00917

Zimbardo, P. G., & Boyd, J. N. (1999). Putting time in perspective: A valid, reliable individual-differences metric. *Journal of Personality and Social Psychology, 77*(6), 1271–1288. https://doi.org/10.1037/0022-3514.77.6.1271

SECTION 2

DURATION, TEMPO, AND PACING
IN PERFORMANCE AND PERCEPTION

Anchor Chapters

5

What Is Musical Tempo?

Justin London

5.1 Musical Tempo Is Not Speed

Musical tempo is commonly regarded as the 'speed' of the music—we routinely characterize a piece or performance as fast, moderate, or slow, and the traditional tempo terms (e.g. largo, *lentement*, and *langsam*) reflect this characterization, at least in musical contexts.[1] However, if speed is the relationship between units of distance travelled per some unit of time (i.e. the physicist's $v = d/t$),[2] then when we talk about musical tempo as speed, we have some problems. The first has to do with distance: how does one measure the 'distance' travelled between successive notes? Intuitively, we might think of distance in terms of melodic intervals—small/short stepwise distances, versus larger/longer skips. But what actually moves? A change in frequency of vibration is not equivalent to a change in spatial position. And another obvious problem here is that we can discern the musical tempo of non-pitched music, as in the case of drumming.

Even if we set those caveats aside and accept pitch intervals as a measure of distance (and leaving aside complications due to harmony and polyphony), matters are still not straightforward. For as intervallic distance between successive pitches increases, so too does the potential for auditory streaming (Bregman, 1990). Thus, when presented with a rapid series of alternating melodic skips, rather than hearing a series of wide distances travelled in quick succession, we tend to hear two interleaved, slower auditory streams/melodies (i.e. each with longer inter-onset intervals), each of which travels in a narrower melodic compass. Similarly, Boltz (1998) found that melodies that contained many changes in pitch direction and/or wider intervals were perceived as moving slower in comparison to a standard with fewer changes in pitch direction and/or smaller intervals. In other words, melodic distance is not a straightforward measurement under the best of circumstances.

There are similar constraints on our perception of time. There is a relatively limited range in which we are able to make reliable judgements of duration and in which we can perceive a beat or pulse (for summaries, see Levitin et al., 2018; London, 2012). Successive events can only become so fast before we hit a trill/subitizing threshold (approximately 100 ms/10 Hz) beyond which events/notes become difficult to separate or count. Likewise, for most listeners a sense of temporal continuity is lost if events are more than 1.5–2.0 s apart (0.75–0.5 Hz), and durational discrimination

Justin London, *What Is Musical Tempo?* In: *Performing Time.* Edited by: Clemens Wöllner and Justin London, Oxford University Press.
© Oxford University Press 2023. DOI: 10.1093/oso/9780192896254.003.0006

becomes appreciably poorer. Thus, there are difficulties in determining both the numerator and denominator of the equation $v = d/t$ for music.

We might at this point admit that rather than velocity or speed—concepts that are at best metaphorically applied to music—we should think of musical tempo as a 'rate of activity'. This is an improvement, but perceptual hazards are still present.

5.2 Musical Tempo Is Not Beats per Minute

If we approach tempo as a 'rate of activity', then a question arises: what is the relevant activity to whose rate we attend? The most common answer in musical contexts would be 'the beat', and hence beat rate, expressed in beats per minute (BPM), would be the index of tempo. And indeed, musicians, DJs, and music psychologists often use BPM rates this way. While most listeners have an intuitive notion of beat, a precise definition is difficult to pin down. A practical/operational definition for beat is 'the rate at which you tap your foot or finger in listening along to the music'—that is, a comfortable rate of periodic motor engagement, which usually falls within or near to 100–120 BPM for most listeners. If one has two melodies, both consisting of isochronous note durations, one note per beat, then within a moderate range of tempo differences, BPM would suffice as a measure of speed.

Things are rarely so musically simple. The first problem has to do with the relationship between notes and beats. Consider the two versions of Beethoven's 'Ode to Joy' given in Figure 5.1.

The melody is the same in both cases, but the tempos are different. In the first, at 78 quarter notes per minute, we are likely to tap our feet/feel the tactus at that same rate—the notes correspond to BPM rate, and we will hear every second or fourth note as a metrically accented downbeat ('D' in Figure 5.1). In the second, sped up to 138 quarter notes per minute, most listeners are likely to tap along/feel the beat every other note, and therefore hear each individual note as a subdivision ('SD' in Figure 5.1) of a beat at 69 BPM. If tempo were simply a matter of beat rate, then for many listeners, the second performance of 'Ode to Joy' (at 138 BPM) would be perceived as *slower* than the first—but it is not. Many if not most melodies and rhythms afford multiple modes of rhythmic engagement and beat perception (see London,

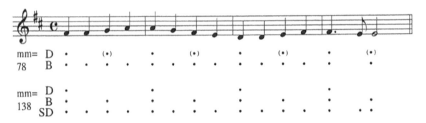

Figure 5.1 Different metrical hierarchies in the opening measures of Beethoven's 'Ode to Joy' (Ninth Symphony, fourth movement) when played at two different tempos.

2012; Martens, 2011, 2012; Palmer, 2013). Thus differences in the 'surface activity' in a melody or rhythm do not always directly correspond to beat rate, but may correspond to different levels of the metric hierarchy—downbeat to downbeat, beat to beat, or beat subdivision to beat subdivision (see London, 2012).

Why not just look at the rate of surface activity, rather than worry about beats? As noted above, there are perceptual limits on our apprehension of successive events. Very fast activity does not equal speed—trills, tremolo, and vibrato, for example, are more aptly regarded as timbre-like qualities of a sustained tone, rather than individual, successive tones. Moreover, most melodies are not like the 'Ode to Joy', which is composed almost entirely of notes of equal duration (i.e. an 'isochronous' rhythm). Rather, most melodies contain a mixture of notes of different lengths— and as a result, the perceived beat cannot be ignored. Consider the melody from Brahms' Fourth Symphony, first movement, given in Figure 5.2. Since the durations vary, a plausible approach is to calculate the average note duration, or more precisely, the average note inter-onset interval duration (allowing for the same calculation whether the melody is played legato or staccato). In Figure 5.2, this would be a half note. However, Brahms' melody seems faster than an isochronous series of half notes. Its short–long rhythm does instil a sense of beat on the level of the notated half note, even though many of these beats are not articulated in the melody at all. But the short–long rhythm also marks a latent level of beat subdivision (corresponding to the notated quarter note), given a sense of more activity than just at the beat (half-note) and downbeat (whole note) periodicity—and thus the passage seems faster.

Finally, in Figure 5.2, the beat is not continuously present in the melody, but must be interpolated by the listener. This illustrates the fact that beats are endogenous aspects of rhythm perception, a series of temporal articulations that are felt by the listener but are not necessarily acoustically articulated by the music.

Thus beat rate (which may or may not correspond to the BPM in relation to a particular rhythmic value, such as a quarter note) and the rate of surface activity— subdivisions in duplets, triplets, quadruplets, and so on—both contribute to our sense of tempo (Drake et al., 1999; London, 2006). Additional musical factors can influence perceived tempo. Composers and musicians have recognized that the pacing of harmonic activity—so-called harmonic rhythm—can affect the perceived sense of musical motion and speed (Rothstein, 1989; Swain, 2002). Boltz (2011) found that register and timbre can affect perceived tempo, with higher pitches and brighter timbres conveying a faster tempo. Burger and colleagues (2013, 2018) found that

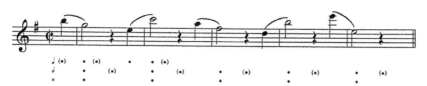

Figure 5.2 Opening melody of Brahms' Fourth Symphony, first movement; interpolated beats are in parenthesis (corresponding to the notated half note).

low-frequency spectral flux and the percussiveness of articulation can also affect one's sense of movement and tempo. Furthermore, as a cautionary tale, Eitan and Granot (2006) found that different parameters (duration, register, loudness, etc.) combine in complex ways to produce perceptions of intensification or abatement, which affect perceived tempo.

5.3 Cross-Modal Complications: Musical Tempo Involves More Than Audition

Even if one could sort out all the cues from the auditory/musical signal, and how they are to be combined and weighted, this would still not suffice to fully explain our sense of tempo. For in addition to what we hear, what we see and what we already know also affect tempo perception. Schutz and Lipscomb (2007) discovered that a performer's physical gesture could affect the listener's perception of the duration of the resulting sound. Specifically, the kind of gesture a marimba player made after striking the instrument with a mallet—either a long, fluid motion, or a short, sharper motion—could make the tone seem longer or shorter. The change in duration is illusory, but tellingly, the illusion only works with the right kind of sounds, and the right kind of gestures—if one sees the gesture characteristic of striking a marimba and hears the sound of violin, for example, the illusion does not occur (Armontrout et al., 2009). Schutz and Kubovy (2009) noted that 'integrating across these modalities makes sense only when the perceptual system has evidence that the sights and the sounds originated from a common event' (p. 1792), which led them to their *binding by causality* hypothesis: 'sounds have a propensity to bind with the visible movements that could have caused them' (p. 1793).

Inspired by the work of Schutz and his co-workers, my colleagues and I examined the effect of visual information on the perception of tempo in a similarly ecologically valid manner (London et al., 2016). Using a motion capture system, we asked participants to freely dance to a selection of Motown R&B songs, chosen for their tempo range (all had a clear periodicity between 100 and 130 BPM), high level of beat salience (Stupacher et al., 2016), and sense of 'groove', affording/inviting rhythmic movement (Janata et al., 2012). We asked participants to produce two different dance interpretations to each song, a smooth/'relaxed' interpretation, and a 'vigorous' interpretation; vigorous interpretations were jerkier and had higher overall levels of acceleration. From these motion capture trials we were able to generate stimuli for a perceptual experiment, in which animated stick-figure dancers were presented with audio stimuli, chosen to ensure that visual and auditory cues were matched (same dancer for each dance condition) and synchronized to the dominant periodicities in the auditory/musical signal.

Our results are given in Figure 5.3a. When asked to rate the tempo of the music on a 7-point scale while watching the dancer animations, participants consistently rated

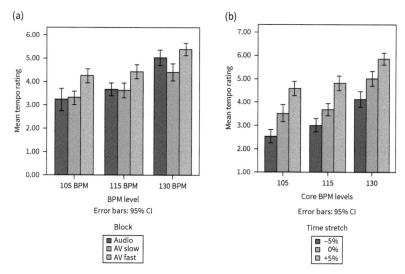

Figure 5.3 Results from London et al. (2016). (a) The effect of visual motion for tempo judgements for stimuli at three fixed tempo levels. Bar colours indicate baseline (audio-only) condition (blue), relaxed/slow dance condition (green), and vigorous/fast dance condition (tan). (b) Tempo anchoring effect (TAE) at three core tempo levels (green), with digitally decreased (blue) and increased (tan) tempos; veridical tempo judgements would be a monotonic increase from left to right. AV, audiovisual; CI, confidence interval.

the 'vigorous' interpretations as faster than both the 'relaxed' interpretations and an audio-only baseline condition.

We argued that, analogously to the binding by causality hypothesis, the higher tempo ratings for the 'vigorous' dance animations are due to people's perceptual systems integrating the information from the 'common event' of seeing someone dancing to the music they are hearing—and that while people sometimes dance slowly to vigorous/fast music, fast/vigorous dancing is only appropriate when the music itself is fast and vigorous. In integrating the auditory and visual information in the most plausible way, people integrate the virtual speed/movement cues in the auditory domain with the actual speed/movement cues in the visual modality—and so the music seems faster.

We also found an unexpected result (London et al., 2016), one revealing another factor which influences our judgements of musical tempo: prior knowledge of a song/ recording can anchor one's perception of subsequent encounters with it. In our baseline listening condition, we presented participants with just the audio portion of the Motown dance songs, and asked them to give tempo ratings to each song (again, on a 7-point scale). To ensure that participants were attentive, and to ensure that they did not reflexively associate a fixed tempo with each stimulus, we told them that sometimes stimuli would be digitally sped up or slowed down. We were expecting in the audio-only condition we would see a more or less veridical set of tempo judgements, reflecting the monotonic increase in tempo across all of our stimuli. The results we obtained are given in Figure 5.3b. As can be seen, participants accurately sorted out tempos for the various presentations of each stimulus (note the ranking within each core BPM level), but overestimated the extent to which tempos were increased or decreased. We dubbed this the *tempo anchoring effect* (TAE), and we were able to replicate it in several subsequent studies (Hammerschmidt et al., 2021; London, Burger, et al., 2019; London, Thompson, et al., 2019). In one set of studies (London, Thompson, et al., 2019), in addition to the original Motown stimuli, an analogous set of disco songs also gave rise to the TAE—but an analogous set of drum stimuli did not.

There are several implications from these studies of the TAE. One is that the TAE is perhaps related to studies of the negative mean asynchrony, that is, the tendency to tap slightly ahead of a click when synchronizing to a metronome, but not when synchronizing to music (Repp, 2005; Repp & Su, 2013). Perhaps there is a sense of 'tonal movement' that is present in melodies/full-blooded songs that is lacking in percussive stimuli, even complex percussive stimuli. Thus, melodic patterns are subject to the TAE while purely percussive patterns are not. Alternatively, this could be an effect of memory encoding. It is well known that it is easier to remember melodies that combine a degree of rhythmic variety/structure along with pitch patterning (e.g. Jones, 1993). If the tempo of the normative version of a song/recording is well encoded (Halpern, 1988; Jakubowski et al., 2015; Levitin & Cook, 1996), the TAE may be an example of *perceptual sharpening*, where the low-level feature differences are exaggerated. As noted by London, Thompson, et al. (2019):

> The digitally sped-up or slowed-down stimuli, however, did present a conflict between absolute and relative judgments, as the robust memory for the tempo of these musically rich stimuli provided a basis for a relative judgment, but rather than more accurate responses relative to the absolute scale, those responses were exaggerated—which is to say, sharpened. The TAE-as-a-form-of-perceptual-sharpening makes sense both in terms of our having robust, high-level object representations of music . . . and in characterizing tempo as a low-level feature of our auditory perception. (p. 38)

Finally, to study the effect of low-level versus higher-level perception of tempo, in a separate study (London, Thompson, et al., 2019) we presented listeners with the original and time-shifted stimuli in two different movement conditions: tapping along and not tapping along. Our hypothesis was that active motor engagement should have eliminated the TAE, as previous studies found that overt movement improved beat finding (Su & Pöppel, 2012) and asynchrony detection (Manning & Schutz, 2016), and that beat-based rhythm perception actively involves the sensorimotor system (e.g. Chen et al., 2008; Maes et al., 2014; Ross et al., 2018). Surprisingly, tapping did not help—the TAE persisted in both tapping and non-tapping conditions. Thus, and consistent with our account of the TAE as a form of perceptual sharpening, the lack of an effect of tapping suggests that while sensorimotor synchronization and asynchrony detection involve relatively low-level sensory processes, a tempo judgement or characterization involves higher-level cognitive processes.

5.4 The Energetics of Action (and Action Perception)

Humans are very sensitive to the energetic cost of their actions and activities, most especially walking and running. Indeed, walking and running are astonishingly efficient ways to move; at optimal walking rates, humans use very little metabolic energy, exploiting the pendular dynamics of bipedal striding that developed through millions of years of evolution. Walking and running are two distinctly different modes of bipedal motion, each of which exploits properties of human biomechanics and pendular dynamics:

> In walking, the body behaves like an inverted pendulum, yielding highly conservative exchanges of kinetic and potential energy. In running, the body behaves like a bouncing ball, in which kinetic energy is converted to elastic energy stored in the tendons and muscles of the stance leg. (Diedrich & Warren, 1995, p. 183)

Bertram (2005) mapped the metabolic costs of walking at various speeds and various step rates by having participants walk on a treadmill at a fixed rate, and matching their step rate to a metronome (NB: this then also forces changes in step length, as one matches the step rate to the treadmill speed). He found that the lowest metabolic cost occurred between 1.7 and 2.0 steps per minute (i.e. 100–120 BPM) at a walking pace of about 1.1 m/s (see also Faraji et al., 2018). Bertram also found that either going faster or slower at the same step rate (i.e. shortening or lengthening one's stride), or maintaining the same speed but with an increased or decreased step rate (and keeping stride length constant), incurred sharply higher metabolic costs. Of interest to music perception researchers is that the range of maximally efficient walking maps closely onto the range of preferred tempo/maximal pulse salience (Fraisse, 1982; London, 2012; McAuley, 2010; see also Hammerschmidt, this volume; Henry & Kotz, this volume); it is not surprising that our preferred tempos correspond to the walking rates that are most comfortable, that is, those with the lowest metabolic cost.

5.5 So, What *Is* Musical Tempo?

Thus far, this chapter has made the following observations regarding our grasp of musical tempo:

1. Tempo is not a direct analogue to speed or velocity, as there are problems in our grasp of both musical 'distance' and musical 'time' that pre-empt any simple relation between the two.
2. Tempo is more than simply beat rate, or the rate of events per unit time (or the average thereof), though these are highly salient cues for our sense of tempo.

3. Additional auditory/musical cues for tempo include loudness, register, timbre, articulation, and dynamic envelope.
4. There are important non-auditory/non-musical inputs to our sense of tempo, most especially visual cues, but also aspects of musical enculturation and memory.
5. While active movement can enhance some aspects of rhythm perception and judgement, such as event timing and synchronization (Manning & Schutz, 2016; Su & Pöppel, 2012), it does not directly influence tempo judgements (London, Thompson, et al., 2019).

From these observations, one can conclude that tempo is not a simple characterization of an auditory or visual stimulus. Rather, it is a kind of 'summary judgement' that involves a multimodal set of perceptual inputs, as well as our background of musical and non-musical experience. Thus, a tempo judgement involves *reducing* this constellation of cues to a single dimension of 'speed'. In this fashion, tempo is akin to pitch, as our perceptual systems make a similar reduction regarding the complex pattern of energies present in a periodic sound to a single 'virtual pitch' (Terhardt et al., 1982). As with pitch, almost all listeners make judgements of tempo very quickly; we are able to make both relative and absolute judgements of tempo; and tempo judgements fall on a single dimension—given two different tempos, we can readily say that one is either faster or slower than another.

Damasio (Bechara & Damasio, 2005: Damasio, 1996, 1999) has explored the ways that cognitive judgements and their accompanying affective-emotional responses/characterizations are intimately intertwined. Moreover, these judgements and their affective aspects are also enmeshed in our bodily actions, from the high-level, deliberate actions to the lowest levels of homeostatic regulation. Damasio proposed his *somatic marker hypothesis* (SMH) as a framework for understanding these interrelationships:

> The key idea in the hypothesis is that 'marker' signals influence the processes of response, at multiple levels of operation, some of which occur overtly (consciously, 'in mind') and some covertly (non-consciously, in a non-minded manner). The marker signals arise in bioregulatory processes, including those which express themselves in emotions and feelings, but are not necessarily those alone. This is the reason why the markers are termed somatic: they relate to body-state and regulation even when they do not arise in the body proper but rather in the brain's representation of the body. (Damasio, 1996, p. 1413)

Damasio developed the SMH to explain the role that emotions play in decision-making and other forms of ratiocination: 'Human reasoning and decision making depend on many levels of neurobiological operation, some of which occur in the mind (i.e., are conscious, overt, cognitive) and some of which do not' (Damasio, 1996, p. 1414). A key element of the SMH is that of *sensorimotor simulation*, an embodied mechanism through which sensory-motor resources are recruited for cognitive purposes through their partial neural activation. This has its origins in the discovery of mirror neurons (Gallese et al., 1996), though it is also related to Damasio's 'as if body loop' in which somatosensory cortices respond 'as if' there were actual bodily responses to some stimulus, even when the bodily response is absent (Damasio, 1996, p. 1415). Similarly, Gallese (2002), who explicitly acknowledges the influence of Lipps (see below), argues for the importance of 'embodied simulation' which 'mediates our capacity to share the meaning of actions, intentions, feelings, and emotions with others' (p. 519).

Damasio's account of sensorimotor simulation is remarkably similar to the notion of 'metakinesis' developed by John Martin (1933/1989). Drawing upon the idea of 'inner imitation' developed by Lipps (1903/1935), which for Lipps was the foundation of our sense of empathy, Martin aimed to give an account for the expressive properties of 'modern' (early 20th century) dance. According to Martin (1933/1989), metakinesis is the 'psychic accompaniment' that is correlated with our perception of movement, which allows for 'the transference of an aesthetic and emotional concept from the consciousness of one individual to that of another' (p. 13). As Martin notes: 'Through kinesthetic sympathy you respond to the impulse of the dancer which has expressed itself by means of a series of movements. Movement, then, is the link between the dancer's intention and your perception of it' (p. 12).

5.6 Conclusion

To summarize, rhythm perception strongly engages our sensorimotor system, if not in terms of actual, overt movement, then in terms of imagined/covert self-movements. Sensorimotor activity—whether our own, or what we observe in others—inherently has an affective character to it. We speak of rhythmic and melodic sequences as 'musical gestures', and not merely because we may be able to see or imagine the physical actions a musician must perform in order to produce them. While Cox (2011) has emphasized this aspect of 'musical gesture' (and hence embodied cognition), one must note that musical instruments are technological artefacts that allow small actions/low-energy inputs to produce much bigger outputs—not just in terms of volume (think of the electric guitar), but in terms of speed and agility, as their ergonomics have evolved over centuries of evolution and refinement. Thus, our grasp of the embodied aspects of a musical gesture involves more than understanding the finger motions or breathing that is involved in musical tone production.

Therefore, if we consider the sensorimotor aspects of rhythm perception in terms of Damasio's SMH, and keep in mind that tempo is a distillation from a constellation of cues, we are now in a position to understand what tempo really is. If pitch is the distillation of the pattern of higher-frequency auditory energy in order to discern its source, tempo is a distillation of lower-frequency auditory energy in order to discern what that source is doing. In non-musical contexts it involves a grasp of the intensity, force, extent, and rate of some activity of some agent. In non-musical contexts, we transparently grasp the ecological significance of pitch and rhythm/tempo cues to gain information about sound sources in our environment (Clarke, 2001). In musical contexts, these same perceptual mechanisms are engaged, but with some (but not all) of the ecological significance of those sounds suppressed. The art of harmony is that of creating chords—that is, multiple voices or instruments which fuse into the appearance of a virtual auditory object. Similarly, the art of rhythm is to create the sense of the action(s) and motion of a virtual musical agent.

Tempo, then, is an energistic assessment of the activity of some agent—whether actual (as in observing someone doing something) or virtual (as in listening to a piece of music). Tempo is correlated with loudness (Eitan & Granot, 2006; Küssner et al., 2014), as well as timbre and register (Boltz, 2011). It is of course related to the rate of activity of the perceived agent, but that percept is 'filtered' through our embodied grasp of what is involved in performing that activity. This is why the most salient rates of rhythmic activity—the rate of the beat or tactus—coincide with those rates that best afford human motor action, including synchronized action. As such, it also allows our somatic markers for such actions to be involved in higher-level judgements/characterizations of that activity, which we often reduce to the single dimension of 'tempo'. This is how and why 'tempo' can be related to our sense of the metabolic cost of those actions—whether we are doing those activities ourselves, or perceiving someone else performing those actions—and thus our real or imaginary sensorimotor engagement with music inherently involves the same kinds of energistic awareness.

What I have proposed here is not the first energistic account of music. Ernst Kurth, in his *Musikpsychologie* (1931/1947), explicitly speaks of musical motion as *Bewegungsenergie*, 'energy of motion'. As Tan (2013) notes, 'Force, Space, and Matter' were metaphors for musical experience (p. 100); and for Kurth, *Bewegungsenergie* was a form of psychic/mental energy, and not a physical force, for many of the same reasons articulated at the beginning of this chapter. Indeed, Kurth's description of the mental grasp of musical motion is tantalizingly similar to a mirror neuron system account of action perception, an 'inner energy of motion' (see Tan, 2013, pp. 102–113). Kurth does not, however, connect *Bewegungsenergie* to real or imagined motor behaviour, or other bodily manifestations of action and motion. My claim here is that musical *Bewegungsenergie* is not metaphorical, but corporal and concrete, and (following Damasio) just as palpable in our experience of music as is our affective responses, motor behaviours, and cognitive awareness.

For all its complexity, what is both amazing and perfectly ordinary is that listeners readily, easily, and quickly make accurate tempo judgements. Within less than a second, we can judge if a piece is fast, moderate, or slow. Our motor system is intimately linked to affective and metabolic systems, and rhythm judgements are deeply entangled in these other aspects of perception. Tempo is a summary judgement of energistic cost(s) of musical behaviour, or more precisely, of the effort involved in moving in a manner analogous to the way the music seems to move. We do this in large part by mirroring/simulating those movements as we listen. Thus, tempo is not simply 'How fast does the music go?' but rather, 'How much energy and effort is re-quired for me to keep up with it?'

Notes

1. Notably, the common Italian terms do not literally refer to speed—allegro is 'lively', and largo con-notes 'wide'. See Fallows (2001) for more on the history and etymology of tempo terms.
2. More precisely, v is a vector which has both magnitude and direction, whereas speed is a scalar with only magnitude. While mostly we speak of musical tempo independent of direction (i.e. it does not matter if the melody is going up or down), when direction is included, one can properly speak of a musical velocity—provided one can accurately calculate the scalar component, upon which this chapter casts doubt.

References

Armontrout, J., Schutz, M., & Kubovy, M. (2009). Visual determinants of a cross-modal illusion. *Attention, Perception & Psychophysics, 71*(7), 1618–1627.

Bechara, A., & Damasio, A. R. (2005). The somatic marker hypothesis: A neural theory of economic decision. *Games and Economic Behavior, 52*(2), 336–372.

Bertram, J. E. (2005). Constrained optimization in human walking: Cost minimization and gait plas-ticity. *Journal of Experimental Biology, 208*(6), 979–991.

Boltz, M. G. (1998). Tempo discrimination of musical patterns: Effects due to pitch and rhythmic struc-ture. *Perception & Psychophysics, 60*(8), 1357–1373.

Boltz, M. G. (2011). Illusory tempo changes due to musical characteristics. *Music Perception, 28*(4), 367–386.

Bregman, A. S. (1990). *Auditory scene analysis: The perceptual organization of sound.* MIT Press.

Burger, B., Thompson, M. R., Luck, G., Saarikallio, S., & Toiviainen, P. (2013). Influences of rhythm- and timbre-related musical features on characteristics of music-induced movement. *Frontiers in Psychology, 4*, 183.

Burger, B., Thompson, M. R., Luck, G., Saarikallio, S., & Toiviainen, P. (2014). Hunting for the beat in the body: On period and phase locking in music-induced movement. *Frontiers in Human Neuroscience, 8*, 903.

Burger, B., London, J., Thompson, M., & Toiviainen, P. (2018). Synchronization to metrical levels in music depends on low frequency spectral components and tempo. *Psychological Research, 82*(6), 1195–1211.

Chen, J. L., Penhune, V. B., & Zatorre, R. J. (2008). Listening to musical rhythms recruits motor regions of the brain. *Cerebral Cortex, 18*(12), 2844–2854.

Clarke, E. F. (2001). Meaning and the specification of motion in music. *Musicae Scientiae, 5*(2), 213–234.

Cox, A. (2011). Embodying music: Principles of the mimetic hypothesis. *Music Theory Online, 17*(2).

Damasio, A. R. (1996). The somatic marker hypothesis and the possible functions of the prefrontal cortex. *Philosophical Transactions of the Royal Society of London. Series B, 351*(1346), 1413–1420.

Damasio, A. R. (1999). *The feeling of what happens: Body and emotion in the making of consciousness.* Harcourt College Publishers.

Diedrich, F. J., & Warren, W. H. (1995). Why change gaits? Dynamics of the walk-run transition. *Journal of Experimental Psychology: Human Perception and Performance, 21*(1), 183–202.

Drake, C., Gros, L., & Penel, A. (1999). How fast is that music? The relation between physical and per-ceived temp. In S. W. Yi (Ed.), *Music, mind, and science* (pp. 190–203). Seoul National University.

Eitan, Z., & Granot, R. Y. (2006). How music moves: Musical parameters and listeners' images of mo-tion. *Music Perception, 23*(3), 221–247.

Fallows, D. (2001). Tempo and expression marks. *Grove Music Online.* Retrieved 18 Jun. 2021, from https://www.oxfordmusiconline.com

Faraji, S., Wu, A. R., & Ijspeert, A. J. (2018). A simple model of mechanical effects to estimate metabolic cost of human walking. *Nature Scientific Reports, 8*(11), 10998.

Fraisse, P. (1982). Rhythm and tempo. In D. Deutsch (Ed.), *The psychology of music* (pp. 149–180). Academic Press.

Gallese, V. (2002). Mirror neurons, embodied simulation, and the neural basis of social identification. *Psychoanalytic Dialogues, 19*(5), 519–536.

Gallese, V., Fadiga, L., Fogassi, L., & Rizzolatti, G. (1996). Action recognition in the premotor cortex. *Brain, 119*(2), 593–609.

Halpern, A. R. (1988). Perceived and imagined tempos of familiar songs. *Music Perception, 6*(2), 193–202.

Hammerschmidt, D., Wöllner, C., London, J., & Burger, B. (2021). Disco time: The relationship between perceived duration and tempo in music. *Music & Science, 4,* 1–11.

Hansen, E. A., Kristensen, L. A. R., Nielsen, A. M., Voigt, M., & Madeleine, P. (2017). The role of stride frequency for walk-to-run transition in humans. *Nature Scientific Reports, 7*(1), 2010.

Iacoboni, M. (2009). Imitation, empathy, and mirror neurons. *Annual Review of Psychology, 60,* 653–670.

Jakubowski, K., Farrugia, N., Halpern, A. R., Sankarpandi, S. K., & Steweart, L. (2015). The speed of our mental soundtracks: Tracking the tempo of involuntary musical imagery in everyday life. *Memory & Cognition, 43*(8), 1229–1242.

Janata, P., Tomic, S. T., & Haberman, J. M. (2012). Sensorimotor coupling in music and the psychology of the groove. *Journal of Experimental Psychology: General, 141*(1), 54–75.

Jones, M. R. (1993). Dynamics of musical patterns: How do melody and rhythm fit together? In T. J. Tighe & W. J. Dowling (Eds.), *Psychology and music: The understanding of melody and rhythm* (pp. 67–92). Lawrence Erlbaum.

Kurth, E. (1947). *Musikpsychologie.* Krompholz. (Original work published 1931)

Küssner, M. B., Tidhar, D., Prior, H. M., & Leech-Wilkinson, D. (2014). Musicians are more consistent: Gestural cross-modal mappings of pitch, loudness, and tempo in real-time. *Frontiers in Psychology: Auditory Cognitive Neuroscience, 5,* 789.

Levitin, D. J., & Cook, P. R. (1996). Memory for musical tempo: Additional evidence that auditory memory is absolute. *Perception and Psychophysics, 58*(6), 927–935.

Levitin, D. J., Grahn, J., & London, J. (2018). The psychology of music: Rhythm and movement. *Annual Review of Psychology, 69*(1), 13.1–13.25.

Lipps, T. (1903). Einfühlung, innere Nachamung, und Organemfindungen (empathy, inner imitation and sense-feelings). In *Asthetik: Psychologie des Schönen und der Kunst,* vol. I, Leopold Voss; translation in Rader, M. (1935). *A modern book of esthetics* (pp. 291–304). Henry Holt & Co.

London, J. (2006). Musical rhythm: Motion, pace, gesture. In A. Gritten & E. King (Eds.), *Music and gesture* (pp. 126–141). Ashgate.

London, J. (2012). *Hearing in time* (2nd ed.). Oxford University Press.

London, J., Burger, B., Thompson, M., & Toiviainen, P. (2016). Speed on the dance floor: Auditory and visual cues for musical tempo. *Acta Psychologica, 164,* 70–80.

London, J., Burger, B., Thompson, M., Hildreth, M., Wilson, J., Schally, N., & Toiviainen, P. (2019). Motown, disco, and drumming: An exploration of the relationship between beat salience, melodic structure, and perceived tempo. *Music Perception, 37*(1), 26–41.

London, J., Thompson, M., Burger, B., Hildreth, M., Wilson, J., & Toiviainen, P. (2019). Tapping doesn't help: Synchronized self-motion and judgments of musical tempo. *Attention, Perception, and Psychophysics, 81*(7), 2461–2472.

Maes, P.-J., Leman, M., Palmer, C., & Wanderley, M. M. (2014). Action-based effects on music perception. *Frontiers in Psychology, 4,* 1008.

Manning, F. C., & Schutz, M. (2016). Trained to keep a beat: Movement-related enhancements to timing perception in percussionists and non-percussionists. *Psychological Research, 80*(4), 532–542.

Martens, P. (2011). The ambiguous tactus: Metric structure, subdivision benefit, and three listener strategies. *Music Perception, 28*(5), 433–448.

Martens, P. (2012). Tactus in performance: Constraints and possibilities. *Music Theory Online, 18*(1), 5.

Martin, J. (1989). *The modern dance*. Princeton Book Company/Dance Horizons. (Original work published 1933)

McAuley, J. D. (2010). Tempo and rhythm. In M. R. Jones, R. R. Fay, & A. N. Popper (Eds.), *Music perception* (pp. 165–199). Springer Science.

Molnar-Szakacs, I., Kaplan, J., Greenfield, P. M., & Iacoboni, M. (2006). Observing complex action sequences: The role of the fronto-parietal mirror neuron system. *NeuroImage, 33*(3), 923–935.

Molnar-Szakacs, I., & Overy, K. (2006). Music and mirror neurons: From motion to 'e'motion. *Social Cognitive and Affective Neuroscience, 1*(3), 235–241.

Ocampo, B., & Kritikos, A. (2011). Interpreting actions: The goal behind mirror neuron function. *Brain Research Reviews, 67*(1–2), 260–267.

Overy, K., & Molnar-Szakacs, I. (2009). Being together in time: Musical experience and the mirror neuron system. *Music Perception, 26*(5), 489–504.

Palmer, C. (2013). Music performance: Movement and coordination. In D. Deutsch (Ed.), *The psychology of music* (3rd ed., pp. 405–422). Academic Press.

Pires, N. J., Lay, B. S., & Rubeson, J. (2014). Joint-level mechanics of the walk-to-run transition in humans. *Journal of Experimental Biology, 217*(19), 3519–3527.

Poppa, T., & Bechara, A. (2018). The somatic marker hypothesis: Revisiting the role of the 'body loop' in decision making. *Current Opinion in Behavioral Sciences, 19*, 61–66.

Repp, B. H. (2005). Sensorimotor synchronization: A review of the tapping literature. *Psychonomic Bulletin & Review, 12*(6), 969–992.

Repp, B. H., & Su, Y. H. (2013). Sensorimotor synchronization: A review of recent research (2006–2012). *Psychonomic Bulletin & Review, 20*(3), 403–452.

Ross, J., Iversen, J., & Balasubramaniam, R. (2018). Dorsal premotor contributions to auditory rhythm perception: Causal transcranial magnetic stimulation studies of interval, tempo, and phase. *bioRxiv*, 368597. https://doi.org/10.1101/368597

Rothstein, W. N. (1989). *Phrase rhythm in tonal music*. Schirmer Books.

Schutz, M., & Kubovy, M. (2009). Causality and cross-modal integration. *Journal of Experimental Psychology: Human Perception and Performance, 35*(6), 1791–1810.

Schutz, M., & Lipscomb, S. (2007). Hearing gestures, seeing music: Vision influences perceived tone duration. *Perception, 36*(6), 888–897.

Scruton, R. (1997). *The aesthetics of music*. Oxford University Press.

Stupacher, J., Hove, M. J., & Janata, P. (2016). Audio features underlying perceived groove and sensorimotor synchronization in music. *Music Perception, 33*(5), 571–589.

Su, Y.-H., & Pöppel, E. (2012). Body movement enhances the extraction of temporal structures in auditory sequences. *Psychological Research, 76*(3), 373–382.

Swain, J. (2002). *Harmonic rhythm: Analysis and interpretation*. Oxford University Press.

Tan, D. (2013). *Ernst Kurth at the boundary of music theory and psychology* [Doctoral dissertation, University of Rochester].

Terhardt, E., Stoll, G., & Seewann, M. (1982). Pitch of complex signals according to virtual-pitch theory: Tests, examples, and predictions. *Journal of the Acoustical Society of America, 71*(3), 671–678.

6
Telling Time

Dancers, Dancemakers, and Audience Members

Renee M. Conroy

6.1 Introduction

It is a truism that the arts of dance trade in time. Yet as musicologist Célestin Deliège observes, 'forms of art that need duration for their accomplishment are the most apt at abolishing our usual perception of time and leading it towards an experience of time that is richer, more complex, less easily analysable' (Deliège, as cited in Paddison, 2019, p. 285). Of philosophical interest, then, is how works of dance art can harness their temporal nature in ways that are artistically rich and reflectively rewarding.

To examine how danceworks can be temporally revealing, I propose a minimal conceptual framework with two elements: a basic distinction between danced time and clock time, and a tripartite classification of danced time. These emphasize perspectival positions that influence how the passage of time might present itself to dancers, dancemakers, and audience members in their various engagements with danceworks, thereby giving rise to experiential discontinuities I will call temporal disconnect and temporal dissonance. Whereas the former is an intrapersonal phenomenon, the latter occurs when there is a time-based experiential gap between various participants during a live dance performance.

For clarity, I develop this conceptual framework independent of theoretical work undertaken by other dance writers and philosophers who have scrutinized the complexities of time, acknowledging that the categories I sketch overlap to some degree with those recommended by experts in these fields. To facilitate the investigation, I consider three dance art cases that promote edifying encounters with the subjectively slippery human experience of time's passage: Daniel Nagrin's *Indeterminate Figure* (1957), Merce Cunningham's *Walkaround Time* (1968), and Jérôme Bel's *Véronique Doisneau* (2004).

6.2 Clock Time and Temporal Disconnect

The difference I mark between danced time and clock time is intuitive: it tracks a 'loose and popular', rather than 'strict and philosophical', way of thinking about time

Renee M. Conroy, *Telling Time* In: *Performing Time*. Edited by: Clemens Wöllner and Justin London, Oxford University Press.
© Oxford University Press 2023. DOI: 10.1093/oso/9780192896254.003.0007

(Chisholm, 1969). Danced time is temporal passage *as experienced by* participants in a dance art context from a first-person perspective. There are many people with an active artistic stake in every live dance performance—including musicians, lighting technicians, costume designers, and stage managers—and their temporal perspectives on the same performance may vary. In this chapter, I focus on danced time only as it pertains to dancers, dancemakers, and audience members.

While danced time is temporal *passage* as assessed from the internal point of view of someone actively engaged in a dance art performance, clock time, as I am using the term here, is temporal *duration* as registered from some external perspective or by appeal to an external framework (cf. Kozak, this volume; Wittmann, this volume; Wöllner, this volume). This could be time from the standpoint of a person in the ticket booth who does not watch the show but attends to whether it exceeds its designated length. More typically, it is time as calculated by a formal device, such as a stopwatch. One way a dance art performance can be artistically rich and reflectively rewarding is by drawing attention to the fact that a person's sense of clock time may be appreciably inconsistent with his or her sense of danced time. I call this temporal disconnect.

The generalized version of temporal disconnect is common: sitting in gridlocked traffic, minutes pass sluggishly; during a good conversation, they fly by. There are, however, numerous examples of danceworks designed to foster it. For instance, some pieces—such as those that embrace choreographic minimalism or challenge traditional dance art conventions—are crafted to incite boredom for some artistic purpose (see Pakes, this volume). These works are organized choreographically to induce audience members to experience time as dragging or plodding, often to lay bare unexamined theatrical expectations. By contrast, danceworks made to inspire meditative or transcendental experiences in audiences—such as Laura Dean's trance dances or Myriam Gourfink's hypnotic yoga-based works (see Joufflineau, this volume)—are carefully structured to generate in viewers the sense that time has flown, been arrested, or disappeared entirely.

Dancers' subjective experiences of time during performance also regularly diverge from what an external timekeeping mechanism would report, and there are many *non-dance* reasons for which temporal disconnect might occur during a dance art event. However, dance performers fall into the phenomenological fissure between clock time and danced time for reasons that regularly differ from those that explain why the standard audience member does because dancers and dance art observers have profoundly different artistic relationships to clock time. For dancers, clock time is directly implicated in common activities such as counting movement phrases to synchronize them with fixed musical structures or internalizing the length of a designated temporal span within which a sequence of steps must be performed to stay *in* time with other dancers or hit a choreographic mark. Thus, mastery of clock time is a fundamental part of all dance technique and most artistic dance performance, and attention to it is often crucial for executing a choreographed work safely and with aplomb.

Indeed, developing an acute awareness of clock time in terms of various external parameters, such as the length of a classroom exercise or where the 'beats and limits of . . . musical phrases are' (Bresnahan, 2017, p. 340), is a foundational part of dance art training. Furthermore, repetition of a choreographic work aims to 'groove in' awareness of relevant temporal limits so that 'once . . . [the dancer] has performed the same dance numerous times . . . she can move within the correct parameters in a faster way and need not be as *reflectively conscious* of particular temporal and spatial markers' (Bresnahan, 2017, p. 341, emphasis added; cf. Shusterman, 2009). Even when the requisite habit has become second nature, reliance on external indicators of time remains an indispensable element of the dancer's implicit conceptual-kinetic framework, especially if she elects to play with prescribed temporal durations for an artistic reason, such as to imbue a choreographic moment with dramatic power by extending it or to enhance the expressive content of a phrase by sustaining one movement and hastening others (see Bresnahan, 2014).

The average dance audience member does not engage with clock time in a similarly nuanced or focused manner, counting along or marking musical measures in her mind. Most often, she simply looks at her watch from time to time to see how *much* time has elapsed when her attentions flag. And there is no particular reason she should do more than this. Attending to the precise details of choreographic timing or very finely articulated temporal units is often not necessary for serious appreciative engagement with a dance art performance. To the contrary, in many cases absorption in the minute temporal details that permeate dancers' attentions would be deleterious to a productive appreciation of the *artistic whole*. One might argue that, while dance performers must be implicitly or explicitly aware of clock time at almost all times, dance observers should typically be attuned to pacing.

What is the difference between these forms of attention? While grasping clock time requires overt or covert appeal to temporal metrics (beats per minute, metronome markings, sweeps of the clock hand), perceiving pacing need not. Instead, recognizing the pace of a temporally extended artistic creation often involves qualitative, rather than quantitative, considerations. An audience member might have no idea how long a film's run time is, yet correctly describe it as *a slow film* and use this as a reasonable, though incomplete, basis for evaluating its cinematic success or failure. The slowness in question is not a matter of measurable speed, such as frames per second or how quickly the actors speak their lines. Nor is it a matter of the film's clocked length: even a short art house flick can drag. It is, instead, the perceived rate at which the film transitions from one significant plot point or narrative landmark to the next. The pace of a temporally extended artwork is primarily a matter of its *development over* time rather than a function of its actual duration or some objectively quantifiable speed.

Suppose dance audiences are customarily invited to attend to pacing rather than clock time. Also presume dancers are typically required to attend to clock time (to some more or less conscious degree) because this substantively affects their individual and group performance and, thereby, influences audience members' sense of the pace of the work. Appreciative invitations and performative prescriptions both implicate *the dancemaker*: in different ways, they reflect his or her artistic efforts understood against the backdrop of norms, values, and expectations of the dance art community in which he or she creates. This suggests another avenue for exploring how works of dance art might be temporally revealing, one that attends to divergent perspectives on artistic pacing.

6.3 Danced Time and Temporal Dissonance

There are three kinds of pacing perspectives—or forms of 'danced time'—that can pull apart in live theatrical contexts, thereby creating what I call temporal dissonance. Whereas temporal disconnect occurs when there is an *intrapersonal* schism between an individual's subjective experience of danced time and awareness of clock time, temporal dissonance occurs when there is an *interpersonal* rift between the dancer's, dancemaker's, or audience member's experience of danced time, for example, between different participants' sense of the work's artistic pace or narrative development. Just as choreographers can design danceworks with the aim of eliciting appreciatively important temporal disconnects, they can also attempt to generate temporal dissonance to provoke reflection on human relationships to time.

First, consider *projective danced time*. This is time from the point of view of the appreciative audience member, which primarily involves audiovisual pacing. It is the rate at which the narrative or abstract structure of a dancework is perceived to unfold given what is presented to viewers in a particular theatrical context. 'Projective' refers to the two sense modalities regarded universally as central to dance art appreciation—sight and hearing (see McFee, 1992, 2011, 2018)—and highlights the degree to which the audience member's mode of apprehending the dance is conceptually active but nonetheless importantly 'distanced' from the performance, being neither physically constitutive of the actual dancing nor metaphysically constitutive of any works the dancers might instantiate.

The experience of projective danced time may have a kinaesthetic aspect if a viewer finds their overall engagement with a dance art creation affected by how it resonates in their body. This can be manifested in unconscious physical activities (toe-tapping or bopping one's head) or in physical sensations not exhibited in behaviour (a feeling of relentless tension in the limbs or a visceral impression of fleeting weightlessness). Hence, to describe the audience member's form of danced time as projective does not rule out the possibility that there could be somatic features of the experience that influence or reflect an appreciator's sense of time. It merely highlights the fact that the *source* of the experience is watching (and hearing) other people dance.

Following John Martin's philosophically pregnant suggestions about metakinesis as a crucial element in correct dance art appreciation (Martin, 1965, pp. 17–25; Van Camp & Conroy, 2013), there is much lively debate about whether kinaesthetic aspects of an observer's experience can contribute positively to *understanding* a choreographic creation or apprehending its aesthetic properties (see Carroll-Seeley, 2013; Conroy, 2013, 2020; Davies, 2013; McFee, 2013, 2018, pp. 206–262; Montero, 2013, 2016, pp. 192–209; Seeley, 2020, pp. 141–162). In this context, I claim only that somatic resonances are often *relevant to* the qualitative character of the viewing experience and, to that extent, have the potential to affect an observer's perception of a work's pacing. I do not assess whether such perceptions are artistically apt or can capture objective features of the work itself.

Second, consider *kinetic danced time*. This is time from the perspective of the dance performer. It involves ways of controlling physical pacing without relying on awareness of clock time by, for example, counting to oneself to stay in step with the music or other performers. Instead, kinetic danced time emerges from the kinematic resources dancers utilize to modify movements in the attempt to generate projective danced time, sometimes to foster perceptual illusions, as when a ballerina skilfully suspends a leap at its peak or a danseur holds the end of the last revolution of a multiple pirouette, thereby elongating the moment as perceived by the audience.

Relevant activities include cycling or adjusting the breath; expending exceptional but imperceptible effort to maintain a prolonged pose or execute a phrase in slow motion; and the ordered activation of integrated bodily systems (skeletal, muscular, and neurological) to embody prescribed dynamics or expressive qualities. Attention to rhythm—understood as 'order in movement . . . [that] arises when *accents* are imposed on a sequence of regular sounds or movements' (Hamilton, 2019, p. 167, emphasis added)—is a central part of every dancer's temporal experience in performance. However, *tracking* a prescribed trajectory of accents within a choreographed work relies on focused attention to some form of clock time. By contrast, kinetic danced time refers to the myriad ways a dancer might regulate rhythm—thereby manipulating perceived pacing—*in her body* independent of reference to, or reliance on, any outside timekeeper or external temporal parameter. If a dancer has fully metabolized awareness of the clock time appropriate to a given dancework through rehearsal, she can devote much more conscious attention to kinematics than to counts. Indeed, this form of movement mastery is desirable because it allows the dancer to 'get out of her head and into her body', a state widely claimed to enhance the aesthetic and artistic qualities of any movement performance (cf. Bläsing, this volume).

Having this kind of 'insider knowledge' is also frequently the reason dancers experience temporal disconnect: they become so absorbed by kinematics that their fine-tuned awareness of clock time functions largely or wholly *sub rosa*. What was temporally 'obtrusive foreground' when the choreography was new becomes 'unobtrusive background' (Carlson, 1979) as focus on the phenomenology of moving and executing specific movement sequences takes attentional centre stage. Theorists characterize this phenomenon in different ways: as exhibiting expertise in a physical domain (see Montero, 2016), as being in a state of flow (see Csikszentmihalyi, 1991), or as involving an overlapping experience of somaesthetic perception and somaesthetic reflection (Shusterman, 2009, p. 194).

Because projective danced time relies on an external (visual-aural) source, and kinetic danced time emerges from internal regulation of the body, the two regularly pull apart, creating temporal dissonance between performer and viewer. A dancer might experience a choreographically complicated or physically tiring movement phrase as long, while an audience member might register the same phrase as relatively short because its movements look simple when executed with ease, or are captivating in their complexity. Alternatively, a dancer engrossed in unobservable kinematic adjustments and fine motor details might perceive as brief a performance observers experience as interminable (see Joufflineau, this volume). The latter form of temporal dissonance typically occurs when viewers cannot find a way into the 'logic' of the choreography and lack conceptual or perceptual benchmarks for acquiring a sense of the work's artistic pace, which requires recognizing the dance events unfolding on stage as ongoing *developments* rather than inchoate successions of movement or extended periods of apparent stasis.

There is also, of course, the possibility that dancers may experience temporal dissonance with one another during a performance. This is, perhaps, most common when dancers are given markedly different choreographic tasks, a situation explored briefly in the last section in this chapter in connection with Bel's work. It may also occur, however, because the same choreographic passage requires dancers with different body types or technical facilities to call on different kinematic means to execute the movement sequences correctly. While a full treatment of 'dissonance between dancers' is warranted, it is beyond the scope of this chapter (see Section 3 on synchrony, this volume).

Third, consider *reflective danced time*. This is time as engineered and envisioned by the dancemaker and is concerned with the overall pacing and artistic purpose of the work. It involves mechanisms utilized by the choreographer to affect audience members' experience of projective time. As a practical consequence, generating reflective danced time always affords dancers unique opportunities to explore kinetic danced time. In addition, dance design tools can be used to foster temporal dissonance between viewer and performer. In such cases, the work's underlying choreographic structure invites dancers and audience members to *reflect on the character of time* itself.

Dance art creators manipulate participants' perception of time in many ways. They can create a prolonged opening section in which little to nothing happens, leaving audiences in a state of artistic suspense while the dancers work slowly and quietly into well-known physical contours of the work's style (e.g. the opening section of George Balanchine's *Serenade* (1933–1934)). They might instruct dancers to improvise at various speeds at once, thereby orchestrating visual cacophonies that disorient the viewer's sense of order and rhythm while engaging dancers in hyperawareness of spatial and temporal parameters that must be respected to prevent collisions and injuries (e.g. the second section of Ralph Lemon's *How Can You Stay in the House All Day and Not Go Anywhere?* (2010)). Or they may employ extended passages of repetition that can be registered by the dancer or viewer either as unpleasantly monotonous or delightfully meditative (e.g. Lucinda Childs's per-ambulation solo *Katema* (1976)). Such strategies inform the design of the work and create broad opportunities for viewers to reflect on time's passage in both the actual world and the fictional world portrayed on stage. They also create opportunities for dancers to embroil themselves in multifaceted confrontations with kinetic danced time. In addition, because reflective danced time emerges from choreographic fea-tures of the work, it may diverge from both projective and kinetic danced time, cre-ating another layer of temporal dissonance that can involve everyone in the theatre.

6.4 Examples of Dance Art Creations

To explore these ideas more fully, I consider three examples of how dance art cre-ations play with these forms of danced time and, thereby, encourage reflection on the vicissitudes of 'telling time' in dance art and life.

6.4.1 Nagrin's *Indeterminate Figure* (1957)

Nothing bends one's sense of time like waiting. It can make minutes feel infinite and turn months into moments. Daniel Nagrin's 1957 solo *Indeterminate Figure*[1] ex-plores how the passage of time can become wildly distorted in the suspended state of protracted waiting for 'the end'. The dancework is an imagistic, provocatively in-verted countdown. Its underlying, largely implicit, narrative framework is the pri-vate experience of a sequestered person who anticipates imminent eradication by the hydrogen bomb. As viewers, we may be nonplussed by the solo's bland begin-nings (which can seem unduly long because the dancer's movements initially appear nonsensical), engaged by its ecstatic middle section (which takes an abruptly spir-itual turn that is emotionally recognizable and choreographically compelling), and surprised by its seemingly swift and frenetic conclusion (which engenders feelings of panic and doom as the fictional clock time of the character's world is announced in actual 10-s increments). By virtue of its choreographic design, *Indeterminate Figure* effectively undermines the audience member's conviction that his or her experience of its projective time tracks the actual clock time of the work's performance by re-peatedly stretching and shortening the viewer's sense of how long a minute really is. It readily engenders temporal disconnect in spectators, particularly those seeing the work for *the first time*.

  Indeterminate Figure also has the choreographic means to encourage temporal dissonance between viewer and dancer. The first section of the solo may 'feel long' to the uninitiated audience member because it contains only a modest amount of movement and Nagrin's choreographic sequences do not follow the 'logic' of any traditional dance technique. Hence, it is difficult for the inexpert viewer to follow the phrases as visual *developments* of recognizable physical patterns or as part of an unfolding narrative. However, for this very reason the opening section may 'fly by' for the dancer: he must call on a range of kinematic skills to make the relatively slow and often quirky choreography appear organic and well motivated.

In addition, the soloist—but not the audience member—knows how each unusual move is connected to the next and can anticipate how broken sequences of poses foreshadow later movement phrases and the dramatic events portrayed by the work as a whole. Hence, what appears inexplicable, and may feel uncomfortably voyeur- istic, to the audience member is experienced as artistically rational, and comfort- ably orchestrated, by the performer. This may make the projective time of the work longer than its kinetic time, in many cases, because the *pacing of the piece as a whole is understood* by the dancer from the inside-out, but is not obvious to the viewer from the outside-in.

The reflective time of *Indeterminate Figure* is the most complex and least ame- nable to satisfactory analysis. It does not map onto the actual duration of the solo or any of its recognizable parts, whether these are considered from the perspective of the dancer or the appreciator. This is, in part, because the length of time impli- cated by the work seems to extend beyond the end of the solo in virtue of its affec- tive and cognitive resonance. Nagrin's movement designs viewed in concert with the score—which concludes with a telephone operator intoning, '11:59 and 40 seconds. 11:59 and 50 seconds. 12 exactly', followed by the whistling sound of a plummeting bomb—engages everyone in the theatre in an unsettling experience of 'time out of time', in which the speed of passing moments is both accelerated and elongated by the dancing character's confrontation with, and denial of, impending death. Hence, no one can be certain whether the fictional time of the work is the last second of a person's life in which a series of recent events 'passes before his eyes', or if Nagrin's creation represents the doomed man's entire 'last night on earth' presented in a the- atrically truncated temporal form.

That the reflective time of *Indeterminate Figure* was crafted deliberately to force audiences and performers to contemplate the differences between appearances and reality is suggested by the solo's framing epigraph: 'Our vanities seduce us into ideal images of what to be and do with our floundering selves. Humans select the sounds and sights which support their illusions *and try to ignore all else*.' As a result, Nagrin's complex way of 'telling time' in this work both advances the aim of fostering ex- tended reflection on time's illusory qualities and fractures any presumption that there might be consistency between the character's, the dancer's, and the audience member's understanding of *Indeterminate Figure*'s actual time, artistic pacing, or even its reflective content.

6.4.2 Cunningham's *Walkaround Time* (1968)

Dancemakers play with time in other ways that disrupt expectations and in- vite us to reconsider what kinds of danced time are possible. For example, Merce

Cunningham's 1968 *Walkaround Time*,[2] an homage to Marcel Duchamp's famous unfinished work known popularly as *The Glass Piece* (1915–1923), invites us to look both at and through the space-time of the work as it unfolds. The dancework is a reflection on the famous early 20th-century artist's most (in)famous creation, which is a static installation piece. But *Walkaround Time* is also preoccupied with temporality, as Cunningham attests:

> The main thing, I think, is the tempo. Marcel always gave one the sense of a human being who is ever calm, a person with an extraordinary sense of calmness, as though days could go by, and minutes could go by. And I wanted to see if I could get that—that sense of time. (Cited in Vaughn, 1992, p. 68)

Cunningham's desire to play with time is evident from the title of the commissioned score by David Behrman . . . *for nearly an hour* . . . This is accurate to the clock time of the 48-min dancework, but arguably does not reflect its projective, kinetic, or reflective time, given that Cunningham's non-narrative homage contains many design features likely to produce temporal disconnect or dissonance, such as extended periods of stillness and slow-motion running. Much could be said about the ways the choreographed sections of *Walkaround Time* highlight the three kinds of danced time articulated thus far and aim to foster a 'Duchampian' sense of time. However, a distinctive feature of Cunningham's creative derivation deserves special attention: its intermission.

In *Walkaround Time* the designed dance sections flank a 7-min entr'acte in which the dancers amble about the stage in rehearsal attire interacting with one another as they would in the studio while cocktail party music plays in the background, a nod to Duchamp's famous ready-mades. This unexpected disruption of theatrical convention enjoins audiences to physically inhabit the kind of 'walkaround time' to which Cunningham's title refers, an ambulatory respite in which computer programmers engaged in the 1960s during which they waited for their latest bit-and-byte creations to finish 'running' or processing.

Cunningham's conscientious shift in the norms associated with intermissions encourages audience members to explore the creation of shared danced time in the theatre. They can choose to continue watching the dancers' informal activities as a kind of improvised everyday movement performance, to engage in genuine walkaround time by perambulating the auditorium during the obligatory 'waiting period', or to pursue personal interactions with the only people in the theatre who are on a literal dance-break, though they remain visible on stage.

Thus, Cunningham turns the customary situation on its head since intermissions are typically a time in the programme during which performers are sequestered from audience members and, therefore, likely to experience the qualitative character of temporal passage quite differently from those in the audience. In standard cases, intermissions often feel rushed and frenetic for dancers attempting to change costumes quickly or warm-up for the next number, while audience members tend to experience the mid-show pause as a serene opportunity to stretch one's legs and chat with friends. *Walkaround Time*'s unusual entr'acte—a recognized part of the dancework—provides an uncommon opportunity for experiential coalescence between projective, kinetic, and reflective danced time insofar as Cunningham has given up directorial control and temporarily eradicated the traditional distance between the performer and the viewer. By reorganizing traditional theatrical roles and dispensing with the 'closed curtain' convention, Cunningham affords an opportunity for everyone to share a calm and common temporal perspective.

Hence, the two formally danced halves of *Walkaround Time* are rife with Cunninghamesque choreographic features that engender both temporal disconnect and dissonance. But it is the special opportunity he affords for generating a shared perspective on temporal passage, and time in the theatre space, that is reflectively significant and pays special homage to Duchamp. The unique intermission not only effectively erases the line between kinetic and projective time: it directly challenges everyone's sense of the typical disconnect between theatre time and the temporal character of real life.

6.4.3 Bel's *Véronique Doisneau* (2004)

In a different way, contemporary choreographer Jérôme Bel's theatrical production *Véronique Doisneau* (2004)[3] also upends traditional theatre time. This work, a poignant autobiography of an ageing Paris Opera *sujet* (a middle-rank dancer) on the eve of her retirement, underscores how significant, yet unnoticed, the conventional demarcation between performer and audience member is in many classical dance art forms. To achieve this reflective aim, Bel demonstrates viscerally one way kinetic time and projective time regularly pull apart in service of a dancemaker's goals (i.e. to generate both the perceived pacing and reflective time of the work). Whereas Cunningham's *Walkaround Time* creates an opportunity for uncommon temporal coalescence between performers and viewers, Bel's work reveals how commonly temporal disconnect may be experienced by corps dancers in ballets, thereby highlighting one regular source of temporal dissonance between audiences and dancers. It simultaneously emphasizes how regularly some forms of choreography, particularly those created for companies in which performers are 'ranked' in a hierarchical artistic structure, give rise to temporal dissonance between dancers on stage.

Véronique Doisneau is a striking recounting of Paris National Opera *sujet* Véronique Doisneau's career, emphasizing its highlights and disappointments. In Bel's multimedia work—in which dramatic dialogue, singing, and dance art are married seamlessly—Véronique performs excerpts from several classic danceworks (including *La Bayadere*, *Giselle*, and Cunningham's *Points in Space*), revealing her personal connections to each and inviting audiences into her experiences as a dancer who was never promoted to a lead position in the company.

The closing section of this theatre piece, which is the most stunning and difficult to watch, offers the audience a 10-min journey into what it is like—from the dancer's point of view—to be a 'human backdrop' to the beloved *pas de deux* from Act II of *Swan Lake*. Alone on the cavernous Paris Opera stage, the diminutive Veronique holds uncomfortable cygnet poses in near-perfect stillness for what seems like an interminable period (the longest interval is approximately 5 min), moving intermittently only to resume a similar statue-like position for another uncomfortably extended duration. While the fact that the *sujet* is visibly 'swallowed' by the stage space may contribute to the viewer's discomfort, Bel's reflective focus is revealing unnoticed temporal discontinuities between performers and appreciators.

This section of Bel's work is revelatory for audience members familiar with *Swan Lake* because it highlights the substantive gap that can exist between projective and kinetic time in service of reflective time, particularly as this schism is experienced by dancers who perform revered works created in Romantic or Classical ballet traditions. For, as Veronique attests, what the classical ballet-maker has designed to seem like mere moments to audience members who are called to revel in the prima ballerina's supported penchés and multiple pirouettes, *most*—though certainly not all—dancers on stage experience as a protracted exercise in physical and artistic torture of seemingly endless duration.

6.5 Conclusion: 'Telling Time'

The lessons of this chapter are simple but substantive. When we consider the various ways tempo and pacing can figure in the perception of dance art performances, we should always keep in mind the varied perspectives of dancers, dancemakers, and audience members to ensure our philosophical work respects their differences, celebrates their continuities, and articulates clearly which *kind* of 'telling time' is at stake in our analyses.

The audience member typically 'tells time' projectively (from the outside-in), while the dancer does so kinematically (from the inside-out) and the dancemaker artistically (by creating choreographic designs with reflective content). This reaffirms, and perhaps sheds some dance-related light on, Deliège's claim that 'forms of art that need duration for their accomplishment are the most apt at abolishing our usual perception of time and leading it towards an experience of time that is richer' (Deliège, cited in Paddison, 2019, p. 285). Some of that richness may come from personal reflection on the intrapersonal experience of temporal disconnect and its sources for an individual in a particular dance art context. But much will emerge from communal discussion of the various ways danceworks can elicit temporal dissonance, sometimes simply in service of immediate artistic ends and sometimes, as in the cases discussed in this chapter, in service of promoting longer-term philosophical reflection on the nature of time itself.

Notes

1. Analysis of *Indeterminate Figure* based on viewing Daniel Nagrin's 1957 performance, posted publicly by the Daniel Nagrin Foundation (2014).
2. No public video available: the work was filmed in 16 mm 1973 by Charles Atlas, and is available for purchase as an HD video from Electronic Arts Intermix (2022). Analysis based on descriptions from Carroll and Banes (1999), Mueller (2011), and Vaughn (1992).
3. Analysis of *Véronique Doisneau* based on viewing Doisneau's 2004 performance filmed under the direction of Jérôme Bel (tatsumi14, 2009).

References

Bresnahan, A. (2014). Improvisational artistry in live dance performance as embodied and extended agency. *Dance Research Journal, 46*(1), 85–94.

Bresnahan, A. (2017). Dancing in time. In I. Phillips (Ed.), *The Routledge handbook of philosophy of temporal experience* (pp. 339–348). Routledge.

Carlson, A. (1979/2004). Appreciation and the natural environment. In A. Carlson and A. Berleant (Eds.), *The aesthetics of natural environments* (pp. 63–74). Broadview Press. (Original work published 1979)

Carroll, N., & Banes, S. (1999). Cunningham and Duchamp. In G. Celant (Ed.), *Merce Cunningham* (pp. 179–185). Edizioni Charta.

Carroll, N., & Seeley, W. (2013). Kinesthetic understanding and appreciation in dance. *Journal of Aesthetics and Art Criticism, 71*(2), 177–186.

Chisholm, R. (1969). The loose and popular and the strict and philosophical senses of identity. In N. S. Care & R. H. Grimm (Eds.), *Perception and personal identity* (pp. 82–106). Press of Case Western Reserve University.

Conroy, R. (2013). Responding bodily. *Journal of Aesthetics and Art Criticism, 71*(2), 201–210.

Conroy, R. (2020). Kinesthetic imagining and dance appreciation. In K. Moser & A. Sukla (Eds.), *Imagination and art: Explorations in contemporary theory* (pp. 621–645). Brill/Rodopi.

Csikszentmihalyi, M. (1991). *Flow: The psychology of optimal experience*. Harper Collins.

Daniel Nagrin Foundation. (2014, 6 June). *Indeterminate Figure 1957 indoor* [Video]. YouTube. https://www.youtube.com/watch?v=8mR88jSuOZs

Davies, D. (2013). Dancing around the issues: Prospects for an empirically grounded philosophy of dance. *Journal of Aesthetics and Art Criticism, 71*(2), 195–202.

Electronic Arts Intermix. (2022). Walkaround Time. https://www.eai.org/titles/walkaround-time/ordering-fees#terms

Hamilton, A. (2019). Rhythm and movement: The conceptual interdependence of music, dance, and poetry. *Midwest Studies in Philosophy, XLIV*, 161–182.

Martin, J. (1965). *The dance in theory*. Dance Horizons-Princeton Book Co. (Original work published 1939)

McFee, G. (1992). *Understanding dance*. Routledge.

McFee, G. (2011). *The philosophical aesthetics of dance: Identity, performance and understanding*. Dance Books Ltd.

McFee, G. (2013). Defusing dualism: John Martin on dance appreciation. *Journal of Aesthetics and Art Criticism, 71*(2), 187–194.

McFee, G. (2018). *Dance and the philosophy of action: A framework for the aesthetics of dance*. Dance Books Ltd.

Montero, B. (2013). The artist as critic: Dance training, neuroscience, and aesthetic evaluation. *Journal of Aesthetics and Art Criticism, 71*(2), 167–175.

Montero, B. (2016). *Thought in action: Expertise and the conscious mind*. Oxford University Press.

Mueller, J. (2011). *Merce Cunningham's Walkaround Time*. The Ohio State University. https://political science.osu.edu/faculty/jmueller/WALKARN2.pdf

Paddison, M. (2019.) Time, rhythm, and subjectivity: The aesthetics of duration. In P. Cheyne, A. Hamilton, & M. Paddison (Eds.), *The philosophy of rhythm: Aesthetics, music, poetics* (pp. 272–290). Oxford University Press.

Seeley, W. (2020). *Attentional engines: A perceptual theory of the arts.* Oxford University Press.

Shusterman, R. (2009). Body consciousness and performance: Somaesthetics east and west. *Journal of Aesthetics and Art Criticism, 67*(2), 133–145.

tatsumi14. (2009, 11 April). *Veronique Doisneau 3* [Video]. YouTube. https://www.youtube.com/watch?v=L10LlVPE-kg

Van Camp, J., & Conroy, R. (2013). Introduction: Dance art and science. *Journal of Aesthetics and Art Criticism, 71*(2), 167–168.

Vaughn, D. (1992). 'Then I thought about Marcel . . .' Merce Cunningham's *Walkaround Time.* In R. Kostelanetz (Ed.), *Merce Cunningham: Dancing in space and time* (pp. 66–70). Chicago Review Press.

7

Preferred Tempo and Its Relation to Personal and Shared Senses of Time and Temporal Flow

Molly J. Henry and Sonja A. Kotz

7.1 Introduction

Our own personal sense of time is highly context dependent. The old adages say that 'time flies when you're having fun', but by contrast, 'a watched pot never boils'. The context dependence of our personal time sense has perhaps never been so apparent on such a large scale as during the COVID-19 pandemic, during which 'Time has slowed to a crawl. The days are a blur. Two weeks ago feels like two years ago' (Holman & Grisham, 2020). Individuals report that time passes in slow motion during near-death experiences such as car accidents (Eagleman, 2008) or frightening experiences such as free fall (Campbell & Bryant, 2007; Stetson et al., 2007). However, context-based time distortions also take place during positive-valence experiences such as music making or during altered states of consciousness (Wittmann, 2015). For example, some jazz musicians enjoy cannabis because of its ability to stretch time so that they can 'work in about twice as much music between the first note and the second note' in order to 'jazz things up' (Dr James Munch, as cited in Fachner, 2009). Our personal sense of time may also depend on factors that are specific to us as individuals. Here, we discuss *preferred rate*, which is the rate at which an individual prefers to rhythmically move their body (Bolton, 1892; Fraisse, 1982; Wallin, 1911). An idiosyncratic preference for a certain rate (tempo) implies that different individuals will preferentially or more easily engage with some rhythmic stimuli, that is, those that closely match their preferred rate, in contrast to stimuli with rates far from their preference (Scheurich et al., 2018).

Our goal was to examine the relationship of preferred rate to our personal sense of time and to the experience of 'temporal flow', which we define as the experience of time's passing *as it passes*. We focus on two dimensions of studying personal time sense. The first is experiential: can a personal sense of time be shared with others? What forms of interpersonal coupling are more or less likely to support shared time sense with another person? The second is methodological: how do we measure and

Molly J. Henry and Sonja A. Kotz, *Preferred Tempo and Its Relation to Personal and Shared Senses of Time and Temporal Flow*
In: *Performing Time*. Edited by: Clemens Wöllner and Justin London, Oxford University Press. © Oxford University Press 2023.
DOI: 10.1093/oso/9780192896254.003.0008

quantify personal sense of time? What are the measurable versus unmeasurable aspects of personal time sense? Finally, we discuss how we might develop a neuroscience of shared personal time and temporal flow, and what pitfalls should be avoided as we do so. We begin by providing background on preferred rate and by previewing the difficulty of studying temporal flow in real time; in the latter case we make an analogy to the study of flow states, where empirical research struggles with many of the same issues that we will encounter, in particular related to measurement.

7.1.1 Preferred Rate

When asked to move their bodies rhythmically at a rate that is most comfortable for them, individuals will spontaneously move at an idiosyncratic rate—their *preferred rate* (Fraisse, 1982; see also Hammerschmidt, this volume). The average preferred rate for adults is approximately 500 ms, 2 Hz, or 120 beats per minute (BPM), strikingly near the modal beat rate of Western pop music (van Noorden & Moelants, 1999). However, there is large interindividual variability, and preferred rates can range from as fast as 200 ms (5 Hz, 300 BPM) to as slow as 2000 ms (0.5 Hz, 30 BPM; Hammerschmidt et al., 2021; McAuley et al., 2006). Interestingly, the preferred rate is stable from day to day, meaning that an individual will produce the same rate tomorrow as they did today (Harrell, 1937), and regardless of whether they use their hand or foot (Rose et al., 2020). Although the specific brain and body factors that determine an individual's preferred rate are unknown, individuals prefer to both produce and listen to rhythms and are better at perceiving rhythms presented at their preferred rate (McAuley et al., 2006).

7.1.2 Flow States During Music Making

Flow is defined as total involvement in a task that leads to a loss of self-awareness (Csikszentmihalyi, 1990). An individual is most likely to achieve a flow state when there is a balance between the difficulty of the task and the skill level of the individual—a 'sweet spot' in terms of challenge, where the task is not difficult enough to be frustrating, and not so easy as to be boring (Nakamura & Csikszentmihalyi, 2002). One of the defining elements of flow is time distortion (Hancock et al., 2019), where individuals experience a subjective speeding or slowing of time's passing during the activity, most commonly in the form of 'lost time' (Nuyens et al., 2020). Flow states are well documented during music making (Sinnet et al., 2020; Wrigley & Emmerson, 2011), but notoriously difficult to study in real time, as directing attention to the experience annihilates the flow state (Hancock et al., 2019). Here, we have opted to discuss the experience of time's passing during a flow state as an analogy to what we have defined above as 'temporal flow'.

7.2 The Experiential Dimension of Personal Time Sense

Here we explore the question of whether and how people can share their personal time senses in social contexts, like two people talking about terrible weather or two street musicians jamming together. These two simple examples make it clear that sharing personal time senses via temporal coordination may be necessary in such social interactions. The former requires that both individuals are sensitive to each other's verbal and non-verbal timing cues that allow for respectful turn-taking (Kotz et al., 2018; Richardson et al., 2008), while the latter necessitates synchronous behaviour in time (Goebl & Palmer, 2009; Pecenka & Keller, 2011). Most likely, both dyads depend on each individual's capacity to temporally *anticipate* one's own and others' turns and actions, and to *adapt* to each other (Jordan, 2009; Sebanz et al., 2006). This may be easiest when two people share a similar time sense. Imagine a guitar player jamming in the street—someone spontaneously joins in with vocals. Now that the music making involves another person, the guitarist must respond to the singer to ensure that the vocals and their guitar playing temporally align. In turn, the vocalist will adapt what they are producing to the pacing of the guitar player. Does a successful shared music-making experience necessitate that the two individuals come to share a personal time sense? And will a merging of time sense lead to more fluid and reciprocal switching between who leads and who follows? In order to explore how these questions might be further studied, we review what we consider to be a critical differentiation among levels of interpersonal coupling that may occur under different social circumstances.

7.2.1 Levels of Coupling

A recent article on the pillars of social interaction proposed that the coupling of two individuals, such as the guitarist and singer in our example, needs to be differentiated at multiple, interrelated levels that explain how and why they can engage in reciprocal timely behaviour (Dumas & Fairhurst, 2021). Four different coupling levels each may give temporal social interaction a distinct flavour.

Spurious coupling arises when two or more people watch a film or listen to an album together. Here, the shared sensory experience does not necessarily imply temporal *coordination* between the two individuals. Rather, measurable behavioural and neural alignment may simply result from two people reacting similarly to sensorial events in their shared environment (Hasson et al., 2004). In that sense two individuals may respond at the same time to an unexpected event like a scream or a high-pitched laugh in a film or a mode change in music, just as each individual would respond to those same events on their own. That two individuals passively respond similarly to the same physical input in no way mandates a shared time sense.

Physiological coupling is quite comparable to spurious coupling, in that two individuals may react similarly and synchronously to information in their shared environment. However, physiological coupling arises from unconscious reactions to mood or state changes in the shared context, and as such may lead to 'affective' coordination. As each person reacts emotionally to, for example, a mode change in a musical piece, their heart and respiration rates will adapt synchronously (Benardi et al., 2009; Gomez & Danuser, 2007). Like spurious coupling though, physiological coupling does not have to rely on a shared time sense, and like spurious coupling, involves each individual physiologically responding to the same information/events in their shared environment. However, physiological coupling may provide the common affective ground for shared temporal flow in music making and listening.

Spontaneous motor coupling involves actions such as rocking or swaying at a concert in time with others or walking in step together. For example, two listeners will synchronously respond to the beat in music by swaying their bodies (Richardson et al., 2008), clapping their hands (Néda et al., 2000), or tapping their feet (Dumas & Fairhurst, 2021). Here the individuals are responding to both an external rhythmic stimulus (the music) as well as each other (e.g. their clapping). Spontaneous motor coupling is likely preceded by spurious and/or physiological coupling, but still may be considered unconscious and non-communicative (though spontaneous synchrony could certainly reach awareness; Dumas & Fairhurst, 2021), and as such we hypothesize that shared time is still unlikely.

Sensorimotor coupling extends motor coupling to a situation where at least two individuals are aware of and intentionally coordinate their actions together. In order to compare to spontaneous motor coupling, imagine two musicians jamming together. They share knowledge about the musical style and each other's musical skills, and they share an intention to play music together. In ensemble performance, for example, each musician must not only respond to music as a shared external stimulus, but also must anticipate when the other will, for example, accentuate a beat or change tempo and adapt accordingly (Fairhurst et al., 2014; Gallotti et al., 2017). Thus, the kind of coupling that benefits successful joint music making requires shared intention and planning as well as anticipation of and adaptation to each other in real time. Here, we do expect that a shared time sense facilitates joint action.

7.2.2 The Role of Preferred Rate in Shared Time Sense and Joint Music Making

How does each musician's personal time sense affect the likelihood that they will come to share a time sense during music making? Tantamount to this discussion is an assumption that sensorimotor coupling is foundational to successful joint music making: experiencing successful interpersonal synchrony encourages affiliation in adults and children (Cirelli, 2018), and blurs the distinction between self and other (Novembre et al., 2016). Thus, we propose that individuals who easily perform in synchrony are more likely to share their personal time sense, and challenges to attaining synchrony among individuals who do not share their personal time sense are likely to be frustrating. Given that individuals synchronize better to stimuli with rates near their preference (Scheurich et al., 2018), it is a natural hypothesis that interpersonal synchrony will be more successful and easier to accomplish between individuals with more similar preferred rates. Indeed, pianists with similar preferred rates produce better-synchronized duets than pairs with disparate preferred rates (Zamm et al., 2015). Thus, we suggest that individuals with similar preferred rates are more likely to share their personal time sense, and thus may anticipate and adapt better to each other during sensorimotor coupling. By contrast, mismatches in preferred rate have the potential to force a leader–follower relationship that might be inappropriate. When crickets synchronize their chirps, for example, the 'leader' is the cricket with the fastest preferred rate (Nityananda & Balakrishnan, 2007). Thus, one musician—the faster musician—may end up in the leader role. In this case, the leader dictates the tempo and does not adapt much to the input from the other player, while the follower must significantly adapt to the leader's pace (Candidi et al., 2015; Fairhurst et al., 2014; Jacoby et al., 2021). A musician who is being dragged along may not come to share the other's time sense, but two musicians who easily trade back and forth who is leading and who is following, we suggest, are more likely to experience a shared temporal flow. We propose that fluidity in leading–following in music making may better promote or reflect a shared time sense (Clayton et al., 2020) and skill sets. In this case, similar preferred rates would be tantamount.

7.3 The Methodological Dimension of Personal Time Sense

Although personal time sense is phenomenologically interesting, its study is complicated by the problem of accessing and measuring an individual's experience of time. Luckily, this is a classic topic in the time perception literature, and there has been much historical interest in whether and under what conditions perceived time is distorted as opposed to 'veridical'. In particular, on the measurable end of the methodological continuum, extensive psychophysical work has been conducted on temporal illusions and distortions. Here, we provide just a few examples of how perceived duration and rate (tempo) can be distorted in a context-dependent manner, though we note that perception of other temporal features such as order and simultaneity are subject to distortions as well (Eagleman, 2008).

7.3.1 Measurable Quantities of Personal Time Sense

In psychophysical experiments, time intervals are usually marked by two stimuli that signal the start and end of an interval, for example, two tones or flashes of light.

Time intervals that contain additional stimuli between those two markers are perceived as longer than empty intervals of the same physical duration (Grondin, 1993; Wearden & Ogden, 2021). Moving stimuli are perceived as longer in duration than stationary stimuli (Kanai et al., 2006). Complex stimuli are perceived as longer than simple stimuli (Roelofs & Zeeman, 1951). The rate (tempo) of a rhythm is also subject to temporal distortions: rhythms with increasing pitch are heard as speeding up, while rhythms with decreasing pitch are heard as slowing down (Herrmann et al., 2013). These experiments show that the perception of time is labile, and as such personal, and at least in the context of temporal illusions, measurable with a high degree of precision.

Outside of the laboratory, despite methodological challenges, creative experimentation can render less 'psychophysical' time distortions measurable as well. For example, skydivers who were fearful before their jump overestimated the duration of their fall, in line with time slowing down, whereas those who were excited before their jump underestimated the duration of their fall, in line with time speeding up (Campbell & Bryant, 2007). Thus, the skydivers' emotional state affected the way they experienced the passage of time. In another study, participants who fell from a 50-m-high tower into a net overestimated the duration of their own fall relative to others' falls, perhaps accounting for the feeling that time slows down, or moves in slow motion, during frightening events. Importantly, however, the experimenters also tested participants' *temporal acuity during the fall*, and did not find that it was improved. Thus, it seemed that the fall was *remembered* as longer (Stetson et al., 2007).

7.3.2 Unmeasurable Quantities of Personal Time Sense—Time Perception During Flow States

Here, we have chosen to focus on the experience of time during flow states. We believe that time sense during flow states is especially interesting because, on the one hand, well-documented time distortions take place during flow states, but on the other hand, measurement of time sense during flow states creates something of a paradox. Psychometric tools designed to measure the elements of flow explicitly direct participants to examine their own experience. In turn, examination of one's own experience in real time destroys the flow state (Hancock et al., 2019). For this reason, few studies have been able to directly explore time sense *during* the flow state (Hancock et al., 2019; Nuyens et al., 2020). In one study that came close to doing so (Sinnet et al., 2020), musicians' temporal-order judgements were more accurate immediately after rehearsals where flow was experienced. This shows that time did not just fly, but that time perception was actually more accurate as the flow state faded away. Thus, it was not the case that musicians only *remembered* time as being distorted, but changes in their time perception thresholds suggest that their real-time personal time sense was truly altered.

7.3.3 Measuring the Unmeasurable

Naturalistic stimuli are rich, multimodal, and dynamic, and can include film, TV commercials, songs, stories, or lived experiences (Sonkusare et al., 2019). Newly developed neuroscientific techniques are making it possible for the first time to study the real-time neural processing of naturalistic stimuli. Here, we focus on two techniques: neural pattern drift and intersubject correlation (ISC), both measured using functional magnetic resonance imaging. Neural pattern drift quantifies the degree to which spatial neural patterns, that is, patterns of activation across voxels in a particular brain area, change as a function of time. The evolution of neural patterns, and in particular the degree to which neural patterns change over time, seems to provide a map of an individual's temporal flow (Lositsky et al., 2016). Nonetheless, it is still unclear whether the neural timeline may better correspond to remembered temporal flow than to experienced temporal flow.

ISC overcomes one of the primary historical hurdles to studying brain responses to naturalistic stimuli, which is the problem of defining the specific events within a stimulus that should evoke a brain response. For example, should we examine brain responses to sensorial changes such as a scream or a high-pitched laugh in a film, or should we examine brain responses to cognitive changes such as those driven by suspense or plot twists? The basic logic behind ISC is that, if individuals' brains respond similarly to the same naturalistic stimulus, as would be expected in the context of spurious or physiological coupling, then correlating the brain activity of many participants while they experience the same naturalistic stimulus would reveal which brain regions respond consistently across individuals, and what content those brain regions respond to (Lerner et al., 2011). ISC can distinguish between different levels and types of emotional content (Sachs et al., 2020) and gauge audience appeal in a marketing context (Dmochowski et al., 2014). ISC is sensitive to variations in humour and suspense (Sonkusare et al., 2019). Critical for our purposes, ISC has been applied to individuals engaged in social interactions: ISC between a speaker and a listener predicts how well the listener will remember what the speaker says (Stephens et al., 2010), and ISC between teacher and student predicts the student's engagement in the classroom (Dikker et al., 2017). We will return to these social applications of naturalistic neuroscience in the next section of this chapter.

7.4 What Are the Next Steps Towards Developing a Neuroscience of Shared Sense of Time and Temporal Flow?

Given that formerly unmeasurable aspects of experience are now becoming measurable, what are the next steps towards developing a neuroscience of shared time sense and temporal flow? We conclude our chapter by describing what we see as fruitful methodological ways forward as well as some pitfalls to avoid. We also highlight several potential avenues for future work that focus on social situations with potentially more porous boundaries between self and other than what we have described so far.

7.4.1 Methodological Ways Forward and Pitfalls to Avoid

Although 'naturalistic neuroscience' has recently started to deliver techniques to understand neural processing of naturalistic stimuli, experiments using ISC are often conducted under traditional laboratory circumstances, for example, with individual participants laying in the bore of a magnetic resonance imaging scanner (Sonkusare et al., 2019). Even when attempts have been made to add a social element to ISC experiments, many studies nonetheless collected neural data serially from different individuals at different times while, for example, playing a recording of one person's voice while another person's brain activity was measured (Stephens et al., 2010). However, there has been a recent argument for the benefits of so-called hyperscanning (Montague et al., 2002), whereby the brain activity of two or more individuals can be measured simultaneously while they interact in a semi-naturalistic social situation (Babiloni & Astolfi, 2014; Mu et al., 2018). These studies have been made possible by recent advances in technologies that make the 'laboratory' look more like the real world. This includes improvements in 'wearable' devices that can measure brain activity, body movement, and physiological responses of multiple individuals simultaneously while they interact (Hamilton, 2020). Naturally, there are technological hurdles that come with synchronizing data from many recording modalities and analysing high-dimensional data. Nonetheless, we currently see wearables as one of the most promising avenues to be able to measure different aspects of interpersonal coupling and temporal flow in real time and in the wild without disrupting the natural experience of social interaction.

Hyperscanning studies using different brain imaging modalities, including functional magnetic resonance imaging, electroencephalography, and functional near-infrared spectroscopy (Czeszumski et al., 2020), have demonstrated that individual brains become coupled to each other during social interaction. This coupling can be described in terms of synchrony or by using measures that allow for asymmetry or time lag between brains, as would be the case when one person leads and the other follows. What these measures deliver theoretically, however, have to be taken with a grain of salt (Burgess, 2013). This is because analytical tools to measure coupling are descriptive by nature, and thus are blind to the *level* at which coupling is taking place (Dumas & Fairhurst, 2021). Indeed, neural synchrony is just as likely to reflect spurious coupling to shared input(s) as it is a shared time sense. Especially problematic in this regard is that, in many hyperscanning studies, experimental conditions do not facilitate intentional, reciprocal interactions as they occur during full-blown sensorimotor coupling (Hasson et al., 2004). Going forward, hyperscanning studies will benefit from experimental designs that require or manipulate an intentional, adaptive brand of sensorimotor coupling informed by experimental psychology. We are not the first to suggest that neuroscience needs behaviour (Krakauer et al., 2016), and in this case, neuroscience may also need physiology, motion capture, eye tracking, and so on (Gaggioli et al., 2017; Hamilton, 2020). In a multimodal experimental context, ISC likely provides a promising measure to investigate the merging of personal time sense in real time for dyads with similar and dissimilar preferred rates.

7.4.2 Avenues for Future Research on Shared Time Sense and Temporal Flow

The merging of time sense during joint music making and social interaction is an understudied scientific question, but one that will be informed by considering levels of coupling and the possibility of a shared sense of time sense in larger groups. Physiological coupling has been observed between choir members as well as between the choir and their conductor (Müller & Lindenberger, 2011). Moreover, physiological and motor coupling may further arise between performers and their audience (Dumas & Fairhurst, 2021; Labbé & Grandjean, 2014; Trost et al., 2017), where next to physiological changes, synchronized movement may reinforce group cohesion (Fischer et al., 2013) through social bonding (Clayton et al., 2020; Launay et al., 2016) in a concert situation. We suggest that the study of merging time sense could be pushed further by delving into situations that are known to be associated with a breakdown of 'self'. This includes, rituals, festivals, liturgy and prayer, sporting events, and protests (Cummins, 2021; González-Grandón, 2018). Moreover, there is an important social difference between situations in which performers make music for an audience, which is indeed a very Western description, versus when there is no formal distinction between performer and audience. Similar to the blurring between speaker and listener during joint speech in church or during protest (Cummins, 2021), we propose that the blurring of the line between performer and audience is likely to facilitate merging of personal time sense.

7.5 Conclusion

Our personal time sense stretches and shrinks depending on context. Here, we discussed the possibility that personal time sense can be shared between individuals engaged in social interaction. We propose that the likelihood that individuals' time senses can merge depends on the similarity of the preferred rates of the interacting individuals, as well as the level of coupling experienced by the individuals. In particular, a gradient of intentional sensorimotor coupling, as enjoyed during joint music making, is most likely to involve a shared time sense. We discussed the methodological background and emerging technologies that we hope will be useful as we move forward towards developing a neuroscience of shared time sense and temporal flow.

References

Babiloni, F., & Astolfi, L. (2014). Social neuroscience and hyperscanning techniques: Past, present and future. *Neuroscience & Biobehavioral Reviews, 44*, 76–93.

Benardi, L., Porta, C., Casucci, G., Basalmo, R., Bernardi, N. F., Fogari, R., & Sleight, P. (2009). Dynamic interactions between musical, cardiovascular, and cerebral rhythms in humans. *Circulation, 119*(25), 3171–3180.

Bolton, T. L. (1892). On the discrimination of groups of rapid click. *American Journal of Psychology, 5*, 294–310.

Burgess, A. P. (2013). On the interpretation of synchronization in EEG hyperscanning studies: A cautionary note. *Frontiers in Human Neuroscience, 7*, 881.

Campbell, L. A., & Bryant, R. A. (2007). How time flies: A study of novice skydivers. *Behaviour Research and Therapy, 45*(6), 1389–1392.

Candidi, M., Curioni, A., Donnarumma, F., Sacheli, L. M., & Pezzulo, G. (2015). Interactional leader–follower sensorimotor communication strategies during repetitive joint actions. *Journal of the Royal Society Interface, 12*(110), 20150644.

Cirelli, L. K. (2018). How interpersonal synchrony facilitates early prosocial behavior. *Current Opinion in Psychology, 20*, 35–39.

Clayton, M., Jakubowski, K., Eerola, T., Keller, P. E., Camurri, A., Volpe, G., & Alborno, P. (2020). Interpersonal entrainment in music performance: Theory, method and model. *Music Perception, 38*(2), 136–194.

Csikszentmihalyi, M. (1990). *Flow: The psychology of optimal experience*. Harper & Row.

Cummins, F. (2021). On vain repetitions: The enactment of collective subjectivities through speaking in unison. In J. Ponzo, R. A. Yelle, & M. Leone (Eds.), *Mediation and immediacy: A key issue for the semiotics of religion* (pp. 165–178). De Gruyter.

Czeszumski, A., Eustergerling, S., Lang, A., Menrath, D., Gerstenberger, M., Schuberth, S., Schreiber, F., Rendon, Z. Z., & König, P. (2020). Hyperscanning: A valid method to study neural inter-brain underpinnings of social interaction. *Frontiers in Human Neuroscience, 14*, 39.

Dikker, S., Wan, L., Davidesco, I., Kaggen, L., Oostrick, M., McClintock, J., Rowland, J., Michalareas, G., Van Bavel, J. J., Ding, M., & Poeppel, D. (2017). Brain-to-brain synchrony tracks real-world dynamic group interactions in the classroom. *Current Biology, 27*(9), 1375–1380.

Dmochowski, J. P., Bezdek, M. A., Abelson, B. P., Johnson, J. S., Schumacher, E. H., & Parra, L. C. (2014). Audience preferences are predicted by temporal reliability of neural processing. *Nature Communications, 5*, 4567.

Dumas, G., & Fairhurst, M. T. (2021). Reciprocity and alignment: Quantifying coupling in dynamic interactions. *Royal Society Open Science, 8*(5), 210138.

Eagleman, D. M. (2008). Human time perception and its illusions. *Current Opinion in Neurobiology, 18*(2), 131–136.

Fachner, J. (2009). Out of time? Music, consciousness states and neuropharmacological mechanisms of an altered temporality [Paper presentation]. 7th Triennial Conference of European Society for the Cognitive Sciences of Music (ESCOM 2009), Jyväskylä, Finland.

Fairhurst, M. T., Janata, P., & Keller, P. E. (2014). Leading the follower: An fMRI investigation of dynamic cooperativity and leader-follower strategies in synchronization with an adaptive virtual partner. *NeuroImage, 84*, 688–697.

Fischer, R., Callander, R., Reddish, P., & Bulbulia, J. A. (2013). How do rituals affect cooperation? *Nature, 24*(2), 115–125.

Fraisse, P. (1982). Rhythm and tempo. In D. Deutsch (Ed.), *The psychology of music* (pp. 149–180). Academic Press.

Gaggioli, A., Chirico, A., Mazzoni, E., Milani, L., & Riva, G. (2017). Networked flow in musical bands. *Psychology of Music*, 45(2), 283–297.

Gallotti, M., Fairhurst, M. T., & Frith, C. D. (2017). Alignment in social interactions. *Consciousness and Cognition*, 48, 253–261.

Goebl, W., & Palmer, C. (2009). Synchronization of timing and motion among performing musicians. *Music Perception*, 26(5), 427–438.

Gomez, P., & Danuser, B. (2007). Relationships between musical structure and psychophysiological measures of emotion. *Emotion*, 7(2), 377–387.

González-Grandón, X. (2018). How music connects: Social sensory consciousness in musical ritual. *Material Religion*, 14(3), 423–425.

Grondin, S. (1993). Duration discrimination of empty and filled intervals marked by auditory and visual signals. *Perception & Psychophysics*, 54(3), 383–394.

Hamilton, A. F. de C. (2020). Hyperscanning: Beyond the hype. *Neuron*, 109(3), 404–407.

Hammerschmidt, D., Frieler, K., & Wöllner, C. (2021). Spontaneous motor tempo: Investigating psychological, chronobiological, and demographic factors in a large-scale online tapping experiment. *Frontiers in Psychology*, 12, 677201.

Hancock, P. A., Kaplan, A. D., Cruit, J. K., Hancock, G. M., MacArthur, K. R., & Szalma, J. L. (2019). A meta-analysis of flow effects and the perception of time. *Acta Psychologica*, 198, 102836.

Harrell, T. W. (1937). Factors influencing preference and memory for auditory rhythm. *Journal of General Psychology*, 17(1), 63–104.

Hasson, U., Nir, Y., Levy, I., Fuhrmann, G., & Malach, R. (2004). Intersubject synchronization of cortical activity during natural vision. *Science*, 303(5664), 1634–1640.

Herrmann, B., Henry, M. J., Grigutsch, M., & Obleser, J. (2013). Oscillatory phase dynamics in neural entrainment underpin illusory percepts of time. *Journal of Neuroscience*, 33(40), 15799–15809.

Holman, E. A., & Grisham, E. L. (2020). When time falls apart: The public health implications of distorted time perception in the age of COVID-19. *Psychological Trauma: Theory, Research, Practice, and Policy*, 12(S1), S63–S65.

Jacoby, N., Polak, R., & London, J. (2021). Extreme precision in rhythmic interaction is enabled by role-optimized sensorimotor coupling: Analysis and modelling of West African drum ensemble music. *Philosophical Transactions of the Royal Society of London. Series B, Biological Sciences*, 376(1835), 20200331.

Jordan, J. S. (2009). Forward-looking aspects of perception–action coupling as a basis for embodied communication. *Discourse Process*, 46(2–3), 127–144.

Kanai, R., Paffen, C. L., Hogendoorn, H., & Verstraten, F. A. (2006). Time dilation in dynamic visual display. *Journal of Vision*, 6(12), 8.

Kotz, S. A., Ravignani, A., & Fitch, W. T. (2018). The evolution of rhythm processing. *Trends in Cognitive Science*, 22(10), 896–910.

Krakauer, J. W., Ghazanfar, A. A., Gomez-Martin, A., MacIver, M. A., & Poeppel, D. (2016). Neuroscience needs behavior: Correcting a reductionist bias *Neuron*, 93(3), 480–490.

Labbé, C., & Grandjean, D. (2014). Musical emotions predicted by feelings of entrainment. *Music Perception*, 32(2), 170–185.

Launay, J., Tarr, B., & Dunbar, R. I. (2016). Synchrony as an adaptive mechanism for large-scale human social bonding. *Ethology*, 122(10), 779–789.

Lerner, Y., Honey, C. J., Silbert, L. J., & Hasson, U. (2011). Topographic mapping of a hierarchy of temporal receptive windows using a narrated story. *Journal of Neuroscience*, 31(8), 2906–2915.

Lositsky, O., Chen, J., Toker, D., Honey, C. J., Shvartsman, M., Poppenk, J. L., Hasson, U., & Norman, K. A. (2016). Neural pattern change during encoding of a narrative predicts retrospective duration estimates. *eLife*, 5, e16070.

McAuley, J. D., Jones, M. R., Holub, S., Johnston, H. M., & Miller, N. S. (2006). The time of our lives: Life span development of timing and event tracking. *Journal of Experimental Psychology: General*, 135(3), 348–367.

Montague, P. R., Berns, G. S., Cohen, J. D., McClure, S. M., Pagnoni, G., Dhamala, M., Wiest, M. C., Karpov, I., King, R. D., Apple, N., & Fisher, R. E. (2002). Hyperscanning: Simultaneous fMRI during linked social interactions. *NeuroImage*, 16(4), 1159–1164.

Mu, Y., Cerritos, C., & Khan, F. (2018). Neural mechanisms underlying interpersonal coordination: A review of hyperscanning research. *Social and Personality Psychology Compass, 12*(11), e12421.

Müller, V., & Lindenberger, U. (2011). Cardiac and respiratory patterns synchronize between persons during choir singing. *PLoS One, 6*(9), e24893.

Nakamura, J., & Csikszentmihalyi, M. (2002). The concept of flow. In C. R. Snyder & S. J. Lopez (Eds.), *Handbook of positive psychology* (pp. 89–105). Oxford University Press.

Néda, Z., Ravasz, E., Brechet, Y., Vicsek, T., & Barabási, A. L. (2000). The sound of many hands clapping. *Nature, 403*(6772), 849–850.

Nityananda, V., & Balakrishnan, R. (2007). Synchrony during acoustic interactions in the bushcricket Mecopoda 'Chirper' (Tettigoniidae:Orthoptera) is generated by a combination of chirp-by-chirp resetting and change in intrinsic chirp rate. *Journal of Comparative Physiology A: Neuroethology, Sensory, Neural, and Behavioral Physiology, 193*(1), 51–65.

Novembre, G., Sammler, D., & Keller, P. E. (2016). Neural alpha oscillations index the balance between self-other integration and segregation in real-time joint action. *Neuropsychologia, 89*, 414–425.

Nuyens, F. M., Kuss, D. J., Lopez-Fernandez, O., & Griffiths, M. D. (2020). The potential interaction between time perception and gaming: A narrative review. *International Journal of Mental Health and Addiction, 18*(5), 1226–1246.

Pecenka, N., & Keller, P. E. (2011). The role of temporal prediction abilities in interpersonal sensorimotor synchronization. *Experimental Brain Research, 211*(3–4), 505–515.

Richardson, D., Dale, R., & Shockley, K. (2008). Synchrony and swing in conversation: Coordination, temporal dynamics, and communication. In I. Wachsmuth, M. K. Lenzen, & G. Knoblich (Eds.), *Embodied communication in humans and machines* (pp. 75–93). Oxford University Press.

Roelofs, C. O., & Zeeman, W. P. C. (1951). Influence sequences of optical stimuli on the estimation of duration of a given interval of time. *Acta Psychologica, 8*, 89–128.

Rose, D., Cameron, D. J., Lovatt, P. J., Grahn, J. A., & Annett, L. E. (2020). Comparison of spontaneous motor tempo during finger tapping, toe tapping and stepping on the spot in people with and without Parkinson's disease. *Journal of Movement Disorders, 13*(1), 47.

Sachs, M. E., Habibi, A., Damasio, A., & Kaplan, J. T. (2020). Dynamic intersubject neural synchronization reflects affective responses to sad music. *NeuroImage, 218*, 116512.

Scheurich, R., Zamm, A., & Palmer, C. (2018). Tapping into rate flexibility: Musical training facilitates synchronization around spontaneous production rates. *Frontiers in Psychology, 9*, 458.

Sebanz, N., Bekkering, H., & Knoblich, G. (2006). Joint action: Bodies and minds moving together. *Trends in Cognitive Science, 10*(2), 70–76.

Sinnet, S., Jäger, J., Singer, S. M., & Philippe, R. A. (2020). Flow states and associated changes in spatial and temporal processing. *Frontiers in Psychology, 11*, 381.

Sonkusare, S., Breakspear, M., & Guo, C. C. (2019). Naturalistic stimuli in neuroscience: Critically acclaimed. *Trends in Cognitive Sciences, 23*(8), 699–714.

Stephens, G. J., Silbert, L. J., & Hasson, U. (2010). Speaker-listener neural coupling underlies successful communication. *Proceedings of the National Academy of Sciences of the United States of America, 107*(32), 14425–14430.

Stetson, C., Fiesta, M. P., & Eagleman, D. M. (2007). Does time really slow down during a frightening event? *PLoS One, 2*(12), 1295.

Trost, W. J., Labbé, C., & Grandjean, D. (2017). Rhythmic entrainment as a musical affect induction mechanism. *Neuropsychologia, 96*, 96–110.

van Noorden, L., & Moelants, D. (1999). Resonance in the perception of musical pulse. *Journal of New Music Research, 28*(1), 43–66.

Wallin, J. (1911). Experimental studies of rhythm and time. *Psychological Review, 18*(2), 100–133.

Wearden, J. H., & Ogden, R. S. (2021). Filled-duration illusions. *Timing & Time Perception, 10*(2), 97–121.

Wittmann, M. (2015). Modulations of the experience of self and time. *Consciousness and Cognition, 38*, 172–181.

Wrigley, W. J., & Emmerson, S. B. (2011). The experience of the flow state in live music performance *Psychology of Music, 41*(3), 292–305.

Zamm, A., Pfordresher, P. Q., & Palmer, C. (2015). Temporal coordination in joint music performance: Effects of endogenous rhythms and auditory feedback. *Experimental Brain Research, 233*(2), 607–615.

Focus Chapters

8

Time Through the Magnifying Glass of Slowness

A Case Study in Myriam Gourfink's Choreography

Coline Joufflineau

8.1 Introduction

Throughout the history of Western art, from the dialogue of Plato's *Charmide* to the figure of the virtuoso, high speed has been a point of aesthetic interest. Symbols of vivacity, effort, and intensity fascinate and capture the viewer's attention (Orlandi et al., 2020). Yet, since the early 1990s, slowness has also become a major trend in the performing arts, particularly in Western dance. How does it feel to attend and to perform a slow dance for 1 hr?

One of the aims of the Labodanse research project (Joufflineau & Bachrach, 2016) was to study changes in time perception experienced by spectators and dancers in the extremely slow choreographies developed by Myriam Gourfink, bringing together physiological, cognitive, and subjective data. All the Labodanse experiments took place either in theatres or dance studios with a group of spectators observing a live rendition of excerpts from Gourfink's dance pieces.

8.2 Slow Dances: The Case of Myriam Gourfink

By slowness, we mean any gesture and movement whose rhythm or speed is below the spontaneous motor tempo (SMT). The SMT describes the preferred and natural pace of regular and repeated movements, such as walking (see Hammerschmidt, this volume). Despite its individual microvariations, the SMT is relatively stable for each individual, around 2 Hz (120 beats per minute) (Moelants, 2002), regardless of their cultural background or gender (Hammerschmidt et al., 2021). It is also considered transhistorical by anthropologists (Ollivro, 2000), which makes it a particularly relevant average speed for delineating slowness in art perception and production, and for comparing the tempi of movements (musical, theatrical, danced) made in different eras. Thus, one finds forms of slow dances from ancient Greece (e.g. the gymnopaedia), in court ballets in the 16th and 17th centuries (e.g. the pavane or

Coline Joufflineau, *Time Through the Magnifying Glass of Slowness* In: *Performing Time*. Edited by: Clemens Wöllner and Justin London, Oxford University Press. © Oxford University Press 2023. DOI: 10.1093/oso/9780192896254.003.0009 the sarabande), in classical ballet (e.g. the adage), in modern dance (e.g. Doris Humphrey's *Air for the G String* (1928) or Mary Wigman's *Seraphic Song* (1929)), and postmodern dance (e.g. Steve Paxton's *Transit* (1962)).

Slowness is not only quantitative: a whole qualitative palette of the gesture is likely to influence danced slowness—the same slow drawing of the dancer's arm in space will take a very different value depending on how it is executed. For instance, the dance step known as 'slow mo' in hip hop gives the impression of a body floating, without weight, or evolving in a non-gravity space; while some slowness in the Butoh dance can give the impression that the dancer moves in a restrictive environment, such as a snowstorm.

One particularly extreme and singular example of slowness in the performing arts, developed for more than 20 years, is that of the French choreographer Myriam Gourfink. The physical speed of the dancers' movements is so slow that they approach immobility: 'it takes 8 min to cross 10 cm' indicates the choreographer (Gourfink, 2009). To an audience member the perceived tempo is extremely slow, but above all, the movement of the dancers is a continuous flow: at the level of the overall choreography there is no break, no rhythmic variations, and at the level of the movement of the dancers one perceives a continuum without any identifiable rhythmic structure. This extreme slowness cancels out all narrativity and offers the spectacle of a metamorphosis stretched in time.

8.3 What Are the Dancers' Techniques to Slow Down the Spontaneous Tempo of Their Movements and to Shape Different Qualities of Slowness?

Achieving a medium degree of slowness in movement with a regular and repetitive swinging—for example, dancing slowly with a partner or practising meditative walking—does not necessarily require a particular technique, and our attention can be quite focused on our thoughts (mind wandering) or on another task (Larson et al., 2015). But maintaining an extreme slowness in duration, within the framework of complex, non-rhythmic movements, and without external indices is not easy to achieve for dancers. Extreme slowness is an unusual speed, literally 'extra-ordinary'; it involves an approach to movement in dimensions that are neither spontaneous, automatic, nor quotidian. Several experimental studies show that individuals spontaneously prefer to move to tempi close to their SMT or to fast tempi (Van Der Wel et al., 2009).

If someone tries to walk very slowly, they might immediately observe that their attention is directed towards bodily sensations, points of support, the distribution of their weight, and their muscle chains. Conversely, if they pay attention to the smallest detail of their movement, they observe that their movement slows down. This reciprocal action between the inner direction of attention and the speed of body movement is reported in many empirical studies in the field of sport (Vance et al.,

2004) and musical performances (Duke et al., 2011; Allingham & Wöllner, 2022). The slower the movement, the more it involves attention to control the motor temporality (Krampe et al., 2010). Slowness is particularly demanding because it involves control of balance (Ben-Soussan et al., 2019; Burger & Wöllner, 2021).

The shaping of the slow movement developed by Myriam Gourfink consists largely in precisely 'choreographing' the dancers' internal attention through a contemplative practice: the yoga of energy. The basis of the practice consists in performing four actions simultaneously: controlling inspiration and expiration, which are extremely lengthened; slowly contracting and relaxing the deep pelvic floor muscles; performing a physical action, such as a movement of a limb; and a specific act of internal attention (Gourfink, 2020). These include different degrees of inner focus, on distinct body parts and sensory modalities, and several paths of attention tracing lines and spirals in the body. It is the constant combination of these different simultaneous internal tasks, the slowing down of breathing and the internal focus, that slows down the dancers' movement.

8.4 Time Through the Magnifying Glass of Extreme Slowness

8.4.1 Audience's Experience of Time and Body

The experience of time during a choreography by Myriam Gourfink varies considerably from one audience member to another. We distributed a questionnaire to 90 spectators following a live rendition at the theatre of the choreography *Souterrain* (2014), which includes 10 dancers and lasts about 70 min. It appears from the responses of the spectators that some of them did not enjoy the extremely slow speed of the dancers. They did not find the performance engaging; they felt bored and found time went by slowly. This experience of time is linked to an augmented attention to body sensations, which lasts beyond the performance itself. The most frequently reported bodily sensations experienced were those related to breath, weight, and stomach, all with a negative valence. Thus, a spectator reported that she felt 'emptied, exhausted, angry, heavy and out of breath' at the end of the performance. Others, in contrast, related a sensation of time flying. In this case, the spectators reported a feeling of calm, relaxation, and serenity. The bodily sensations experienced were also those related to breath, weight, and stomach, but in this case had a positive valence. A spectator indicated feeling 'Out of time, less rushed, out of step with normal rhythm, physically lighter'. Beyond this effect of relaxation, some feedback from the audience suggested a modified state of consciousness: the terms 'stoned', 'second state', 'weightless', 'elsewhere', or 'leaving on a journey to another galaxy' came back regularly (Joufflineau & Bachrach, 2022).

To quantify these changes in temporal perception, we made use of two cognitive tasks (Joufflineau et al., 2018): SMT and apparent motion (AM) effect before and after a 40-min live performance. AM has been studied in order to understand the structure and the duration of the temporal interval constituting the subjective present moment. It is a visual illusion in which two sequentially presented and spatially separated stimuli give rise to the experience of one moving stimulus (Finlay & von Grünau, 1987). The same temporal tasks were tested with a custom-created control choreography. It had the same length and overall structure of Gourfink's choreography but was not based on a contemplative practice (no voluntary control of breathing or internal attention) and contained various rhythmic variations.

After the performance of Gourfink's choreography, we observed a significant deceleration of SMT and a decrease in its variability, while AM was reported with longer temporal intervals. None of these effects was observed for spectators of a controlled choreography. Furthermore, an increase in perception of AM was correlated with a slower breathing rate after the performance. Investigating whether changes in time perception are associated with the subjective experience of the spectators, we have also found, using a time estimation task of short duration before and after the performance, that the extent of time distortion effects (after vs before the performance) correlated with the degree to which participants attended to their own breathing (Bachrach et al., 2015).

Finally, if slowness, by way of the emotions it may induce, such as boredom, has every chance of giving the viewer the feeling that time passes slowly, it can also produce other affects and lead to different temporal experiences. But one question remains unresolved and rarely explored: what is the experience of dancers, themselves, in such a slow pace?

8.4.2 Dancers' Experience of Time and Body

The choreographer Myriam Gourfink and the dancers reported a series of phenomenological traits. These included changes in body perception in the sense of a dissolution of the perceived boundaries of the body, an extension of the spatial frame of reference beyond the physical body, and a greater porosity of internal and external space (Gourfink, 2009). Alongside these changes in body perception during the dance, they report a strong retrospective contraction of the objective duration of choreography: 'We felt like we danced for an hour after 6 hours' Gourfink points out (2009, p. 135). It seems that the extreme slowness of the dance causes the feeling of being out of objective time for the dancers, or the feeling that time flies during the dance (see Droit-Volet & Martinelli, this volume).

In addition, the choreographer reports an unsuspected experience for an outside observer: although the extreme slowness of the dancers implies a great calm, it rests on an extraordinarily high internal speed. Gourfink says 'from the inside, it feels like things are moving very fast, there are so many micro-events to chain' (2009, p. 135). Similarly, Mikhail Mordkin, former dancer of the Moscow school at the beginning of the century, said about dance steps that:

If you want to be fast, you have to be very slow, because if you go very fast, you mix up all your steps, all your gestures and you get lost. But if you want to go very slowly, you have to have an extraordinarily high speed within yourself to tie all the small parts together. (Andrews, 2017, p. 61, translated from French)

At first glance, the claim of extreme slowness related to 'high internal speed' is contrary to the time-perception timekeeper models—for example, if the internal pacemaker or clock accelerates, subjective time should seem longer (Droit-Volet & Wearden, 2003). But, as part of the attentional model of internal clocks (Droit-Volet & Wearden, 2003), this contraction reported by dancers can be explained by the lack of attention they pay to the passage of time during a dance, which leads to a decrease in the number of pulsations emitted, and thus an underestimation of duration. In fact, Myriam Gourfink's scores contain no indication of time, to such an extent that the overall objective duration of the same choreography varies greatly on each night of the performance (Gourfink, 2009).

Perception of time on the subsecond, second, minute, and hour scales engage different mechanisms (Meck, 1996). In this vein, the feedback of the choreographer and dancers echoes empirical studies on meditation which show, on the one hand, that the contemplative state induces underestimation of the overall duration of the meditative sessions (Thönes & Wittmann, 2016), and, on the other hand, that an expansion of short durations at the millisecond to second scale corresponds to the subjective present moment (Sauer et al., 2012).

8.5 Conclusion

Recent research on time perception suggests that our experience of time is intimately linked to the sense of self and the body because they each share a common underlying neural system: the insular cortex and the interoceptive system (Craig, 2009). The internal techniques of manufacturing slow movement and the subjective reports of the dancers as well as those of the spectators support this hypothesis.

Finally, a fascinating point that remains to be explored is the inversely proportional relationship between the apparent speed of the dancers' movements and the internal speeds they experience. To our knowledge, the high internal speeds underlying the extremely slow movements have not been the subject of any theoretical or empirical studies.

References

Allingham, E., & Wöllner, C. (2022). Effects of attentional focus on motor performance and physiology in a slow-motion violin bow-control task: Evidence for the constrained action hypothesis in bowed string technique. *Journal of Research in Music Education, 70*(2), 68–189. https://doi.org/10.1177/00224294211034735

Andrews, J. (2017). *La danse profonde: De la carcasse à l'extase.* Centre national de la danse.

Bachrach, A., Fontbonne, Y., Joufflineau, C., & Ulloa, J. L. (2015). Audience entrainment during live contemporary dance performance: Physiological and cognitive measures. *Frontiers in Human Neuroscience, 9,* 179.

Ben-Soussan, T. D., Glicksohn, J., De Fano, A., Mauro, F., Marson, F., Modica, M., & Pesce, C. (2019). Embodied time: Time production in advanced Quadrato and Aikido practitioners. *PsyCh Journal, 8*(1), 8–16. https://doi.org/10.1002/pchj.266

Burger, B. & Wöllner, C. (2021). The challenge of being slow: Effects of tempo, laterality, and experience on dance movement consistency. *Journal of Motor Behavior.* https://doi.org/10.1080/00222 895.2021.1896469.

Craig, A. D. (2009). Emotional moments across time: A possible neural basis for time perception in the anterior insula. *Philosophical Transactions of the Royal Society B: Biological Sciences, 364*(1525), 1933–1942.

Deinzer, V., Clancy, L., & Wittmann, M. (2017). The sense of time while watching a dance performance. *SAGE Open, 7*(4), 2158244017745576.

Droit-Volet, S., & Wearden, J. (2003). Les modèles d'horloge interne en psychologie du temps. *L'Année Psychologique, 103*(4), 617–654.

Duke, R. A., Cash, C. D., & Allen, S. E. (2011). Focus of attention affects performance of motor skills in music. *Journal of Research in Music Education, 59*(1), 44–55.

Finlay, D., & von Grünau, M. (1987). Some experiments on the breakdown effect in apparent motion. *Perception & Psychophysics, 42*(6), 526–534.

Gourfink, M. (2009). Temps tiraillés et perceptions infimes [Interview by P. Gioffredi & S. Troche]. *Geste, 6,* 126–138.

Gourfink, M. (2020). *Composer en danse: Un vocabulaire des opérations et des pratiques.* Les presses du reel.

Hammerschmidt, D., Frieler, K., & Wöllner, C. (2021). Spontaneous motor tempo: Investigating psychological, chronobiological, and demographic factors in a large-scale online tapping experiment. *Frontiers in Psychology, 12,* 2338.

Joufflineau, C., & Bachrach, A. (2016). Spectating Myriam Gourfink's dances; Transdisciplinary explorations. In Z. Kapoula & M. Vernet (Eds.), *Aesthetics and neuroscience* (pp. 93–116). Springer.

Joufflineau, C., & Bachrach, A. (2022). *Subjective time and body distortion after spectating an extreme slow dance: an analysis of reports.* Manuscript in preparation.

Joufflineau, C., Vincent, C., & Bachrach, A. (2018). Synchronization, attention and transformation: Multidimensional exploration of the aesthetic experience of contemporary dance spectators. *Behavioral Sciences, 8*(2), 24.

Krampe, R. T., Doumas, M., Lavrysen, A., & Rapp, M. (2010). The costs of taking it slowly: Fast and slow movement timing in older age. *Psychology and Aging, 25*(4), 980–990.

Larson, M. J., LeCheminant, J. D., Carbine, K., Hill, K. R., Christenson, E., Masterson, T., & LeCheminant, R. (2015). Slow walking on a treadmill desk does not negatively affect executive abilities: An examination of cognitive control, conflict adaptation, response inhibition, and post-error slowing. *Frontiers in Psychology, 6,* 723.

Meck, W. H. (1996). Neuropharmacology of timing and time perception. *Cognitive Brain Research, 3*(3–4), 227–242.

Moelants, D. (2002, July). Preferred tempo reconsidered. In C. Stevens, D. Burnham, G. McPherson, E. Schubert, & J. Renwick (Eds.), *Proceedings of the 7th International Conference on Music Perception and Cognition, Sydney, 2002* (pp. 580–583).

Ollivro, J. (2000). *L'homme à toutes vitesses: De la lenteur homogène à la rapidité différenciée.* Presses Universitaires de Rennes.

Orlandi, A., Cross, E. S., & Orgs, G. (2020). Timing is everything: Dance aesthetics depend on the complexity of movement kinematics. *Cognition, 205,* 104446.

Sauer, S., Lemke, J., Wittmann, M., Kohls, N., Mochty, U., & Walach, H. (2012). How long is now for mindfulness meditators? *Personality and Individual Differences, 52*(6), 750–754.

Thönes, S., & Wittmann, M. (2016). Time perception in yogic mindfulness meditation—Effects on retrospective duration judgments and time passage. *Psychology of Consciousness: Theory, Research, and Practice, 3*(4), 316–325.

Vance, J., Wulf, G., Töllner, T., McNevin, N., & Mercer, J. (2004). EMG activity as a function of the performer's focus of attention. *Journal of Motor Behavior, 36*(4), 450–459.

Van Der Wel, R. P., Sternad, D., & Rosenbaum, D. A. (2009). Moving the arm at different rates: Slow movements are avoided. *Journal of Motor Behavior, 42*(1), 29–36.

9

How Long Is 10 Minutes? Exploring Spatiotemporality With a Group of Musicians and Dancers

Alexander Refsum Jensenius

9.1 Why Is Human Standstill Interesting?

One, two, three . . . stand! And off we went, standing still for 10 min, similar to what we had done so many other times during a year of preparing for the final performance of the artistic research project *Sverm*. After a year of explorations into human micromotion—here defined as the smallest producible and perceivable bodily actions—standing still had been a commonplace activity for the team: three musicians, two dancers, and one light designer. What at first had seemed like an odd technical test of the infrared motion capture system had turned into a 1-year-long artistic exploration of involuntary body motion.

Initially, we started with the idea of testing the 'sub-millimetre' accuracy and precision of the new motion capture system. Would we be able to see the tiniest motion of the human body? The short answer is yes. Through several experiments, we have shown that people's *quantity of motion* (QoM) when standing still—measured as the displacement of a marker on top of a person's head—is relatively similar between people and across trials (Jensenius et al., 2014). We have also found that listening to music while standing still makes people move more (González Sánchez et al., 2018). Other studies have found that tempi slightly faster than 120 beats per minute are the most common in dance music (Moelants, 2008) and that groove-based music is particularly movement-inducing (Witek et al., 2014). We found the same effects in our standstill studies, along with the findings that people move more when listening with headphones than with loudspeakers (Zelechowska, González Sánchez, Laeng, & Jensenius, 2020) and that the micromotion patterns have fractal qualities (González Sánchez et al., 2020). Moreover, people who score high on 'empathic concern' generally move more than others (Zelechowska, González Sánchez, Laeng, Vuoskoski, & Jensenius, 2020), supporting other recent studies of relationships between empathy and interpersonal coordination through music (Novembre et al., 2019). In sum, standstill has proven to be a valuable paradigm for studying various musical effects.

Alexander Refsum Jensenius, *How Long Is 10 Minutes? Exploring Spatiotemporality With a Group of Musicians and Dancers*
In: *Performing Time*. Edited by: Clemens Wöllner and Justin London, Oxford University Press. © Oxford University Press 2023.
DOI: 10.1093/oso/9780192896254.003.0010

9.2 Getting Used to Standing Still

Although many scientific results have come out of our standstill studies, the *Sverm* project was primarily artistic in nature. The aim was to develop a 45-min performance piece exploring human micromotion. Musicians and dancers are trained to *do* things: play an instrument or move on stage. What happens, though, if they try *not* to do anything? How does 'not-doing' feel to the performer, and how does an audience experience it? During the 1-year-long development period, the team of musicians and dancers met for weekly rehearsals. We quickly developed the habit of starting each session with a 10-min 'warm-up' exercise: standing still in silence (Figure 9.1). During the year, we explored different types of standstill: standing with open or closed eyes, in different configurations in the space, with different mental foci, and so on.

All the standstill sessions were documented with motion capture of each member of the group's head motion and written notes about the experience. One finding is the lack of correspondence between the QoM and the subjective moving experience. As reported previously (Jensenius et al., 2014), the QoM values turned out to be somewhat similar for each person across trials. This should come as no surprise; the micromotion level is primarily related to body attributes (height and weight) and various bodily processes (respiration and heart rate) that remain relatively similar over time. As Figure 9.2 shows, the displacements of the cumulative distance of head markers of three participants over 48 trials were linear. Exceptions included instances of people starting to sway after feeling dizzy or needing to cough. Still, when we began the exploration, we expected to see more variation in the measurable

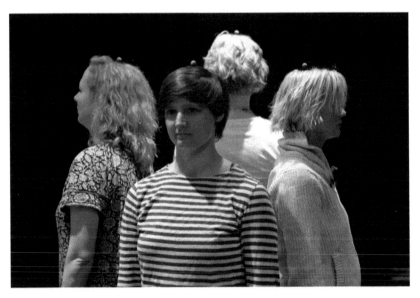

Figure 9.1 Each participant wore a motion capture marker on their head during the 10-min standstill sessions. Photo: A. R. Jensenius.

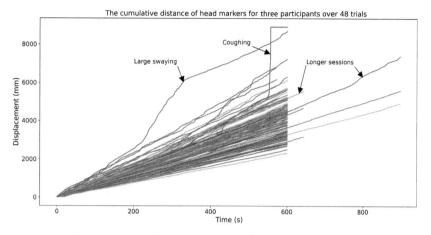

Figure 9.2 Plots of the cumulative distance travelled of markers placed on top of three participants' heads. Most of the 48 standstill sessions were 10 min long (600 s) but the linear trend can also be seen in a couple of longer sessions.

data, especially when someone reported that they felt moving more. For example, we see almost identical QoM values between two sessions described by a participant as being particularly 'good' ('I could have stood there for ten more minutes') or 'bad' ('Today I really had to focus on getting through').

One of the most common comments in the subjective reports is the need to scratch. Other times, the participants reported that it was difficult to concentrate. Still, no one ever stopped early during a standstill session. This was probably due to the collective nature of the task. It felt like we supported each other in making it through the 10 min. The majority of reports indicate a feeling of well-being after a standstill session. This resonates with findings from studies on meditation and well-being practices (Kerr et al., 2013).

9.3 The Experience of Time During Standstill

Over the years, we have run many seminars and workshops in which we have asked people to stand still for 10 min. Many people's first reaction is that it sounds 'hard'. Ten minutes may feel like an eternity in our rushed society, and *not doing* something is often perceived as stressful. Yet, only a few from among hundreds of participants have quit early. Most have completed the standstill session, and many have commented that it felt shorter than they had thought.

Looking over the hundreds of logs I have collected over the years, people report that 10 min feel both 'short' and 'long'. When someone has said that it felt long, it was usually related to some physical pain or feeling unwell. It could also be connected to one's state of mind and finding a comfortable standing posture. Several times people felt stressed when starting the standstill but reported that they managed to relax by the end of the session.

One participant said, 'I was very stressed and tense for the first half, then everything slowly faded away, and I could enjoy just standing there'. However, can this be seen in the measured data? No: looking at the QoM data of that session reveals no change at any point in time. Thus, the experiential change 'halfways' was psychological, not physical. The *Sverm* group performed some standstill sessions where we tried to identify the 'first half' through a slight nod. The nods were spread over several minutes. Subjective reports also reveal that sometimes the first couple of minutes of a standstill felt the longest; other times, the last minutes felt as though they would never end.

We have also found that performing consecutive standstill sessions affects the experience. Sometimes we did three 10-min standstill sessions in a row. At first, we thought that participants would become tired or bored after a couple of standstill sessions, thus experiencing the latter ones as longer. However, in most cases, the first standstill session of the day was perceived as the longest. If one comes into the laboratory with a busy mind, it takes some time to adjust and relax.

9.4 The Effect of Tasks

Studying the logs of hundreds of standstill sessions, it is clear that having a particular *task* makes the standstill feel shorter. In the *Sverm* project, we experimented with many types of tasks:

- *Focus tasks* included focusing on a particular modality (sight, hearing, or balancing); thinking of a person or thing; or concentrating on an involuntary bodily activity (breathing, swallowing, or blinking).
- *Mental exercises* included counting numbers or 'rolling' a ball within the body.
- *Physical exercises* included continuous micromotion, such as slowly shifting weight between the legs, rotating the head, or moving a finger back and forth. It also included microaction tasks, such as performing three rapid finger taps during a 10-min standstill.

Almost without exception, everyone reported that performing tasks during a standstill made the time pass more quickly. A concrete task removed the focus of 'just' standing there, which is in line with recent time perception models (Ivry & Schlerf, 2008). We turned this to our advantage during the final *Sverm* performances. Because we did eight 45-min performances over 2 weeks, it was important for the performers to develop strategies for maintaining focus. During the training sessions, each performer had experienced which focus tasks and mental exercises worked well for them. They also knew that these tasks would have little influence on their physical standstill, so they could use these tasks when they felt the need to focus.

Many people have asked if we became 'better' at standing still over time. Contrary to our expectations, the average QoM values remained consistent for each person over time. However, the *experience* of standing still changed considerably. After a year of practising standstill, we all came to embrace the experience.

9.5 Time Flies When Performing

The final 45-min *Sverm* performance was divided into seven 'pieces', exploring different types of micromotion and microinteraction (Jensenius, 2017b). Very little happened in each piece. For example, the piece *Head Rotation* consisted of the two dancers turning their heads 90° over 5 min. The piece *Sound Sound* was focused on the violinist and singer performing three short sound events over 8 min. Most of the time, the performers stood still.

At first, we thought that it would be challenging to keep the audience's attention for a full 45 min. That was why we decided to break it up into smaller pieces. Based on reported experiences of inattentiveness during some test performances, we decided to ask the audience to join us in a 3-min standstill at the beginning of the performance. Experiencing micromotion requires a specific level of attention. Fortunately, a 3-min standstill was sufficient to calm the audience down and help them focus. Interestingly, many audience members said that time passed quickly and that they would have wanted both the pre-performance standstill and the performance, itself, to last much longer.

9.6 Conclusion

Our daily lives consist primarily of what can be called *meso-meso* level actions (Jensenius 2017a), that is, actions within both spatial (1–100 cm) and temporal (0.5–5 s) meso ranges. Actions below these levels (micro) will be experienced as small and fast, actions above (macro) as long and sustained. In *Sverm*, we explored different combinations of micro and macro levels in time and space. The oddness of combinations—long/short and small/large—felt unnatural, but it also made them fascinating: 'It felt like an explosion when the dancer moved her finger five centimetres after standing still for several minutes', one audience member reported. Also, the performers found it rewarding, albeit challenging: 'I would never have thought it was so hard to play so little', the violinist commented after the first performance.

After 10 years of exploring and studying human micromotion, we know much more about micromotion levels and how music influences people standing still (González Sánchez et al., 2018, 2020; Zelechowska, González Sánchez, Laeng, & Jensenius, 2020; Zelechowska, González Sánchez, Laeng, Vuoskoski, & Jensenius, 2020). However, there are many unanswered questions regarding the experience of time when standing still. For example, how do different mental or physical exercises alter time perception? There are also many open questions about the interaction of time and space perception at different levels.

References

González Sánchez, V., Zelechowska, A., & Jensenius, A. R. (2018). Correspondences between music and involuntary human micromotion during standstill. *Frontiers in Psychology*, 9, 1382. https://doi.org/10.3389/fpsyg.2018.01382

González Sánchez, V., Zelechowska, A., & Jensenius, A. R. (2020). Analysis of the movement-inducing effects of music through the fractality of head sway during standstill. *Journal of Motor Behavior*, *52*(6), 734–749. https://doi.org/10.1080/00222895.2019.1689909

Ivry, R. B., & Schlerf, J. E. (2008). Dedicated and intrinsic models of time perception. *Trends in Cognitive Sciences*, *12*(7), 273–280. https://doi.org/10.1016/j.tics.2008.04.002

Jensenius, A. R. (2017a). Exploring music-related micromotion. In C. Wöllner (Ed.), *Body, sound and space in music and beyond: Multimodal explorations* (pp. 29–48). Routledge. http://urn.nb.no/URN:NBN:no-62326

Jensenius, A. R. (2017b). Sonic microinteraction in 'the air'. In M. Lesaffre, P.-J. Maes, & M. Leman (Eds.), *The Routledge companion to embodied music interaction* (pp. 431–439). Routledge. http://urn.nb.no/URN:NBN:no-62327

Jensenius, A. R., Bjerkestrand, K. A. V., & Johnson, V. (2014). How still is still? Exploring human standstill for artistic applications. *International Journal of Arts and Technology*, *7*(2/3), 207–222. https://doi.org/10.1504/IJART.2014.060943

Kerr, C., Sacchet, M., Lazar, S., Moore, C., & Jones, S. (2013). Mindfulness starts with the body: Somatosensory attention and top-down modulation of cortical alpha rhythms in mindfulness meditation. *Frontiers in Human Neuroscience*, *7*, 12. https://doi.org/10.3389/fnhum.2013.00012

Moelants, D. (2008, 25–29 August). *Hype vs. natural tempo: A long-term study of dance music tempi* [Paper presentation]. 10th International Conference on Music Perception and Cognition. Sapporo, Japan.

Novembre, G., Mitsopoulos, Z., & Keller, P. E. (2019). Empathic perspective taking promotes interpersonal coordination through music. *Scientific Reports*, *9*(1), 12255. https://doi.org/10.1038/s41598-019-48556-9

Witek, M. A., Clarke, E. F., Wallentin, M., Kringelbach, M. L., & Vuust, P. (2014). Syncopation, body-movement and pleasure in groove music. *PloS One*, *9*(4), e94446. https://doi.org/10.1371/journal.pone.0094446

Zelechowska, A., González Sánchez, V. E., Laeng, B., & Jensenius, A. R. (2020). Headphones or speakers? An exploratory study of their effects on spontaneous body movement to rhythmic music. *Frontiers in Psychology*, *11*, 698. https://doi.org/10.3389/fpsyg.2020.00698

Zelechowska, A., González Sánchez, V. E., Laeng, B., Vuoskoski, J. K., & Jensenius, A. R. (2020). Who moves to music? Empathic concern predicts spontaneous movement responses to rhythm and music. *Music & Science*, *3*, 2059204320974216. https://doi.org/10.1177/2059204320974216

10

Spontaneous Motor Tempo

A Window Into the Inner Sense of Time

David Hammerschmidt

10.1 What Is Spontaneous Motor Tempo?

Spontaneous motor tempo (SMT) describes the tempo of self-paced regular and repeated movements, such as walking, hand clapping, or swimming. It can be observed when carrying out these and other periodic motor actions at an unconsciously chosen preferred pace; it is also sometimes referred to as internal tempo (Boltz, 1994). The initial conception of this idea leads back to William Stern's 'das psychische Tempo', proposing a preferred pace for mental as well as motoric activities (Stern, 1900, p. 115). SMT is typically measured with a finger-tapping paradigm, whereby people tap with the index finger of their preferred hand at a pace that feels most natural and comfortable. It is crucial that no external rhythmical events like music are present, because the tempo of these external events may carry the periodic motor actions away from one's SMT. In such sensorimotor synchronization situations, individuals eventually fall back into their SMT when the external rhythmic events are no longer present (Bove et al., 2009; McAuley et al., 2006). The SMT indicates preferences of internal time processes as well as motoric activity, and investigating it may provide further insights into inter- and intra-individual differences in the perception and performance of music and dance.

10.2 SMT as an Estimate of the Intrinsic Timekeeper

In the psychophysics of time, SMT can be seen as a central feature for the perception of time (e.g. time judgements) and the timing of events (e.g. finger tapping). Internal clock models can be classified into interval-based and entrainment-based models (McAuley & Jones, 2003). Interval-based models assume a central mechanism constantly producing pulses (i.e. pacemaker) that are stored (i.e. accumulated), and when a time judgement is made, these accumulated pulses are compared to a reference memory. The neurophysiological plausibility of these models has been called into question, and recent studies point towards the role of neural oscillations in these

David Hammerschmidt, *Spontaneous Motor Tempo* In: *Performing Time*. Edited by: Clemens Wöllner and Justin London, Oxford University Press. © Oxford University Press 2023. DOI: 10.1093/oso/9780192896254.003.0011 processes (Allman & Meck, 2012). Entrainment-based models also include an intrinsic timekeeper or endogenous rhythm, using a dynamic approach compared to the linear properties of interval-based models (for a review, see Wang & Wöllner, 2020). The SMT is thought to be an estimate of this intrinsic timekeeper in both theoretical frameworks, thus representing the internal tempo (Boltz, 1994; McAuley et al., 2006).

The SMT typically clusters around 2 Hz (500 ms) and 4 Hz (250 ms) for finger tapping (Collyer et al., 1994; Fraisse, 1982; Hammerschmidt, Frieler, & Wöllner, 2021), and around 2 Hz for walking (MacDougall & Moore, 2005) as well as toe tapping and stepping on the spot (Rose et al., 2021). These results suggest a base frequency of around 4 Hz (Ding et al., 2017). Based on a sample with $N = 3{,}576$ participants, a recent study suggests that mostly lower modes of this base frequency are used for SMT finger tapping (Figure 10.1), the second mode (2 Hz, 500 ms) being the most common one (Hammerschmidt, Frieler, & Wöllner, 2021). Regarding these SMT measures, different kinematics of cyclic movements may cause these differences in the base frequency due to anatomical and biomechanical properties of the body (Goodman et al., 2000; Todd et al., 2007). Figure 10.1 also shows that a large variability in the pace of the SMT can be observed, indicating that other factors may play an important role for the pace of SMT, as well.

The assumption of the SMT as an estimate of an intrinsic timekeeper finds further support from studies proposing the same underlying mechanism for perceptual and rhythmic motor behaviours. This *preferred period hypothesis* suggests that each individual has a preferred and characteristic rhythm in perception and production (Amrani & Golumbic, 2020; McAuley et al., 2006; Provasi et al., 2014). For example, the SMT correlates with the preferred perceptual tempo (PPT) for auditory rhythmic structures (Amrani & Golumbic, 2020; McAuley et al., 2006), and shares the same

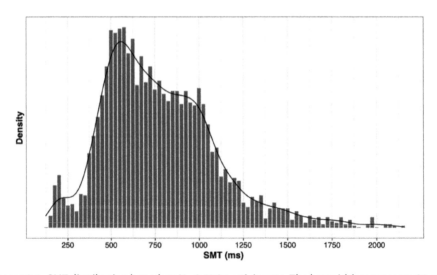

Figure 10.1 SMT distribution based on $N = 3{,}576$ participants. The bar width represents 25 ms. Data from a study by Hammerschmidt, Frieler, and Wöllner (2021).

perceptual preference for musical tempo (Moelants, 2002; van Noorden & Moelants, 1999) and language (Ding et al., 2017). At the PPT, processing and temporal discrimination abilities are regarded as optimal. Furthermore, the SMT of finger tapping and the spontaneous production rates of music, which involves a rhythmical component, are correlated as well (Pfordresher et al., 2021). Musicians perform most consistently at their spontaneous production rate (Zamm et al., 2018) and synchronization with external rhythmical auditory events is most accurate at this rate (Scheurich et al., 2018). The SMT, PPT, and spontaneous production rate may therefore reflect the most stable state of movement trajectories, requiring the least physiological and neurological energy (Poeppel & Assaneo, 2020).

Further support for the assumption that the SMT is an estimate of the intrinsic timekeeper stems from research on time judgements. Studies have shown that higher arousal increases the rate of the intrinsic timekeeper, leading to durations being perceived as longer. This has been shown to be the case in both the visual and the auditory domains, including music (Droit-Volet et al., 2013; Ortega & López, 2008; Wearden, 2008). Furthermore, higher physiological arousal also speeds up the PPT, suggesting a close relationship between tempo and arousal (Jakubowski et al., 2015). Evidence of this relationship is strengthened by findings showing that durations are judged longer when people synchronize their movement with faster rhythmic events (Allingham et al., 2021; Droit-Volet et al., 2013; Hammerschmidt, Wöllner, et al., 2021) or when they attend to different metrical levels (i.e. different tapping tempi) within the same tempo (Hammerschmidt & Wöllner, 2020). Yet, in the context of music, this effect might be primarily driven by tempo and other factors such as perceived event density, and less so by perceived arousal (Wöllner & Hammerschmidt, 2021).

10.3 Factors Influencing the SMT

10.3.1 The Arousal Effect

The SMT tends to cluster around 2 and 4 Hz (250 and 500 ms), yet it is not fixed at a certain tempo; rather, it is subject to inter- and intra-individual changes. Accordingly (as Figure 10.1 shows), studies found a large variability of SMTs ranging from 150 to over 1,000 ms (Collyer et al., 1994; Hammerschmidt, Frieler, & Wöllner, 2021). Thus, one of the main research questions is which factors influence the SMT. The PPT has been shown to increase with higher arousal (Jakubowski et al., 2015) and in accordance with the *preferred period hypothesis* this seems also to be the case for the SMT (Boltz, 1994; Hammerschmidt, Frieler, & Wöllner, 2021; Hammerschmidt & Wöllner, 2022). Physiological changes in the body (e.g. heart rate, cortical blood flow) affect arousal level (Fisher, 2014), yet the relationship between increased physiological states and SMT is not entirely understood, since studies have yielded contrasting results: higher physiological states evoked by physical activity caused SMT to speed up in a study using a cycling task (Dosseville et al., 2002), whereas no changes were measured in a study using swimming, running, or wrestling (Sysoeva et al., 2013). These contrasting results might be explained by biomechanics: the optimal stride rate in running and the optimal stroke rate in swimming are strongly constrained, whereas, in cycling, the bicycle mechanism affords a wider range of pedalling rates.

10.3.2 The Age Effect

Perhaps the most frequently studied factor influencing the SMT is age. Children (2–7 years) have an average SMT around 300–450 ms, which is faster than adults (whose SMT averages around 500–600 ms) (McAuley et al., 2006; Provasi & Bobin-Bègue, 2003; Vanneste et al., 2001). SMT slows down even more (1,050–1,125 ms) for the elderly (66–94 years), suggesting a slowing-with-age effect (Baudouin et al., 2004; McAuley et al., 2006). This slowing might also start earlier in adults; recent studies have found this effect in samples with an age range between 7–49 years (Hammerschmidt, Frieler, & Wöllner, 2021), and 20–82 years (Signori et al., 2017). Which mechanism causes this slowing is a current subject of debate. It might be that an actual slowing of internal time processes (i.e. a slower intrinsic timekeeper) slow down the SMT, as well; it may also reflect a decline in cognitive functions like memory and attention. Research on age-related changes in time perception mostly refers to retrospective time judgements of long durations (e.g. years, decades), whereas prospective interval timing (milliseconds to minutes) seems to be less or not at all affected by age (Turgeon et al., 2016). Thus, these studies do not support a slowing of the intrinsic timekeeper. Another explanation for the slowing of the SMT is based on cognitive functions. Ageing leads to a decline in processing, mental, and behavioural speed (Salthouse, 2010), as well as reduced muscle strength and endurance due to changes in the neuromuscular system (Baudouin et al., 2004). Furthermore, a large study on time perception failed to find an age effect of time judgements when controlling for cognitive capabilities (Bartholomew et al., 2015). For the elderly, motor control relies in greater measure on the prefrontal cortex and basal ganglia networks, which are brain regions that are often impaired with higher age (Seidler et al., 2010). Hence, it seems likely that the slowing of the SMT represents a reduction of processing speed and a weakening of the neuromuscular system, rather than a slowing of the intrinsic timekeeper.

10.3.3 The Circadian Rhythm Effect

A growing body of chronobiological research points towards the relationship between SMT and our body's biological clock. The circadian rhythm describes the 24-hr cycle regulating the sleep–wake cycle. This cycle has been shown to affect musicians' performance tempo as well as multiple cognitive and physiological functions, including motor processes, reaction times, time judgements, and memory (Valdez et al., 2012; Wright & Palmer, 2020). Consequently, studies investigating the SMT at different times during the day found intra-individual changes in SMT resembling circadian fluctuations. It has been shown that the SMT of finger tapping and cycling sped up during the day and slowed down again during the evening (Moussay et al., 2002). Two recent studies using finger tapping found a similar effect of the time of the day. In a large-scale online study, results showed that the earlier the time of test participation, the slower SMT was (Hammerschmidt, Frieler, & Wöllner, 2021); and, in a study measuring the SMT four times a day over 7 consecutive days, SMT was also slowest in the morning and sped up during the day (Hammerschmidt & Wöllner, 2022). Furthermore, the latter study showed that these circadian fluctuations were dependent on individuals' chronotype. The chronotype describes individual preference in the sleep–wake cycle, meaning the phase reference or midpoint between sleep onsets (Roenneberg et al., 2003). The study showed that the SMT of morning types was faster in the morning compared to evening types. Over the course of the day, the SMT of morning types remained relatively constant, whereas the SMT of evening types became faster. These results are in line with other chronotype-dependent performance differences like attention (Matchock & Mordkoff, 2009), as well as sensorimotor and timing tasks (Tamm et al., 2009; van Vugt et al., 2013). Thus, these studies show that the biological clock influences the SMT.

10.3.4 The Musical Experience Effect

The effect of musical experience on SMT has also been investigated. Children with musical training had a slower SMT than children with no training, yet these differences were absent among adults (Drake et al., 2000). Two other studies investigated the relationship between musical experience and SMT: one study did find differences in SMT, yet its findings were inconclusive because different analytical approaches yielded divergent results (Hammerschmidt, Frieler, & Wöllner, 2021); the other one did not find any differences in the pace of the SMT based on the Goldsmiths Musical Sophistication Index (Hammerschmidt & Wöllner, 2022). It is unclear that the enhanced cognitive abilities gained from musical training would transfer to the relatively simple and low-level SMT tapping task; it seems more likely that musical training and experience have no general effect on the SMT, and that their effects are limited to more complex and domain-specific musical tasks, such as sensorimotor synchronization.

10.4 Conclusion

This chapter argued that the SMT may be regarded as an estimate of an intrinsic timekeeper, representing its base frequency. Since it is directly linked to the preferred tempo in the perception/production of both music and language, SMT offers valuable insights into the underlying mechanisms of intrinsic time processes. This assumed link between SMT and the internal clock is further supported by the effects influencing SMT (i.e. SMT slows down with age, speeds up with higher arousal, and fluctuates according to the biological clock), all of which are in accordance with the prevalent internal clock models. Taken together, the research summarized here emphasizes the benefits of investigating the SMT in the context of time-related processes. Clear predications regarding internal time processes can be drawn from these theories and investigated by measuring the SMT, especially from the suggested shared mechanism for perceptual and rhythmic motor behaviours. For example, does the proposed influence of the circadian rhythm transfer to music- and dance-specific temporal preferences in perception and performance? Furthermore, the discussed factors influencing the pace of the SMT may guide future research in time-related fields, since SMT indicates a 'sweet spot' between temporal predictability and temporal preference.

References

Allingham, E., Hammerschmidt, D., & Wöllner, C. (2021). Time perception in human movement: Effects of speed and agency on duration estimation. *Quarterly Journal of Experimental Psychology, 74*(3), 559–572. https://doi.org/10.1177/1747021820979518

Allman, M. J., & Meck, W. H. (2012). Pathophysiological distortions in time perception and timed performance. *Brain, 135*(Pt 3), 656–677. https://doi.org/10.1093/brain/awr210

Amrani, A. K., & Golumbic, E. Z. (2020). Spontaneous and stimulus-driven rhythmic behaviors in ADHD adults and controls. *Neuropsychologia, 146*, 107544. https://doi.org/10.1016/j.neuropsychologia.2020.107544

Bartholomew, A. J., Meck, W. H., & Cirulli, E. T. (2015). Analysis of genetic and non-genetic factors influencing timing and time perception. *PloS One, 10*(12), e0143873. https://doi.org/10.1371/journal.pone.0143873

Baudouin, A., Vanneste, S., & Isingrini, M. (2004). Age-related cognitive slowing: The role of spontaneous tempo and processing speed. *Experimental Aging Research, 30*(3), 225–239. https://doi.org/10.1080/03610730490447831

Boltz, M. G. (1994). Changes in internal tempo and effects on the learning and remembering of event durations. *Journal of Experimental Psychology: Learning, Memory, and Cognition, 20*(5), 1154–1171. https://doi.org/10.1037/0278-7393.20.5.1154

Bove, M., Tacchino, A., Pelosin, E., Moisello, C., Abbruzzese, G., & Ghilardi, M. F. (2009). Spontaneous movement tempo is influenced by observation of rhythmical actions. *Brain Research Bulletin, 80*(3), 122–127. https://doi.org/10.1016/j.brainresbull.2009.04.008

Collyer, C. E., Broadbent, H. A., & Church, R. M. (1994). Preferred rates of repetitive tapping and categorical time production. *Perception & Psychophysics, 55*(4), 443–453. https://doi.org/10.3758/bf03205301

Ding, N., Patel, A. D., Chen, L., Butler, H., Luo, C., & Poeppel, D. (2017). Temporal modulations in speech and music. *Neuroscience and Biobehavioral Reviews, 81*(Pt B), 181–187. https://doi.org/10.1016/j.neubiorev.2017.02.011

Dosseville, F., Moussay, S., Larue, J., Gauthier, A., & Davenne, D. (2002). Physical exercise and time of day: Influences on spontaneous motor tempo. *Perceptual and Motor Skills, 95*(3 Pt 1), 965–972. https://doi.org/10.1177/003151250209500301

Drake, C., Jones, M. R., & Baruch, C. (2000). The development of rhythmic attending in auditory sequences: Attunement, referent period, focal attending. *Cognition, 77*(3), 251–288. https://doi.org/10.1016/S0010-0277(00)00106-2

Droit-Volet, S., Ramos, D., Bueno, J. L. O., & Bigand, E. (2013). Music, emotion, and time perception: The influence of subjective emotional valence and arousal? *Frontiers in Psychology, 4*, 417. https://doi.org/10.3389/fpsyg.2013.00417

Fisher, J. P. (2014). Autonomic control of the heart during exercise in humans: Role of skeletal muscle afferents. *Experimental Physiology, 99*(2), 300–305. https://doi.org/10.1113/expphysiol.2013.074377

Fraisse, P. (1982). Rhythm and tempo. In D. Deutsch (Ed.), *The psychology of music* (pp. 149–180). Academic Press.

Goodman, L., Riley, M. A., Mitra, S., & Turvey, M. T. (2000). Advantages of rhythmic movements at resonance: Minimal active degrees of freedom, minimal noise, and maximal predictability. *Journal of Motor Behavior, 32*(1), 3–8. https://doi.org/10.1080/00222890009601354

Hammerschmidt, D., Frieler, K., & Wöllner, C. (2021). Spontaneous motor tempo: Investigating psychological, chronobiological, and demographic factors in a large-scale online tapping experiment. *Frontiers in Psychology, 12*, 677201. https://doi.org/10.3389/fpsyg.2021.677201

Hammerschmidt, D., & Wöllner, C. (2020). Sensorimotor synchronization with higher metrical levels in music shortens perceived time. *Music Perception, 37*(4), 263–277. https://doi.org/10.1525/mp.2020.37.4.263

Hammerschmidt, D., & Wöllner, C. (2022). Spontaneous motor tempo over the course of a week: The role of the time of the day, chronotype, and arousal. *Psychological Research*, 1–12. Advance online publication. https://doi.org/10.1007/s00426-022-01646-2

Hammerschmidt, D., Wöllner, C., London, J., & Burger, B. (2021). Disco time: The relationship between perceived duration and tempo in music. *Music & Science, 4*, 205920432098638. https://doi.org/10.1177/2059204320986384

Jakubowski, K., Halpern, A. R., Grierson, M., & Stewart, L. (2015). The effect of exercise-induced arousal on chosen tempi for familiar melodies. *Psychonomic Bulletin & Review, 22*(2), 559–565. https://doi.org/10.3758/s13423-014-0687-1

MacDougall, H. G., & Moore, S. T. (2005). Marching to the beat of the same drummer: The spontaneous tempo of human locomotion. *Journal of Applied Physiology, 99*(3), 1164–1173. https://doi.org/10.1152/japplphysiol.00138.2005

Matchock, R. L., & Mordkoff, J. T. (2009). Chronotype and time-of-day influences on the alerting, orienting, and executive components of attention. *Experimental Brain Research, 192*(2), 189–198. https://doi.org/10.1007/s00221-008-1567-6

McAuley, J. D., & Jones, M. R. (2003). Modeling effects of rhythmic context on perceived duration: A comparison of interval and entrainment approaches to short-interval timing. *Journal of Experimental Psychology: Human Perception and Performance, 29*(6), 1102–1125. https://doi.org/10.1037/0096-1523.29.6.1102

McAuley, J. D., Jones, M. R., Holub, S., Johnston, H. M., & Miller, N. S. (2006). The time of our lives: Life span development of timing and event tracking. *Journal of Experimental Psychology: General, 135*(3), 348–367. https://doi.org/10.1037/0096-3445.135.3.348

Moelants, D. (2002). Preferred tempo reconsidered. In C. Stevens, D. Burnham, G. McPherson, E. Schubert, & J. Renwick (Eds.), *Proceedings of the ICMPC 7: 7th International Conference on Music Perception & Cognition* (pp. 580–583). Causal Productions.

Moussay, S., Dosseville, F., Gauthier, A., Larue, J., Sesboüe, B., & Davenne, D. (2002). Circadian rhythms during cycling exercise and finger-tapping task. *Chronobiology International, 19*(6), 1137–1149. https://doi.org/10.1081/cbi-120015966

Ortega, L., & López, F. (2008). Effects of visual flicker on subjective time in a temporal bisection task. *Behavioural Processes, 78*(3), 380–386. https://doi.org/10.1016/j.beproc.2008.02.004

Pfordresher, P. Q., Greenspon, E. B., Friedman, A. L., & Palmer, C. (2021). Spontaneous production rates in music and speech. *Frontiers in Psychology, 12*, 611867. https://doi.org/10.3389/fpsyg.2021.611867

Poeppel, D., & Assaneo, M. F. (2020). Speech rhythms and their neural foundations. *Nature Reviews Neuroscience, 21*(6), 322–334. https://doi.org/10.1038/s41583-020-0304-4

Provasi, J., Anderson, D. I., & Barbu-Roth, M. (2014). Rhythm perception, production, and synchronization during the perinatal period. *Frontiers in Psychology*, 5, 1048. https://doi.org/10.3389/fpsyg.2014.01048

Provasi, J., & Bobin-Bègue, A. (2003). Spontaneous motor tempo and rhythmical synchronisation in 2½- and 4-year-old children. *International Journal of Behavioral Development*, 27(3), 220–231. https://doi.org/10.1080/01650250244000290

Roenneberg, T., Wirz-Justice, A., & Merrow, M. (2003). Life between clocks: Daily temporal patterns of human chronotypes. *Journal of Biological Rhythms*, 18(1), 80–90. https://doi.org/10.1177/0748730402239679

Rose, D., Ott, L., Guérin, S. M. R., Annett, L. E., Lovatt, P., & Delevoye-Turrell, Y. (2021). A general procedure to measure the pacing of body movements timed to music and metronome in younger and older adults. *Scientific Reports*, 11(1), 3264. https://doi.org/10.1038/s41598-021-82283-4

Salthouse, T. A. (2010). Selective review of cognitive aging. *Journal of the International Neuropsychological Society*, 16(5), 754–760. https://doi.org/10.1017/S1355617710000706

Scheurich, R., Zamm, A., & Palmer, C. (2018). Tapping into rate flexibility: Musical training facilitates synchronization around spontaneous production rates. *Frontiers in Psychology*, 9, 458. https://doi.org/10.3389/fpsyg.2018.00458

Seidler, R. D., Bernard, J. A., Burutolu, T. B., Fling, B. W., Gordon, M. T., Gwin, J. T., Kwak, Y., & Lipps, D. B. (2010). Motor control and aging: Links to age-related brain structural, functional, and biochemical effects. *Neuroscience and Biobehavioral Reviews*, 34(5), 721–733. https://doi.org/10.1016/j.neubiorev.2009.10.005

Signori, A., Sormani, M. P., Schiavetti, I., Bisio, A., Bove, M., & Bonzano, L. (2017). Quantitative assessment of finger motor performance: Normative data. *PLoS One*, 12(10), e0186524. https://doi.org/10.1371/journal.pone.0186524

Stern, W. (1900). *Über Psychologie der individuellen Differenzen: Ideen zu einer 'Differentiellen Psychologie'*. Johann Ambrosius Barth.

Sysoeva, O. V., Wittmann, M., Mierau, A., Polikanova, I., Strüder, H. K., & Tonevitsky, A. (2013). Physical exercise speeds up motor timing. *Frontiers in Psychology*, 4, 612. https://doi.org/10.3389/fpsyg.2013.00612

Tamm, A. S., Lagerquist, O., Ley, A. L., & Collins, D. F. (2009). Chronotype influences diurnal variations in the excitability of the human motor cortex and the ability to generate torque during a maximum voluntary contraction. *Journal of Biological Rhythms*, 24(3), 211–224. https://doi.org/10.1177/0748730409334135

Todd, N. P. M., Cousins, R., & Lee, C. S. (2007). The contribution of anthropometric factors to individual differences in the perception of rhythm. *Empirical Musicology Review*, 2(1), 1–13. https://doi.org/10.18061/1811/24478

Turgeon, M., Lustig, C., & Meck, W. H. (2016). Cognitive aging and time perception: Roles of Bayesian optimization and degeneracy. *Frontiers in Aging Neuroscience*, 8, 102. https://doi.org/10.3389/fnagi.2016.00102

Valdez, P., Ramírez, & García, A. (2012). Circadian rhythms in cognitive performance: Implications for neuropsychological assessment. *ChronoPhysiology and Therapy*, 2, 81–92. https://doi.org/10.2147/CPT.S32586

van Noorden, L., & Moelants, D. (1999). Resonance in the perception of musical pulse. *Journal of New Music Research*, 28(1), 43–66. https://doi.org/10.1076/jnmr.28.1.43.3122

van Vugt, F. T., Treutler, K., Altenmüller, E., & Jabusch, H.-C. (2013). The influence of chronotype on making music: Circadian fluctuations in pianists' fine motor skills. *Frontiers in Human Neuroscience*, 7, 347. https://doi.org/10.3389/fnhum.2013.00347

Vanneste, S., Pouthas, V., & Wearden, J. H. (2001). Temporal control of rhythmic performance: A comparison between young and old adults. *Experimental Aging Research*, 27(1), 83–102. https://doi.org/10.1080/03610730125798

Wang, X., & Wöllner, C. (2020). Time as the ink that music is written with: A review of internal clock models and their explanatory power in audiovisual perception. *Jahrbuch Musikpsychologie*, 29, Article e67. https://doi.org/10.5964/jbdgm.2019v29.67

Wearden, J. H. (2008). Slowing down an internal clock: Implications for accounts of performance on four timing tasks. *Quarterly Journal of Experimental Psychology, 61*(2), 263–274. https://doi.org/10.1080/17470210601154610

Wöllner, C., & Hammerschmidt, D. (2021). Tapping to hip-hop: Effects of cognitive load, arousal, and musical meter on time experiences. *Attention, Perception & Psychophysics, 83*(4), 1552–1561. https://doi.org/10.3758/s13414-020-02227-4

Wright, S. E., & Palmer, C. (2020). Physiological and behavioral factors in musicians' performance tempo. *Frontiers in Human Neuroscience, 14*, 311. https://doi.org/10.3389/fnhum.2020.00311

Zamm, A., Wang, Y., & Palmer, C. (2018). Musicians' natural frequencies of performance display optimal temporal stability. *Journal of Biological Rhythms, 33*(4), 432–440. https://doi.org/10.1177/0748730418783651

11

An Embodied Perspective on Rhythm in Music–Dance Genres

Mari Romarheim Haugen

11.1 Experienced Rhythm and Music Culture

It is commonly understood that the experience of musical rhythm encompasses the interaction between *sonic rhythm* and *endogenous reference structures* such as *meter* (e.g. Danielsen, 2010; London, 2012). Musical meter, then, may or may not be represented by the sonic events but, nevertheless, always supplies the temporal framework against which we perceive them. Essential to the present perspective is the notion that we understand both the sonic rhythm and the meter as aspects of the *experienced rhythm*. The meter, therefore, is not derived from the sonic rhythm; instead, the two *interact*. Our perception of that interaction is conditioned by our previous experiences and our *musical enculturation*, here understood as the sonic rhythm–meter interactions that we have encountered most frequently. Even though any sonic rhythm could, in theory, be perceived in multiple metrical contexts (see, e.g. London, 2012, on *metric malleability*), most music cultures feature specific sonic rhythm–meter interactions such that rhythm will be experienced within a consistent metrical context by insiders. In other words, a culture-specific meter is not the *only* perceivable meter possible, but it is likely to be quite consistent among the people conversant with the music culture in question.

11.2 Experienced Rhythm and Motion

The literature frequently highlights the intimate relationship between experienced rhythm and motion in music (see London, this volume; Maes & Leman, this volume; Stuphacher, Hove, & Vuust, this volume). Embodied perspectives on perception point out that we use multiple senses simultaneously when we perceive our environment, and these multimodal experiences, in turn, influence how we perceive the world (e.g. Gibson, 1966). Perception, then, is considered an active process—it is something that we *do* that is related to sense-making and based on our previous multimodal experiences (e.g. Noë, 2004; Thompson, 2007; Varela et al., 2016). Sound perception, for example, includes not only auditory input but also an understanding

Mari Romarheim Haugen, *An Embodied Perspective on Rhythm in Music–Dance Genres* In: *Performing Time*. Edited by: Clemens Wöllner and Justin London, Oxford University Press. © Oxford University Press 2023. DOI: 10.1093/oso/9780192896254.003.0012 of the source or the action that we attribute to the sound (e.g. Berthoz, 2000; Clarke, 2005; Cox, 2016; Godøy, 2010; Jensenius, 2007; Liberman & Mattingly, 1985).

Periodic body motions such as foot tapping, body swaying, head nodding, and dance moves are often described as entrained motion that follows the perceived meter (e.g. Dahl et al., 2010; Jensenius, 2007; Merchant et al., 2015). I would argue, however, that such meter-related motions are not only externalizations of a perceived meter but also the means through which we both learn and shape that meter. Just as we make sense of perceived sounds based on our previous experience with how sounds are produced (i.e. source/action–sound relationships), we also make sense of musical meter based on our previous experiences involving meter-related bodily motion. In other words, we do not perceive the meter as one thing and meter-related movements as something else. Instead, we understand meter–motion relationships as meaningful wholes, and our meter perception therefore encompasses our embodied knowledge of the related motion (Chemero, 2009; Clarke, 2005; Toiviainen et al., 2010). When we perceive a meter and its corresponding motion, their relationship makes sense to us because of our previous embodied experiences. This insight also resonates with Blom's (2006) *Motor Theory of Rhythm*, which suggests that meter obtains its specific motion patterns (in, for example, a corresponding dance) from the tacit knowledge of style that is shared by those familiar with the music genre in question. In what follows, I will discuss examples of this embodied perspective on meter via genres in which music and dance are intrinsically related.

11.3 Meter in Music–Dance Genres

I refer to music cultures wherein music and dance have developed together under conditions of mutual influence as *music–dance* genres (Haugen, 2016b, 2021). This balanced relation describes not only genres whose music and dance are always performed together but also ones where dance is integral to the musical experience even when there is no actual dancing (Blom, 2006; Haugen, 2016b; Zbikowski, 2012).

The meter in music–dance genres must be understood in relation to the corresponding dance. In a study of Brazilian drum patterns, for example, Kubik (1990) observes that the percussionists' 'inner pulsation' is often not present in the sound but can be discerned in the body motion of the performers and dancers. The literature also locates the intimate relationship between meter and dance in so-called *time-line* music—that is, genres characterized by the interaction between specific sonic rhythms, or time-lines, and the endogenous meter. Such rhythmic patterns, often played on high-pitched instruments such as claves or a bell, can specify a culture-specific meter without directly aligning with it. Time-lines are used in much West and Central African music/dance, as well as some Afro-Cuban and Afro-Brazilian music/dances (see, e.g. Agawu, 2006; Anku, 2000; Peñalosa, 2009; Stover, 2009). Agawu (2003) also notes that, in many time-line genres in West and Central Africa, the music and the dance took shape together, and the main 'beat' in performance is often expressed by the dancers' feet. For cultural insiders, then, the perception of the time-line (or *topos*, in Agawu's terminology) will instinctively and spontaneously incorporate either the actual dancers' feet or a motor image of their movement. Agawu explains that people unfamiliar with the corresponding dance may have trouble perceiving the meter based on the sounding music alone because it does not necessarily convey the intended way of moving.

Studies of Afro-Brazilian samba have also highlighted the intimate relationship between music and dance in this genre, as well as the need to consider dance motions when examining its rhythm (Haugen, 2016b; Naveda, 2011). Interestingly, recent research has revealed that, in samba, the 16th notes are uneven in duration—that is, they include two to four distinct durational categories and the fourth 16th note in a given beat is always longer than the others, and this systematic duration pattern is a prominent feature of this groove (e.g. Gouyon, 2007; Haugen & Danielsen, 2020; Naveda et al., 2009). Moreover, scholars note that this rhythm pattern should not be understood as a systematic deviation from even metrical 16th notes but that the meter is uneven, or *non-isochronous*, in and of itself (Gerischer, 2006; Haugen, 2016b; see also Polak & London, 2014, on non-isochronous subdivisions in dance music from Mali). In other words, in samba, not only the sonic rhythm but also the meter itself is non-isochronous. This conclusion was supported by a motion capture study that found that the same non-isochronous duration pattern at the 16th-note level (*medium–medium–medium–long*) was found in both the sonic rhythm of samba and the musicians' and dancers' periodic body motions (Haugen & Godøy, 2014). In another study, Haugen and Danielsen (2020) investigated the effect of tempo on the non-isochronous 16th notes (*medium-long–short–medium-short–long*) in performed samba. They found that the duration pattern at this level was maintained across tempi, even when the durational categories became very similar (the difference between the *medium-long* and the *medium-short*, for example, was only 6–15 ms). This study concluded that humans are capable of differentiating between very similar durations, and that even very finely meshed rhythmic patterns can be perceived and reproduced with high accuracy, depending on the musical context. Considering the close relationship between meter and motion, it might be difficult for people unfamiliar with samba and its intrinsic way of moving to perceive the genre's precise and accurate non-isochronous meter and, in turn, how it interacts with the sonic rhythm. For example, one might perceive that the sonic events are played systematically 'ahead' of isochronous metrical 16th notes instead of 'on' the non-isochronous meter. Along these lines, Naveda (2011) observes that the Europeans' early descriptions of Afro-Brazilian music as 'more or less in time' reveal a poor understanding of the relationship between music and dance in these styles: 'Participants without the tacit knowledge of how movements are related to sonic patterns will listen, move and understand it differently' (Naveda, 2011, p. 51).

The intimate relationship between music and dance is also frequently mentioned in rhythm studies of specific styles of traditional Scandinavian music–dance genres (e.g. Bengtsson, 1987; Blom, 1981; Kaminsky, 2014; Kvifte, 2007), including the genre of folk music and dance from Norway called *telespringar*. Telespringar is normally notated in 3/4 meter, but cultural insiders understand that its beats themselves are uneven in duration, forming what is often referred to as *asymmetrical triple meter*. In telespringar, that is, the beats follow a *long–medium–short* beat duration pattern (e.g. Blom, 1981; Groven, 1971; Kvifte, 1999), and this meter must be understood in relation to the corresponding dance (see, e.g. Bakka, 1978; Blom, 1981; Omholt, 2009), and in particular to the dancers' periodic vertical motion of their center of gravity (e.g. Blom, 1981; Kvifte, 2004). The telespringar couple dance consists of style-specific ways of 'dance walking,' turning, and winding, and it is improvisational in the sense that the order of its style-specific motion patterns is not prescribed. For example, in a situation where multiple couples dance simultaneously, they do not necessarily perform the same moves at the same time. In addition, the way in which the dancers execute the moves can vary considerably (Blom, 1981; Mårds, 1999).

Despite all of this improvisation and variation, however, the vertical movements of the dancers' center of gravity seem to be highly periodic. Blom (1981, 2006) labels this the *patterned libration of the body's center of gravity*, or the *libration curve*. He points out that the shape of this movement curve, the number of oscillations, and the vertical position of their turning points during a given measure of telespringar are all style-specific components of the meter. A motion capture study was devoted to this relationship between the performers' periodic body motions and the meter in telespringar (Haugen, 2016a, 2017). It uncovered an asymmetrical beat-duration pattern in the musician's foot stamping that itself followed a very consistent long–medium–short pattern (Figure 11.1b). The analysis of the dancers' vertical motions also revealed a very regular pattern at both measure and beat levels—namely, a small 'valley-shaped' down-up motion during the long beat 1, a deeper down-up motion during the medium-long beat 2, and a small up-down motion during the short beat 3 (Figure 11.1a).

Even though it is commonly understood that the meter in telespringar is non-isochronous, its performers talk instead about accentuation—as in the experienced force or weight—of the beats. When performers teach telespringar dance, for example, they do not describe a long–medium–short duration pattern but rather a *heavy–heavier–light* pattern (Omholt, 2011). This weight pattern likely derives from the dancers' libration curve since the 'valley-shaped' beats 1 and 2 might feel 'heavier' than beat 3, which has a light up-down motion. The musicians, interestingly, think this way as well. In a study by Johansson (2022), folk musicians explained how their foot tapping influences their playing using terms related to force rather than beat interval. A systematic accentuation pattern was also found in the motion capture study by Haugen (2017). The musician's acceleration curves, based on foot stamping, revealed a high–higher–low pattern (Figure 11.1c) indicating that more power was put into the first two foot stamps than into the third. This pattern also corresponded closely to the dancers' libration pattern and experienced heavy–heavier–light pattern. This suggests that all the performers shared an understanding of the meter, including how it 'feels' in terms of force and weight, and that this metrical feel relates to

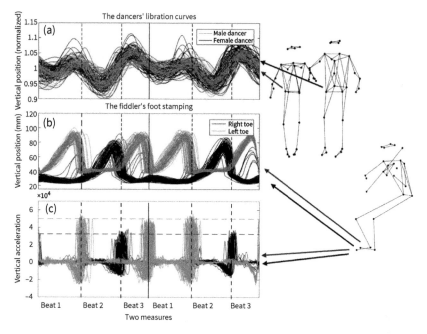

Figure 11.1 Plots showing (a) the dancers' vertical position of the hips (*libration curves*), (b) the fiddler's vertical position of the foot stamping, and (c) and the fiddler's vertical acceleration of the foot stamping during a telespringar performance. All the movement trajectories are chunked into segments of two measures and plotted on the same graph.

embodied sensations of the genre. This distinctive feel does not derive from movements as responses to sound features or sound as a response to motion patterns in actual performance, but rather from an embodied experience of the music–dance, as a whole, within a tradition wherein the music and dance have developed in tandem over time. People who are not conversant with this genre and its intrinsic way of moving will probably experience the rhythm differently than insiders do.

11.4 Conclusion

In this chapter, I have highlighted the intimate relationship between meter and motion, in general, and between meter and dance, in particular. My point of departure was that meter-related motions are not only responses to a perceived meter; they are also the means through which meter is learned and shaped. In other words, the perceived meter and the corresponding meter-related motion are *intrinsically* related—they are essentially the same. Moreover, musical meter is conditioned by musical enculturation, by the ways in which cultural insiders learn to move, and by each person's embodied experience with that culture's and that genre's ways of moving. Consequently, individuals with different embodied experiences will perceive the musical meter, and thus the rhythm, differently. Music–dance genres make ideal cases for investigating these relationships since the meter of music–dance genres exemplify the embodied knowledge of performers and cultural insiders— knowledge that has developed over time through music and dance interactions, and that relates to the periodic motions of the corresponding dance. In other words, in music–dance genres, the experienced rhythm requires an understanding of the corresponding dance. What's more, this insight might pertain to other music genres as well: we might get a deeper understanding of a particular musical rhythm if we have some embodied experience with the genre's associated ways of moving.

References

Agawu, K. (2006). Structural analysis or cultural analysis? Competing perspectives on the 'standard pattern' of West African rhythm. *Journal of the American Musicological Society, 59*(1), 1–46. https://doi.org/10.1525/jams.2006.59.1.1

Agawu, V. K. (2003). *Representing African music: Postcolonial notes, queries, positions*. Routledge.

Anku, W. (2000). Circles and time: A theory of structural organization of rhythm in African music. *Music Theory Online, 6*(1), 1–9. https://mtosmt.org/issues/mto.00.6.1/mto.00.6.1.anku.html

Bakka, E. (1978). *Norske dansetradisjonar* (Vol. 15). Samlaget.

Bengtsson, I. (1987). Notation, motion and perception: Some aspects of musical rhythm. In A. Gabrielsson (Ed.), *Action and perception in rhythm and music* (Vol. 55, pp. 69–80). Royal Swedish Academy of Music.

Berthoz, A. (2000). *The brain's sense of movement*. Harvard University Press.

Blom, J.-P. (1981). The dancing fiddle: On the expression of rhythm in hardingfele slåtter. In J. P. Blom, S. Nyhus, & R. Sevåg (Eds.), *Norsk folkemusikk* (Vol. VII, pp. 305–312). Universitetsforlaget.

Blom, J.-P. (2006). Making the music dance: Dance connotations in Norwegian fiddling. In I. Russell & M. A. Alburger (Eds.), *Play it like it is: Fiddle and dance studies from around the North Atlantic* (Vol. 5, pp. 75–86). Elphinstone Institute, University of Aberdeen.

Chemero, A. (2009). *Radical embodied cognitive science*. MIT Press.

Clarke, E. F. (2005). *Ways of listening: An ecological approach to the perception of musical meaning*. Oxford University Press.

Cox, A. (2016). *Music and embodied cognition: Listening, moving, feeling, and thinking*. Indiana University Press.

Dahl, S., Bevilacqua, F., Bresin, R., Clayton, M., Leante, L., Poggi, I., & Rasamimanana, N. (2010). Gestures in performance. In R. I. Godøy & M. Leman (Eds.), *Musical gestures: Sound, movement, and meaning* (pp. 36–68). Routledge.

Danielsen, A. (2010). *Musical rhythm in the age of digital reproduction*. Ashgate.

Gerischer, C. (2006). O suingue baiano: Rhythmic feeling and microrhythmic phenomena in Brazilian percussion. *Ethnomusicology, 50*(1), 99–119.

Gibson, J. J. (1966). *The senses considered as perceptual systems*. Houghton Mifflin.

Godøy, R. I. (2010). Gestural affordances of musical sound. In R. I. Godøy & M. Leman (Eds.), *Musical gestures: Sound, movement, and meaning* (pp. 103–125). Routledge.

Gouyon, F. (2007). Microtiming in 'Samba de Roda': Preliminary experiments with polyphonic audio [Presentation]. XII Simpósio da Sociedade Brasileira de Computação Musical (SBCM), São Paulo, Brazil.

Groven, E. (1971). Musikkstudiar—ikkje utgjevne før. 1. Rytmestudiar. In O. Fjalestad (Ed.), *Eivind Groven. Heiderskrift til 70-årsdagen 8. oktober 1971* (pp. 93–102). Noregs boklag.

Haugen, M. R. (2016a). Investigating periodic body motions as a tacit reference structure in Norwegian telespringar performance. *Empirical Musicology Review, 11*(3–4), 272–294. https://doi.org/10.18061/emr.v11i3-4.5029

Haugen, M. R. (2016b). *Music–Dance: Investigating rhythm structures in Brazilian samba and Norwegian telespringar performance* [PhD thesis, University of Oslo]. 07 Oslo Media, Oslo. http://urn.nb.no/URN:NBN:no-56252

Haugen, M. R. (2017). Investigating musical meter as shape: Two case studies of Brazilian samba and Norwegian telespringar. In E. Van Dyck (Ed.), *Proceedings of the 25th Anniversary Conference of the European Society for the Cognitive Sciences of Music* (pp. 67–74). University of Ghent.

Haugen, M. R. (2021). Investigating music–dance relationships: A case study of Norwegian telespringar. *Journal of Music Theory, 65*(1), 17–38. https://doi.org/10.1215/00222909-9124714

Haugen, M. R., & Danielsen, A. (2020). Effect of tempo on relative note durations in a performed samba groove. *Journal of New Music Research, 49*(4), 349–361. https://doi.org/10.1080/09298215.2020.1767655

Haugen, M. R., & Godøy, R. I. (2014). Rhythmical structures in music and body movement in samba performance. In M. K. Song (Ed.), *Proceedings of the ICMPC-APSCOM 2014 Joint Conference: 13th Biennial International Conference for Music Perception and Cognition and 5th Triennial Conference of the Asia Pacific Society for the Cognitive Sciences of Music* (pp. 46–52). College of Music, Yonsei University.

Jensenius, A. R. (2007). *Action–sound: Developing methods and tools to study music-Related body movement.* [PhD thesis, University of Oslo].

Johansson, M. (2022). Timing-Sound Interactions. Groove-Forming Elements in Traditional Scandinavian Fiddle Music. *PULS, 7.*

Kaminsky, D. (2014). Total rhythm in three dimensions: Towards a motional theory of melodic dance rhythm in Swedish polska music. *Dance Research, 32*(1), 43–64. https://doi.org/10.3366/drs.2014.0086

Kubik, G. (1990). Drum patterns in the 'Batuque' of Benedito Caxias. *Latin American Music Review/Revista de Música Latinoamericana, 11*(2), 115–181.

Kvifte, T. (1999). Fenomenet 'asymmetrisk takt' i norsk og svensk folkemusikk. *Studia Musicologica Norvegica, 25,* 387–430.

Kvifte, T. (2004). Description of grooves and syntax/process dialectics. *Studia Musicologica Norvegica, 30,* 54–77.

Kvifte, T. (2007). Categories and timing: On the perception of meter. *Ethnomusicology, 51*(1), 64–84. http://www.jstor.org/stable/20174502

Liberman, A. M., & Mattingly, I. G. (1985). The motor theory of speech perception revised. *Cognition, 21*(1), 1–36. http://doi.org/10.1016/0010-0277(85)90021-6

London, J. (2012). *Hearing in time: Psychological aspects of musical meter.* Oxford University Press.

Mårds, T. (1999). *Svikt, kraft og tramp: En studie av bevegelse og kraft i folkelig dans* [MA thesis, Norges Idrettshøgskole, Oslo].

Merchant, H., Grahn, J., Trainor, L., Rohrmeier, M., & Fitch, W. T. (2015). Finding the beat: A neural perspective across humans and non-human primates. *Philosophical Transactions of the Royal Society of London B: Biological Sciences, 370*(1664), 20140093. https://doi.org/10.1098/rstb.2014.0093

Naveda, L. (2011). *Gesture in samba: A cross-modal analysis of dance and music from the Afro-Brazilian culture* [PhD thesis, Faculty of Arts and Philosophy, Ghent University, Belgium].

Naveda, L., Gouyon, F., Guedes, C., & Leman, M. (2009, 7–9 September). *Multidimensional microtiming in samba music* [Presentation]. 12th Brazilian Symposium on Computer Music, Recife, Brazil.

Noë, A. (2004). *Action in perception.* MIT Press.

Omholt, P. Å. (2009). *Regional og typologisk variasjon i norsk slåttemusikk: En kvantitativ tilnærming med et historisk perspektiv* [PhD thesis, University of Bergen].

Omholt, P. Å. (2011). Rytmen i kryllingspringar. *Musikk og tradisjon, 25,* 47–65.

Peñalosa, D. (2009). *The clave matrix: Afro-Cuban rhythm: Its principles and African origins.* Bembe Books.

Polak, R., & London, J. (2014). Timing and meter in Mande drumming from Mali. *Music Theory Online, 20*(1). https://mtosmt.org/issues/mto.14.20.1/mto.14.20.1.polak-london.html

Stover, C. (2009). *A theory of flexible rhythmic spaces for diasporic African music* [PhD thesis, University of Washington].

Thompson, E. (2007). *Mind in life: Biology, phenomenology, and the sciences of mind*. Harvard University Press.

Toiviainen, P., Luck, G., & Thompson, M. R. (2010). Embodied meter: Hierarchical eigenmodes in music-induced movement. *Music Perception: An Interdisciplinary Journal, 28*(1), 59–70. https://doi.org/10.1525/mp.2010.28.1.59

Varela, F. J., Thompson, E., & Rosch, E. (2016). *The embodied mind: Cognitive science and human experience* (Rev. ed.). MIT Press.

Zbikowski, L. M. (2012). Music, dance, and meaning in the early nineteenth century. *Journal of Musicological Research, 31*(2–3), 147–165. https://doi.org/10.1080/01411896.2012.680880

SECTION 3

SYNCHRONY

Keeping Together in Time

Anchor Chapters

12

Moving Together in Music and Dance

Features of Entrainment and Sensorimotor Synchronization

Guy Madison

12.1 Introduction

Music and dance are intrinsically social activities, which like drill, ritual, and even encore synchronized handclapping are more meaningful when done together with others (Wilson & Cook, 2016). This indicates an adaptive basis, although no consensus has emerged regarding their possible evolutionary origin, despite the ubiquity of human rhythmic abilities and behaviours (reviews of entrainment from an evolutionary perspective are found in Kotz et al., 2008; Merker et al., 2009; Patel & Iversen, 2014; Ravignani et al., 2014; Ravignani & Madison, 2017).

Music and dance typically involve entrainment, in the sense of the processes by which independent rhythmical systems interact. The classic illustrative example is when two or more pendulum clocks lock their periods to each other, as reported by Christiaan Huygens in 1665. His clocks were coupled through a beam, leading their pendula to swing in anti-phase, while other types of coupling have been shown to render in-phase movement (Willms et al., 2017). This extends the analogy with human entrainment, which may also occur at different phase angles. Entrainment is a broad enough term to include a variety of behaviours that entail some sort of temporal rapport, without necessarily constituting synchronization of physical events (for definitions and discussions of these terms, see Clayton, 2012; Clayton et al., 2020; Madison et al., 2017; Wilson & Cook, 2016). It may thus refer to the synchronization or temporal coordination of body movements, brain activity, or other behaviours, to the period of some external rhythmic process, such as music or another person's movements. In contrast, sensorimotor synchronization refers to actions being temporally coordinated to predictable external events, implying a one-to-one action to stimulus behaviour. Although this frequently occurs, it is far from the most common or even typical form of entrainment in the context of music and dance. Therefore, entrainment will be used as a broad inclusive term, unless the distinction from sensorimotor synchronization or coordination is critical.

The aim of this chapter is to take a broad view on how entrainment is likely to be achieved, building on the assumption that typical features of the behaviours associated with entrainment signify important properties of the underlying

Guy Madison, *Moving Together in Music and Dance* In: *Performing Time*. Edited by: Clemens Wöllner and Justin London, Oxford University Press. © Oxford University Press 2023. DOI: 10.1093/oso/9780192896254.003.0013 mechanisms. Interest in these issues have spawned some of the earliest empirical studies within the field of psychology. Wallin (1911) demonstrated duration specificity, in the sense that listeners prefer sound sequences with intervals within a narrow range around 0.5 s, within which the relative variability of movements is also smallest (Woodrow, 1932). Another feature is subjective rhythmization, the tendency for listeners to spontaneously group successive sounds into chunks that tend to become larger (i.e. have more elements) the shorter the intervals between successive sounds (Dietze, 1885; MacDougall, 1903). This has been related to a window of subjective presence in time (James, 1890; Dunlap, 1911). A third one is negative asynchrony, meaning that movements attempting to synchronize tend to precede the stimulus, and that this is smaller for auditory than for visual stimuli (Dunlap, 1910).

These early studies used simple isochronous stimulus sequences and asked for likewise simple responses. Intriguing as this may be, similar synchronization feats are found in some species with less elaborate neural systems, such as frogs and fireflies (for reviews, see Greenfield, 1994; Wilson & Cook, 2016). The synchronization behaviour of fireflies, for example, has been quite comprehensively modelled (see Ermentrout, 1991). Such modelling is unlikely to capture that of humans, however, even when the task is similar. Human entrainment behaviour is generally more stable, flexible, and versatile, and can deal with complex stimuli and perform complex movements. It has been argued that entrainment is therefore a fruitful window for studying a range of different aspects of human functioning, including cognitive, motor, emotional, and social behaviours (e.g. Clayton, 2012; Iversen & Balasubramaniam, 2016; Merker et al., 2015). Let us list features that a comprehensive model of human entrainment needs to account for, in addition to duration specificity, subjective rhythmization, and negative asynchrony.

12.2 Broad Characteristics of Entrainment

Human entrainment features stability of movement. For example, the intervals between responses are essentially unperturbed when the external signal disappears in the classic synchronization-continuation paradigm (Repp, 2005). The synchronization part is very simple a task inasmuch as there is only and always one stimulus for every response, separated by perfectly isochronous intervals. Real-world signals are typically much more complex, and realistic modelling should be able to account for the fact that overt movement can often proceed seemingly unaffected by dramatic and sudden changes in the external signal.

Another feature is adaptability. People can maintain precise entrainment to signals with a gradually increasing or decreasing period, and can quickly entrain to step changes to the phase or period, and can do all this across a wide range of interval duration and magnitude of change. People can also 'pick up' the tempo and begin synchronizing after hearing only two beats worth of music.

A third feature is flexibility, meaning that almost any type of movement pattern can be entrained to an external signal. This is apparent in regular ensemble performance, where some musicians may be playing eighth- or fourth-note ostinato figures, while other musicians play different syncopated rhythmic patterns. These different voices need not even have any simultaneous sound events, demonstrating how powerful a common temporal model they share. Likewise, dance or other larger-scale movements can be synchronized with every so many sounds, and people can voluntarily stop what they are doing and start doing other things as they see fit.

12.3 1/f Noise and its Possible Causes

Turning to some more specific features, timed behaviour typically exhibits a peculiar form of variability called long-range correlation, 1/f noise, or fractional Gaussian noise. It refers to a certain type of statistical dependency among related data that is common in natural phenomena (Bak, 1997; Gilden, 2001). It is also found in humanly produced sequences of intervals intended to be isochronous, such as playing a uniform rhythm or otherwise 'acting as a metronome' (probably first reported by Musha et al., 1985). Expressed in the frequency domain, 1/f noise is characterized by a non-integer scaling exponent for the spectral density function, somewhere intermediate between white noise and Brownian motion. White noise constitutes a sequence of values that are independently sampled from a certain distribution, and that have, consequently, no serial dependence. In contrast, Brownian motion (more specifically one-dimensional Brownian motion or a Wiener process) consists of random increments, such that the next interval is equal to the previous interval with a random error. In terms of the process for generating such isochronous serial interval sequences, commonly called self-paced tapping, 1/f noise means that the next interval is not a copy of an internal clock or similar process with a random execution error (white noise), as proposed by Wing and Kristofferson (1973). It rather suggests that recent intervals inform the next interval, likely with more weight for more recent intervals. This is consistent with prediction models based on Bayesian approaches (e.g. Cannon, 2021; Vuust & Witek, 2014) This dependency persists across a wide range of inter-onset intervals (IOIs), but is closer to white noise at 0.5 s IOI and closer to Brownian motion at 1.5 s IOI (Madison, 2004b; cf. Gilden et al., 1995), and exhibits a plateau between 0.7 and 1.0 s (Madison, 2006). This plateau might reflect the categorical effect of including a certain number of previous intervals that fit within some temporal limit related to veridical memory of sensory input, like the concept of the phonological loop (Baddeley & Hitch, 2019; cf. Staddon, 2005). Madison and Delignières (2009) tested this hypothesis by comparing self-paced sequence production across a range of intervals with and without auditory feedback, when visual and tactile feedback was minimized. Removing auditory feedback led to stronger serial dependency at 0.5 s, no change at 0.8 s, and weaker dependency at 1.1 and 1.5 s, consistent with the hypotheses. Referring to production of sequences, these examples above would apply to entrainment behaviour only when the external signal is absent, when it suddenly changes, or is too noisy. However, long-range correlation is also found in response sequences during synchronization (Y. Chen et al., 1997; Pressing & Jolley-Rogers, 1997), and is argued to be informative about underlying mechanisms (e.g. Delignières et al., 2009; Hennig, 2014; Torre & Delignières, 2008). This is an understudied phenomenon, partly because most studies feature synchronization sequences too short for calculating their long-range correlation. Nevertheless, it seems that human timing is unable to function as a stationary clock or oscillator. This raises the question whether long-range correlation is a signature of the same underlying mechanisms involved in both production and entrainment, or perhaps an emergent property of these types of processes.

12.4 Duration Specificity

Time-regular behaviours exhibit a sweet spot around 0.4–0.8 s, and deteriorate substantially below 200 ms and above 2 s (Mates et al., 1994; for reviews see, e.g. London, 2012; Madison, 2001a). Half a second corresponds to the preferred tempo (e.g. Moelants, 2002), the average pace of walking (McDougall & Moore, 2005), and to the smallest relative variability at around 3–4% of the interval during both synchronization (e.g. Madison, 2001b) and sequence production (e.g. Madison et al., 2013). Two seconds seems to pose a limit for temporal integration, at least for simple sound sequences (for a review, see Baddeley & Hitch, 2019).

However, duration specificity is also manifest as breaks in the otherwise near-linear increase in variability with longer intervals. This scalar timing property is found across a wide range of IOIs, and is similar across both perceptual and action timing and across both sequences and discrete intervals (for reviews, see Grondin, 2008; Lewis & Miall, 2009). Variability increases much more rapidly from about 1.3 s to 2 s (e.g. Madison, 2001b), where the SD is around 120 ms or 6%. While production is feasible for even longer intervals, synchronization tends to break down at around 2.4–2.8 s (Mates et al., 1994). However, these limits can be overcome when the timed intervals are multiplied or subdivided, whether this is manifest in the external signal or invoked by the listener (e.g. Grondin et al., 1999; Repp, 2010). That is the essence of the metrical structure of music, which is inseparable from the beat. In psychological terms, this duo highlights the distinction between the sensory signal and the percept that it induces.

12.5 The Pulse

The pulse (or beat or tactus) can be described as a neural process that is manifest in a sequence of regular time intervals (e.g. Honing, 2012; Merker, 2000; Todd et al., 1999, 2002; Patel & Iversen, 2014). I will henceforth refer to pulse, not to confuse this neural process with music theoretical concepts. The earliest works inferred the pulse from introspection (Dietze, 1885) and behaviour (Stevens, 1886). Recent technical sophistication has made the pulse objectively observable through electroencephalography and other brain imaging techniques (J. L. Chen et al., 2009; Honing, 2012; Levitin et al., 2018; Merchant et al., 2015; Nguyen et al., 2018). Such analyses demonstrate brain activity that coincides with the subjectively perceived pulse (Jongsma et al., 2005; Nozaradan et al., 2011), even in the absence of coinciding sensory events (Potter et al., 2009; Tal et al., 2017). This ability seems to be present at birth (Honing et al., 2009; Winkler et al., 2009). It is suggested to stem from activating brain areas involved in movement (Cannon & Patel, 2021), consistent with a correlation between preferred pulse rate and anthropometric factors, especially those related to motion of the upper body (Todd et al., 2007). Taken together, this strongly implies an independent 'pulse generator', rather than a process that is passively entrained to external stimuli (Bose et al., 2019; Nozaradan et al., 2011, 2015). To which extent the distinction between these two conceptions are accurate and useful remains an open question. However, an internal, independent oscillatory process would seem to be required when the external signal is noisy or otherwise unreliable, but the entrained behaviour needs to be stable, as well as when the entrained behaviour needs to be flexible in relation to the signal.

The pulse seems to represent a privileged temporal level, such that one cannot perceive more than one pulse percept at a time (London, 2012, pp. 30–32). This is consistent both with the concept of a pulse generator and with the fact that any perception of rhythms, however complex, seems to be processed within a metrical structure (e.g. Grahn, 2012; Repp et al., 2011; Vuust & Witek, 2014). There is growing evidence of neural representations that correspond to the metrical structure of measured music (Grahn & Rowe, 2009; Jongsma et al., 2004; Nozaradan et al., 2011, 2015; Snyder & Large, 2004, 2005). The metrical structure is typically binary, in which case it accommodates all powers of two. It encompasses thereby a very wide range of durations that are all 'time-locked' to the pulse interval (Fitch, 2013). Although binary metres are by far the most common, even across cultures, any combination of subdivisions is in principle possible, including ternary ones. That metres such as 9/8 are nevertheless rare may be because they are less likely to afford maximal pulse salience, as discussed by London (2012, p. 46). However, the crucial point is that hierarchical metrical structures extend the range of durations to both shorter and longer intervals than the pulse, such as half notes, bars, and groups of bars, corresponding to the length of musical phrases. Even outside the context of music, such hierarchical structures afford substantial information reduction, which extends memory and other cognitive constraints, as elaborated elsewhere (Madison et al., 2017; Merker, 2002, 2014).

A rhythmic illusion, first discovered by Risset (1986) and more recently explored by Madison (2009) demonstrates many of the features mentioned so far. It is based on a multilevel temporal pattern that utilizes the interaction of a binary metrical structure and the privileged temporal level of the pulse. First, every other sound event in an isochronous sequence of sounds is made louder, which gives the impression of a second temporal level (2^1) with half the rate of the first one. Increasing the loudness of every other sound of the second level creates a third level (2^2), and so forth. This was extended to nine levels, the slowest having 2^8 or 256 times longer intervals than the fastest, although only six levels fit within the 64 events of the portion of the sequence depicted in Figure 12.1a. Second, this binary structure was then combined with tempo change in such a way that the change would seemingly continue infinitely while the sound pattern essentially remained the same. This is achieved by halving (or doubling) the event rate across a specific number of events, repeating this subsequence without divulging the boundaries between each subsequence. This is illustrated in Figure 12.1b, which shows a 96-interval subsequence with increasing IOIs, and its boundaries with the previous and following subsequence. The more events in a subsequence, the slower the tempo change. Having time rather than sequence index on the abscissa and relative loudness rather than metrical levels on the ordinate reveals that both IOI and loudness increase from left

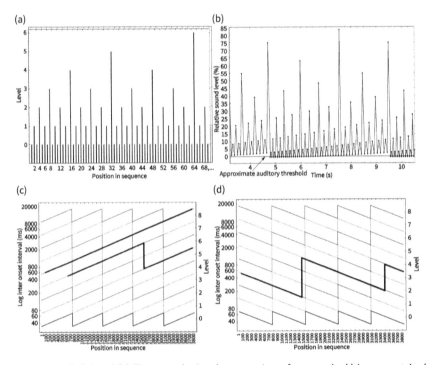

Figure 12.1 Panels (a) and (b) illustrate the implementation of a canonical binary metrical structure, with the addition of tempo change, repetition of tempo change across a certain numbers of events, and concealed boundaries between repetitions. Panels (c) and (d) depict patterns used in an experiment, the actual stimuli for five repeated 768-event patterns shown as medium solid lines (level 0) and alternative perceived IOIs corresponding to each level as discontinuous thin lines (levels 1–8), for both increasing IOIs (c) and decreasing IOIs (d). Examples of typical response sequences are shown as thick solid lines. See text for further explanations.

to right and that this change is exponential rather than linear. Third, the boundary between each subsequence is concealed by a step change in the loudness pattern, such that level 2 assumes the same loudness as level 1, level 3 the same as level 2, and so forth, and by the fact that the suddenly appearing faster events on level 0 are below the auditory threshold and then gradually become perceivable. All these features are simply reversed when IOIs decrease, creating the illusion of infinitely increasing tempo. Altogether, the resulting sequence features many alternative tempi to which one can attribute one's perceived psychological pulse, distinguished only by their relative loudness.

Figure 12.1c and d shows the actual implementation in a synchronization experiment using a subsequence of 768 events, which was repeated five times (Madison, 2009). The medium thick lines for level 0 correspond to the actual sequence of sounds, and the alternating solid and dotted thin lines for levels 1 through 8 illustrate the IOIs that correspond to the metrical structure suggested by the loudness pattern. These graphs represent the IOI as a function of the sequence index for all nine levels on a logarithmic scale, which makes the plotted exponential IOI change appear linear. Listeners were asked to synchronize as they found comfortable, and to adjust their movement cadence accordingly. Figure 12.1c shows the pattern with increasing intervals, and the two most common types of responses. Starting at a comfortable 500–600-ms pulse interval it either continues to the integration limit at around 2 s, and then switches back to the initial tempo two levels below, or continues until the stimulus sequence stops after five levels or 32 times longer IOIs at around 15–20 s. Figure 12.1d exemplifies that decreasing intervals rapidly lead to fast movements that are difficult to perform, and require more frequent switches to higher levels. Thus, human entrainment to these types of sequences exhibits adaptability, flexibility, and duration specificity, and demonstrates the effectiveness of the metrical structure and the privileged temporal level of the pulse. The currently perceived pulse seems to serve as an 'anchor', from which listeners are compelled to follow the gradual change in tempo, even though it brings them outside the comfortable zone and the stimulus pattern remains the same across different perceived metrical levels.

Another effect of metrical structure is decreased variability during sensorimotor synchronization with longer movement intervals, when faster metrical levels are added. This has been done by asking participants to imagine or feel an event in between actual sounds (Repp, 2010). Extending to more than these two metrical levels, Madison (2014) used a metrical sequence similar to that in Figure 12.1a, but with a maximum of four levels and without any tempo change. The variability in participants' responses was around 4% for one-level sequences up to 1 s, and increased rapidly above that, as is typical. In contrast, variability decreased to 3% for two, three, and four levels up to 2 s, and then decreased further to 2% for three and four levels at the longest intervals close to 3-s movement IOIs. Thus, the multilevel pattern sequences yielded lower variability than did single-level sequences at any IOI, and the lowest variability was found for the longest response IOIs, between 2 and 3 s (Madison, 2014). This finding suggests that the metrical structure not only overcomes duration-specific limits, by 'moving' the pulse into the optimal range, but also that the extra information from faster metrical levels is used to improve maximal temporal precision.

12.6 Temporal Variability in Entrainment

Virtually all temporal signals contain deviations from perfect isochrony, at the same time as isochrony is the underlying model for entrainment. So how tolerant is the pulse for temporal variability (see Danielsen, 2018, this volume)? To address this question, listeners heard a nominally isochronous sequence with 600-ms IOI, in which each interval was either longer or shorter by a fixed magnitude, following an unpredictable Kolakoski sequence (Madison & Merker, 2002). Their responses to the statement 'Is there a pulse in this sound sequence, such that I would be able to beat along with it?' (yes/no) determined the deviation magnitude for the next trial, according to an adaptive psychophysiological algorithm. The group mean threshold was 51 ms, or 8.6% of the mean IOI (nominally 600 ms), as compared to 21 ms or 3.5% for detecting a deviation ('Can I hear any irregularity in this sound sequence?' (yes/no)). The latter is essentially the corresponding level of variability in motor behaviour for both sensorimotor synchronization and self-paced generation of isochronous sequences of intervals (e.g. Madison, 2001b; Madison et al., 2013). Thus, the threshold for accepting information for inducing a pulse, in terms of its variability, is more than double that of detecting it.

This can be compared to the magnitude of deviations that is utilized during entrainment. Experiments that manipulate temporal perturbations show that both subliminal (less than approximately 20 ms) and supraliminal perturbations up to about 50 ms are linearly reflected in the immediately following interval, but are weaker and considerably more variable for subsequent intervals (Repp, 2002a, 2002b; as reviewed in Repp & Su, 2013). These reactions are attributed to perceiving asynchronies between one's own actions and the external signal, and should therefore not occur for subliminal perturbations. The distinction between sub- and supraliminal perturbations seems not consistently related to behaviour. Changing the period in the signal leads to gradually increasing asynchronies so long as the response period remains the same, rapidly making even an initially subliminal asynchrony supraliminal. However, monotonically increasing or decreasing each consecutive interval by 1–4 ms did not exhibit any threshold effect when reaching a certain magnitude (Madison & Merker, 2005). Participants' responses were consistently late when stimulus intervals decrease, and early when they increase, even though this change was perfectly predictable. Changing even just one interval in a sequence leads to an involuntary phase correction reaction that makes the subsequent responses asynchronous. One could therefore argue that subliminal shifts might be aggregated to surpass the detection threshold across a few responses. To eliminate this confound, Madison and Merker (2004) devised a sequence of sounds where each interval was either longer or shorter, according to an unpredictable sequence, and showed that the mean response intervals were almost identical to the preceding stimulus interval even when the difference was as small as 1.5 ms. Taken together, these findings are consistent with a mechanism that simply copies the last interval (Staddon, 2005; Wearden, 1999), and does so with a temporal resolution way below the detection threshold.

12.7 Modelling Approaches

Combining these observations from different strands of research, a viable conception of entrainment consists of a neural representation of a hierarchical time structure, as reflected in the metrical structure of music, superimposed on an internally generated regular pulse (as exemplified in Figure 12.1). This structure overcomes natural constraints for perceiving, representing, and acting upon temporal information, and is reflected in sensorimotor synchronization, in terms of the attraction to integer ratios (cf. Bouvet et al., 2019; Repp, 2008; Repp et al., 2008). It provides an optimized representation of both short and long time intervals with sufficient precision for functional synchrony, as well as for complex temporal patterns (cf. Bose et al., 2019; Hardy & Buonomano, 2016; Henry & Grahn, 2017; Large et al., 2015; Madison et al., 2017; Merker, 2002, 2006, 2014; Merker et al., 2009). The pulse seems to have a profound significance as a psychological or internal vehicle for sequential timing in general, enabling a smooth and flexible transition between production of movement and entrainment of movement to external signals. This is demonstrated, for example, by differences in temporal performance as a function of attributing the pulse to different alternative tempi (typically from binary levels with double of half the IOI) (Cannon & Patel, 2021; Chemin et al., 2014; Madison, 2009, 2014; Repp, 2010). When we perceive periodicity in a sound signal, within the range indicated above and with an interval-to-interval variability less than approximately 8–9% of the interval (Madison & Merker, 2002), these mechanisms are automatically and involuntarily invoked, and then sustain themselves at the neural level as long as there is motivation to do so (Wilson & Cook, 2016). They continue their pulse-based and hierarchical temporal-grid mapping of recent and future time, with more long-term correlation drift the less information is available for relating recent and future time, reflecting memory-based rather than beat-based timing (Madison, 2004a, 2004b; Madison & Delignières, 2009; Madison & Merker, 2004, 2005; Staddon, 2005; for discussions of neural substrates, see Balasubramaniam et al., 2021; Malapani & Fairhurst, 2002; Paton & Buonomano, 2018). Also, entrainment seems to adapt to the degree of variability in the signal, in line with the concept of the beat bin (Danielsen, 2010; cf. Danielsen et al., 2019, 2022).

The sketch above encompasses many of the observations that have been noted. However, negative asynchrony seems not to be intrinsic to, or implied by, any family of models below. As reviewed in Repp and Su (2013), negative asynchrony decreases with more complex sound sequences, for example, those with sounds that intervene the responses, and may even disappear for professional musicians. It is also associated with larger variability (Yang et al., 2020). Its origin remains unclear, but some observations suggest that it might be an artefact of unnatural stimuli, like metronome clicks (for reviews, see Aschersleben, 2002; Aschersleben et al., 2004). Likewise, extant models account for only parts of the suite of features observed in entrainment.

Briefly, extant entrainment and synchronization models can be divided into two main families. The first can be referred to as linear, information-processing, or error-correction models (Delignières et al., 2009; Egger et al., 2020; Gonzalez et al., 2019; Harry & Keller, 2019; Hary & Moore, 1985, 1987; Mates, 1994; Michon, 1967; Schulze, 1992; Schulze & Vorberg, 2002; Semjen et al., 1998; van der Steen & Keller, 2013; Vorberg & Schulze, 2002). They are generally flexible but less stable and versatile. Their simple linear functions allows them to quickly correct for large asynchronies and tempo changes, but their strong dependence on feedback makes them unstable, and may, for example, lead them to oscillate in the absence of an external signal (e.g. Mates, 1994). Within the limited parameter space in which they tend to be tested, however, human performance often fits their predictions well (Ezzina et al., 2020; cf. Torre & Balasubramaniam, 2009). They cannot account for how complex stimuli or movements are dealt with, absent a representation of metrical structure. The 'clock' that maintains the specific temporal reference that allows predicting the next interval is abstract and elusive, and does not account for duration specificity or long-range correlation. However, there have been attempts to build models that combine error correction and prediction (van der Steen & Keller, 2013). On a general level, error-correction models seem well suited to account for adaptability, flexibility, and stability of movement, but not for duration specificity, long-range correlation, and subjective rhythmization, or for the emergence of metrical structure. But as has been discussed, long-range correlation can emerge from a linear model if some external source of duration specificity is assumed, such as a temporal limit for retention of sensory input.

The second family is based on the dynamical systems approach, which tends to naturally imply stability and to account for duration specificity in terms of the mass and other movement-relevant parameters of the body and the limbs involved in the behaviour (Schmidt et al., 1991, 1993; Todd et al., 2002; van der Steen & Keller, 2013; for reviews, see Bose et al., 2019). The intrinsic involvement of motor networks also enables perception of the pulse without actual movement, (Clayton et al., 2020; Large et al., 2015), which could, in other words, constitute a pulse generator. These models do not generally emulate human performance very well, however. Because they build on iterative processes that gradually adapt to changing conditions, they tend to be inflexible and to not readily account for human versatility and fast reactions and changes in tempo. By contrast, the dynamical systems approach provide an architecture that lends itself well to include neural and physiological levels of implementation, which may encompass rhythmic structure and long-range correlation (for a discussion, see Large et al., 2015). Thus, the dynamical systems approach seems to naturally entail duration specificity, and its neural network architecture of oscillators is consistent with subjective rhythmization and a metrical structure (Large et al., 2015; Large & Snyder, 2009). By contrast, that same architecture renders such models unable to adapt to sudden tempo changes, as well as making them relatively inflexible with respect to immediately starting, stopping, or changing an entrained movement pattern.

12.8 Conclusion

The pulse phenomenon and its concomitant metrical structure has received attention from music theorists (Lerdahl & Jackendoff, 1983; London, 2012), but given its suggested central role for sequential timing in general, it needs further empirical study. Indeed, it has been noted that most research that makes reference to it treats it as something self-evident (Merker et al., 2009). Conceptualizing the pulse as a self-sustained, internal process makes sense in relation to the general stability of behaviour, and is consistent with seamless switching between production and synchronization, and associated patterns of brain activation (Chauvigné et al., 2014). It may also potentially resolve some apparent inconsistencies between model and human behaviour, such as negative asynchrony, long-range correlation, and differences between period correction and phase correction. Comprehensive reviews of the sensorimotor synchronization literature, with more than 200 (Repp, 2005) and 300 references (Repp & Su, 2013), document many modelling efforts. Yet, none of these models are very successful at accounting for typical features of human entrainment behaviour, and certainly not for the whole array of such features. Moreover, it has proven difficult to discriminate between particular models, at least under the simple performance conditions typically applied (Ezzina et al., 2020; Jacoby & Repp, 2012). This is as it should be. Modelling is an extremely powerful tool, and these efforts have tremendously increased our understanding of these phenomena. The future will show if extensions and development of established types of models or conceptually novel models will prove more successful.

References

Aschersleben, G. (2002). Temporal control of movements in sensorimotor synchronization. *Brain and Cognition, 48*(1), 66–79.

Aschersleben, G., Gehrke, J., & Prinz, W. (2004). A psychophysical approach to action timing. In C. Kaernbach, E. Schröger, & H. Müller (Eds.), *Psychophysics beyond sensation: Laws and invariants of human cognition.* (pp. 117–136). Lawrence Erlbaum Associates, Inc.

Baddeley, A., & Hitch, G. J. (2019). The phonological loop as a buffer store: An update. *Cortex, 112*, 91–106.

Bak, P. (1997). *How nature works.* Oxford University Press.

Balasubramaniam, R., Haegens, S., Jazayeri, M., Merchant, H., Sternad, D., & Song, J.-H. (2021). Neural encoding and representation of time for sensorimotor control and learning. *Journal of Neuroscience*, *41*(5), 866–872.

Bose, A., Byrne, A., & Rinzel, J. (2019). A neuromechanistic model for rhythmic beat generation. *PLoS Computational Biology*, *15*(5), e1006450.

Bouvet, C., Varlet, M., Dalla Bella, S., Keller, P. E., Zelic, G., & Bardy, B. (2019). Preferred frequency ratios for spontaneous auditory-motor synchronization: Dynamical stability and hysteresis. *Acta Psychologica*, *196*, 33–41.

Cannon, J. J. (2021). Expectancy-based rhythmic entrainment as continuous Bayesian inference. *PLoS Computational Biology*, *17*(6), e1009025.

Cannon, J. J., & Patel, A. D. (2021). How beat perception co-opts motor neurophysiology. *Trends in Cognitive Sciences*, *25*(2), 137–150.

Chauvigné, L. A. S., Gitau, K. M., & Brown, S. W. (2014). The neural basis of audiomotor entrainment: An ALE meta-analysis. *Frontiers in Human Neuroscience*, *8*, 776.

Chemin, B., Mouraux, A., & Nozaradan, S. (2014). Body movement selectively shapes the neural representation of musical rhythms. *Psychological Science*, *25*(12), 2147–2159.

Chen, J. L., Penhune, V. B., & Zatorre, R. J. (2009). The role of auditory and premotor cortex in sensorimotor transformations. *Annals of the New York Academy of Sciences*, *1169*, 15–34.

Chen, Y., Ding, M., & Kelso, J.-A. S. (1997). Long memory processes (1/f^a type) in human coordination. *Physical Review Letters*, *79*(22), 4501–4504.

Clayton, M. (2012). What is entrainment? Definition and applications in musical research. *Empirical Musicology Review*, *7*(1–2), 49–56.

Clayton, M., Jakubowski, K., Eerola, T., Keller, P. E., Camurri, A., Volpe, G., & Alborno, P. (2020). Interpersonal entrainment in music performance: Theory, method, and model. *Music Perception*, *38*(2), 136–194.

Danielsen, A. (2010). Here, there and everywhere: Three accounts of pulse in D'Angelo's 'Left and Right'. In A. Danielsen (Ed.), *Musical rhythm in the age of digital reproduction* (pp. 19–35). Ashgate.

Danielsen, A. (2018). Pulse as dynamic attending: Analysing beat bin metre in Neo Soul grooves. In C. Scotto, K. Smith, & J. Brackett (Eds.), *The Routledge companion to popular music analysis* (pp. 1–27). Routledge.

Danielsen, A., Nymoen, K., Anderson, E., Camara, G. S., Langerød, M. T., Thompson, M. R., & London, J. (2019). Where is the beat in that note? Effects of attack, duration, and frequency on the perceived timing of musical and quasi-musical sounds. *Journal of Experimental Psychology: Human Perception and Performance*, *45*(3), 402–418.

Danielsen, A., Nymoen, K., Langerød, M. T., Jacobsen, E., Johansson, M. S., & London, J. (2022). Sounds familiar(?): Expertise with specific musical genres modulates timing perception and micro-level synchronization to auditory stimuli. *Attention, Perception & Psychophysics*, *84*(2), 599–615.

Delignières, D., Torre, K., & Lemoine, L. (2009). Long-range correlation in synchronization and syncopation tapping: A linear phase correction model. *PLoS One*, *4*(11), e7822.

Dietze, G. (1885). Untersuchungen über den Umfang des Bewusstseins bei regelmässig auf einander folgenden Schalleindrucken. *Philosophische Studien*, *2*, 362–393.

Dunlap, K. (1910). Reactions to rhythmic stimuli with attempt to synchronize. *Psychological Review*, *17*(6), 399–416.

Dunlap, K. (1911). Rhythm and the specious present. *Journal of Philosophical, Psychological and Scientific Method*, *8*(13), 348–354.

Egger, S. W., Le, N. M., & Jazayeri, M. (2020). A neural circuit model for human sensorimotor timing. *Nature Communications*, *11*(1), 3933.

Ermentrout, B. (1991). An adaptive model for synchrony in the firefly Pteroptyx malaccae. *Journal of Mathematical Biology*, *29*(6), 571–585.

Ezzina, S., Scotti, M., Roume, C., Pla, S., Blain, H., & Delignières, D. (2020). Interpersonal synchronization processes in discrete and continuous tasks. *Journal of Motor Behavior*, *53*(5), 583–597.

Fitch, W. T. (2013). Rhythmic cognition in humans and animals: Distinguishing meter and pulse perception. *Frontiers in Systems Neuroscience*, *7*, 68.

Gilden, D. L. (2001). Cognitive emissions of 1/f noise. *Psychological Review*, *108*(1), 33–56.

Gilden, D. L., Thornton, T., & Mallon, M. W. (1995). 1/f noise in human cognition. *Science, 267*(5205), 1837–1839.

Gonzalez, C., Bavassi, M. L., & Laje, R. (2019). Response to perturbations as a built-in feature in a mathematical model for paced finger tapping. *Physical Review E, 100*(6–1), 062412.

Grahn, J. A. (2012). Neural mechanisms of rhythm perception: Current findings and future perspectives. *Topics in Cognitive Science, 4*(4), 585–606.

Grahn, J. A., & Rowe, J. B. (2009). Feeling the beat: Premotor and striatal interactions in musicians and nonmusicians during beat perception. *Journal of Neuroscience, 29*(23), 7540–7548.

Greenfield, M. D. (1994). Cooperation and conflict in the evolution of signal interactions. *Annual Review of Ecological Systems, 25*(1), 97–126.

Grondin, S. (2008). *Psychology of time.* Emerald.

Grondin, S., Meilleur-Wells, G., & Lachance, R. (1999). When to start counting in a time-intervals discrimination task: A critical point in the timing process of humans. *Journal of Experimental Psychology: Human Perception and Performance, 25*(4), 993–1004.

Hardy, N. F., & Buonomano, D. V. (2016). Neurocomputational models of interval and pattern timing. *Current Opinion in Behavioral Sciences, 8,* 250–257.

Harry, B., & Keller, P. E. (2019). Tutorial and simulations with ADAM: An adaptation and anticipation model of sensorimotor synchronization. *Biological Cybernetics, 113*(4), 397–421.

Hary, D., & Moore, G. P. (1985). Temporal tracking and synchronization strategies. *Human Neurobiology, 4*(2), 73–77.

Hary, D., & Moore, G. P. (1987). Synchronizing human movement with an external clock source. *Biological Cybernetics, 56*(5–6), 305–311.

Hennig, H. (2014). Synchronization in human musical rhythms and mutually interacting complex systems. *Proceedings of the National Academy of Sciences of the United States of America, 111*(36), 12974–12979.

Henry, M. J., & Grahn, J. A. (2017). Music, brain, and movement. Time, beat, and rhythm. In R. Ashley & R. Timmers (Eds.), *The Routledge companion to music cognition* (pp. 63–74). Routledge.

Honing, H. (2012). Without it no music: Beat induction as a fundamental musical trait. *Annals of the New York Academy of Sciences, 1252,* 85–91.

Honing, H., Ladinig, O., Háden, G., & Winkler, I. (2009). Is beat induction innate or learned? Probing emergent meter perception in adults and newborns using event-related brain potentials. *Annals of the New York Academy of Sciences, 1169,* 93–96.

Iversen, J. R., & Balasubramaniam, R. (2016). Synchronization and temporal processing. *Current Opinion in Behavioral Sciences, 8,* 175–180.

Jacoby, N., & Repp, B. H. (2012). A general linear framework for the comparison and evaluation of models of sensorimotor synchronization. *Biological Cybernetics, 106*(3), 135–154.

James, W. (1890). *The principles of psychology* (Vol. 1). Holt.

Jongsma, M., Desain, P., & Honing, H. (2004). Rhythmic context influences the auditory evoked potentials of musicians and nonmusicians. *Biological Psychology, 66*(2), 129–152.

Jongsma, M., Eichele, T., Jenks, K. M., Desain, P., & Honing, H. (2005). Expectancy effects on omission evoked potentials in musicians and non-musicians. *Psychophysiology, 42*(2), 191–201.

Kotz, S. A., Ravignani, A., & Fitch, W. T. (2008). The evolution of rhythm processing. *Trends in Cognitive Sciences, 22*(10), 896–910.

Large, E. W., Herrera, J. A., & Velasco, M. J. (2015). Neural networks for beat perception in musical rhythm. *Frontiers in Systems Neuroscience, 9,* 159.

Large, E. W., & Snyder, J. S. (2009). Pulse and meter as neural resonance. *Annals of the New York Academy of Sciences, 1169,* 46–57.

Lerdahl, F., & Jackendoff, R. (1983). *A generative theory of tonal music.* MIT Press.

Levitin, D. J., Grahn, J. A., & London, J. (2018). The psychology of music: Rhythm and movement. *Annual Review of Psychology, 69,* 51–75.

Lewis, P. A., & Miall, R. C. (2009). The precision of temporal judgement: Milliseconds, many minutes, and beyond. *Philosophical Transactions of the Royal Society of London B, 354*(1525), 1897–1905.

London, J. (2012). *Hearing in time: Psychological aspects of musical meter* (2nd ed.). Oxford University Press.

MacDougall, R. (1903). The structure of simple rhythm forms. *Psychological Review Supplement, 4*, 309–411.

Madison, G. (2001a). *Functional modelling of the human timing mechanism* [PhD thesis]. Uppsala University Library.

Madison, G. (2001b). Variability in isochronous tapping: Higher-order dependencies as a function of inter tap interval. *Journal of Experimental Psychology: Human Perception and Performance, 27*(2), 411–422.

Madison, G. (2004a). Detection of linear temporal drift in sound sequences: Principles and empirical evaluation. *Acta Psychologica, 117*(1), 95–118.

Madison, G. (2004b). Fractal modeling of human isochronous serial interval production. *Biological Cybernetics, 90*(2), 105–112.

Madison, G. (2006). Duration specificity in the long-range correlation of human serial interval production. *Physica D (Nonlinear phenomena), 216*(2), 301–306.

Madison, G. (2009). An auditory illusion of infinite tempo change based on multiple temporal levels. *PLoS One, 4*(12), e8151.

Madison, G. (2014). Sensori-motor synchronisation variability decreases with the number of metrical levels in the stimulus signal. *Acta Psychologica, 147*, 10–16.

Madison, G., & Delignières, D. (2009). Auditory feedback affects the long-range correlation of isochronous serial interval production. Support for a closed-loop or memory model of timing. *Experimental Brain Research, 193*(4), 519–527.

Madison, G., Karampela, O., Ullén, F., & Holm, L. (2013). Effects of practice on variability in an isochronous serial interval production task: Asymptotical levels of tapping variability after training are similar to those of musicians. *Acta Psychologica, 143*(1), 119–128.

Madison, G., & Merker, B. (2002). On the limits of anisynchrony in pulse attribution. *Psychological Research, 66*(3), 201–207.

Madison, G., & Merker, B. (2004). Human sensorimotor tracking of continuous subliminal deviations from isochrony. *Neuroscience Letters, 370*(1), 69–73.

Madison, G., & Merker, B. (2005). Timing of action during and after synchronization with linearly changing intervals. *Music Perception, 22*(3), 441–459.

Madison, G., Ullén, F., & Merker, B. (2017). Metrically structured time and entrainment. In M. Lesaffre, M. Leman, & P.-J. Maes (Eds.), *The Routledge companion to embodied music interaction* (pp. 22–30). Routledge.

Malapani, C., & Fairhurst, S. (2002). Scalar timing in animals and humans. *Learning and Motivation, 33*(1),156–176.

Mates, J. (1994). A model of synchronization of motor acts to a stimulus sequence: I. Timing and error corrections. *Biological Cybernetics, 70*(5),463–473.

Mates, J., Radil, T., Müller, U., & Pöppel, E. (1994). Temporal integration in sensorimotor synchronization. *Journal of Cognitive Neuroscience, 6*(4), 332–340.

McDougall, H. G., & Moore, S. T. (2005). Marching to the beat of the same drummer: The spontaneous tempo of human locomotion. *Journal of Applied Physiology, 99*(3), 1164–1173.

Merchant, H., Grahn, J. A., Trainor, L. J., Rohrmeier, M., & Fitch, W. T. (2015). Finding the beat: A neural perspective across humans and non-human primates. *Philosophical Transactions of the Royal Society of London. Series B, Biological Sciences, 370*(1664), 20140093.

Merker, B. (2000). Synchronous chorusing and human origins. In N. L. Wallin, B. Merker, & S. W. Brown (Eds.), *The origins of music* (pp. 315–327). MIT Press.

Merker, B. (2002). Music: The missing Humboldt system. *Musicae Scientiae, 6*(1), 3–21.

Merker, B. (2006). Layered constraints on the multiple creativities of music. In I. Deliège & G. Wiggins (Eds.), *Musical creativity: Multidisciplinary research in theory and practice* (pp. 25–41). Psychology Press.

Merker, B. (2014). Groove or swing as distributed rhythmic consonance: Introducing the groove matrix. *Frontiers in Human Neuroscience, 8*, 454.

Merker, B., Madison, G., & Eckerdal, P. (2009). On the role and origin of isochrony in human rhythmic entrainment. *Cortex, 45*(1), 4–17.

Merker, B., Morley, I., & Zuidema, W. (2015). Five fundamental constraints on theories of the origin of music. *Philosophical Transactions of the Royal Society of London. Series B, Biological Sciences, 370*(1664), 20140095.

Michon, J. A. (1967). *Timing in temporal tracking*. Van Gorcum.

Moelants, D. (2002). Preferred tempo reconsidered. In C. Stevens, D. Burnham, G. McPherson, E. Schubert, & J. Renwick (Eds.), *Proceedings of the 7th International Conference on Music Perception and Cognition* (pp. 580–583). Causal Productions.

Musha, T., Katsurai, K., & Teramachi, Y. (1985). Fluctuations of human tapping intervals. *IEEE Transactions on Biomedical Engineering, 32*(8), 578–582.

Nguyen, T., Gibbings, A., & Grahn, J. A. (2018). Rhythm and beat perception. In R. Bader (Ed.), *Springer Handbook of systematic musicology* (pp. 507–521). Springer.

Nozaradan, S., Peretz, I., Missal, M., & Mouraux, A. (2011). Tagging the neuronal entrainment to beat and meter. *Journal of Neuroscience, 31*(28), 10234–10240.

Nozaradan, S., Zarouali, Y., Peretz, I., & Mouraux, A. (2015). Capturing with EEG the neural entrainment and coupling underlying sensorimotor synchronization to the beat. *Cerebral Cortex, 25*(3), 736–747.

Patel, A. D., & Iversen, J. R. (2014). The evolutionary neuroscience of musical beat perception: The Action Simulation for Auditory Prediction (ASAP) hypothesis. *Frontiers in Systems Neuroscience, 8*, 57.

Paton, J. J., & Buonomano, D. V. (2018). The neural basis of timing: Distributed mechanisms for diverse functions. *Neuron, 98*(4), 687–705.

Potter, D. D., Fenwick, M., Abecasis, D., & Brochard, R. (2009). Perceiving rhythm where none exists: Event-related potential (ERP) correlates of subjective accenting. *Cortex, 45*(1), 103–109.

Pressing, J., & Jolley-Rogers, G. (1997). Spectral properties of human cognition and skill. *Biological Cybernetics, 76*(5), 339–347.

Ravignani, A., Bowling, D. L., & Fitch, W. T. (2014). Chorusing, synchrony, and the evolutionary functions of rhythm. *Frontiers in Psychology, 5*, 1118.

Ravignani, A., & Madison, G. (2017). The paradox of isochrony in the evolution of human rhythm. *Frontiers in Psychology, 8*, 1820.

Repp, B. H. (2002a). Automaticity and voluntary control of phase correction following event onset shifts in sensorimotor synchronization. *Journal of Experimental Psychology: Human Perception and Performance, 28*(2), 410–430.

Repp, B. H. (2002b). Phase correction in sensorimotor synchronization: Nonlinearities in voluntary and involuntary responses to perturbations. *Human Movement Science, 21*(1), 1–37.

Repp, B. H. (2005). Sensorimotor synchronization: A review of the tapping literature. *Psychonomic Bulletin and Review, 12*(6), 969–992.

Repp, B. H. (2008). Multiple temporal references in sensorimotor synchronization with metrical auditory sequences. *Psychological Research, 72*(1), 79–98.

Repp, B. H. (2010). Self-generated interval subdivision reduces variability of synchronization with a very slow metronome. *Music Perception, 27*(5), 389–397.

Repp, B. H., Iversen, J. R., & Patel, A. D. (2008). Tracking an imposed beat within a metrical grid. *Music Perception, 26*(1), 1–18.

Repp, B. H., London, J., & Keller, P. E. (2011). Perception–production relationships and phase correction in synchronization with two-interval rhythms. *Psychological Research, 75*(3), 227–242.

Repp, B. H., & Su, Y.-H. (2013). Sensorimotor synchronization: A review of recent research (2006–2012). *Psychonomic Bulletin and Review, 20*(3), 403–452.

Risset, J.-C. (1986). Pitch and rhythm paradoxes: Comments on 'Auditory paradox based on fractal waveform'. *Journal of the Acoustical Society of America, 80*(3), 961–962.

Schmidt, R. C., Beek, P. J., Treffner, P. J., & Turvey, M. T. (1991). Dynamical substructure of coordinated rhythmic movements. *Journal of Experimental Psychology: Human Perception and Performance, 17*(3), 635–651.

Schmidt, R. C., Shaw, B. K., & Turvey, M. T. (1993). Coupling dynamics in interlimb coordination. *Journal of Experimental Psychology: Human Perception and Performance, 19*(2), 397–415.

Schulze, H. H. (1992). The error correction model for the tracking of a random metronome: Statistical properties and an empirical test. In F. Macar, V. Pouthas, & W. J. Friedman (Eds.), *Time, action and cognition* (pp. 275–286). Kluwer.

Schulze, H. H., & Vorberg, D. (2002). Linear phase correction models for synchronization: Parameter identification and estimation of parameters. *Brain and Cognition, 48*(1), 80–97.

Semjen, A., Vorberg, D., & Schulze, H. H. (1998). Getting synchronized with the metronome: Comparisons between phase and period correction. *Psychological Research, 61*(1), 44–55.

Snyder, J. S., & Large, E. W. (2004). Tempo dependence of middle- and long-latency auditory responses: Power and phase modulation of the EEG at multiple time-scales. *Clinical Neurophysiology, 115*(8), 1885–1895.

Snyder, J. S., & Large, E. W. (2005). Gamma-band activity reflects the metric structure of rhythmic tone sequences. *Cognitive Brain Research, 24*(1), 117–126.

Staddon, J. E. R. (2005). Interval timing: Memory, not a clock. *Trends in Cognitive Sciences, 9*(7), 312–314.

Stevens, L. T. (1886). On the time-sense. *Mind, 11*(43), 393–404.

Tal, I., Large, E. W., Rabinovitch, E., Wei, Y., Schroeder, C. E., Pöppel, D., & Zion Golumbic, E. (2017). Neural entrainment to the beat: The 'missing-pulse' phenomenon. *Journal of Neuroscience, 37*(26), 6331–6341.

Todd, N. P. M., Cousins, R., & Lee, C. S. (2007). The contribution of anthropometric factors to individual differences in the perception of rhythm. *Empirical Musicology Review, 2*(1), 1–13.

Todd, N. P. M., Lee, C. S., & O'Boyle, D. J. (2002). A sensorimotor theory of temporal tracking and beat induction. *Psychological Research, 66*(1), 26–39.

Todd, N. P. M., O'Boyle, D. J., & Lee, C. S. (1999). A sensory-motor theory of rhythm, time perception and beat induction. *Journal of New Music Research, 28*(1), 5–29.

Torre, K., & Balasubramaniam, R. (2009). Two different processes for sensorimotor synchronization in continuous and discontinuous rhythmic movements. *Experimental Brain Research, 199*(2), 157–166.

Torre, K., & Delignières, D. (2008). Unraveling the finding of 1/f (beta) noise in self-paced and synchronized tapping: A unifying mechanistic model. *Biological Cybernetics, 99*(2), 159–170.

van der Steen, M. C. M., & Keller, P. E. (2013). The ADaptation and Anticipation Model (ADAM) of sensorimotor synchronization. *Frontiers in Human Neuroscience, 7*, 253.

Vorberg, D., & Schulze, H. H. (2002). Linear phase-correction in synchronization: Predictions, parameter estimation, and simulations. *Journal of Mathematical Psychology, 46*(1), 56–87.

Vuust, P., & Witek, M. A. G. (2014). Rhythmic complexity and predictive coding: A novel approach to modeling rhythm and meter perception in music. *Frontiers in Psychology, 5*, 1111.

Wallin, J. E. W. (1911). Experimental studies of rhythm and time: II. The preferred length of interval (tempo). *Psychological Review, 18*(3), 202–222.

Wearden, J. H. (1999). 'Beyond the fields we know . . .': Exploring and developing scalar timing theory. *Behavioural Processes, 45*(1–3), 3–21.

Willms, A., Kitanov, P., & Langford, W. (2017). Huygens' clocks revisited. *Royal Society Open Science, 4*(9), 170777.

Wilson, M., & Cook, P. F. (2016). Rhythmic entrainment: Why humans want to, fireflies can't help it, pet birds try, and sea lions have to be bribed. *Psychonomic Bulletin and Review, 23*(6), 1647–1659.

Wing, A. M., & Kristofferson, A. (1973). Response delays and the timing of discrete motor responses. *Perception & Psychophysics, 14*(1), 5–12.

Winkler, I., Háden, G., Ladinig, O., Sziller, I., & Honing, H. (2009). Newborn infants detect the beat in music. *Proceedings of the National Academy of Sciences of the United States of America, 106*(7), 2468–2471.

Woodrow, H. (1932). The effects of rate of sequence upon the accuracy of synchronization. *Journal of Experimental Psychology, 15*(4), 357–379.

Yang, J., Ouyang, F., Holm, L., Huang, X., Gan, L., Zhou, L. et al. (2020). Tapping ahead of time: Its association with timing variability. *Psychological Research, 84*(2), 343–351.

13

Joint Shaping of Musical Time

How Togetherness Emerges in Music Ensemble Performance

Werner Goebl and Laura Bishop

13.1 Introduction

Performing music from a notated score, as is standard in some Western music traditions, requires that a musician first develops an individual understanding of the music and then realizes this 'interpretation' through corporeal performance. Performing ensemble music requires that ensemble members adapt their individual understanding to that of the group during rehearsal and performance in order to achieve a cohesive group performance. Both planned and emergent coordination are needed for an ensemble to achieve a shared creative goal (Knoblich et al., 2011). Their interpretations may diverge, due to their personal understanding of the music, but they must also overlap, such that their contributions are complementary (Canonne & Aucouturier, 2016).

During ensemble performance, several online processes operate simultaneously, allowing musicians to maintain synchrony at different timing levels. At the micro timing level of individual performed notes, synchrony occurs within a few tens of milliseconds, while expressive cohesion arises at larger timing levels of phrases and hyper-phrases controlled and mediated through body movements. At the lowest, and largely automatic, cognitive level, error correction processes compensate for asynchronies that may arise at each point in time due to differences in musical interpretation or motor variability (Repp, 2005; Repp & Su, 2013). At higher cognitive levels, more open to deliberate reflection and control, performers constantly adapt their internal notion of the musical tempo to that of their partners (period correction, see below), and they are able to communicate with their ensemble partners and readily diverge from a stable performance idea to settle almost instantly at a new one.

Communication among performers is fundamentally multi modal. The auditory modality as the main carrier of musical information has the highest temporal resolution and allows for precise synchronization of auditory events, while visual communication may serve many different important roles (Bishop & Goebl, 2015): a conductor signalling with body gestures to the orchestra members (Wöllner et al., 2012), ensemble members executing cueing or breathing gestures to coordinate the

Werner Goebl and Laura Bishop, *Joint Shaping of Musical Time* In: *Performing Time*. Edited by: Clemens Wöllner and Justin London, Oxford University Press. © Oxford University Press 2023. DOI: 10.1093/oso/9780192896254.003.0014 simultaneous beginning of a piece or section (Bishop & Goebl, 2018b), or the complex eye gaze patterns during a performance that reflect the rich real-time interaction characteristic of creative and inspired ensemble performance (Bishop et al., 2019a).

Ensembles vary in size and structure and sometimes depend on a leader to help regulate their performance. For large ensembles, like orchestras, a conductor decides how the music will be interpreted and provides visual cues to timing and expressive content during performances. Smaller ensembles may operate more democratically, but leader/follower relationships still often arise, resulting in small signed asynchronies in note onset times and correlations in periodic body motion (Chang et al., 2017; Goebl & Palmer, 2009). Leader/follower relationships sometimes emerge naturally in response to specific musical structures (e.g. melody and harmony parts), and may also facilitate coordination when musical timing is uncertain, for example, at the beginning of a piece.

Playing music with others can be aesthetically and socially rewarding. Feelings of 'musical togetherness' arise as musicians engage in the process of synchronizing their body motion, creating a rhythm together, and collectively setting and achieving artistic goals. The effects of body synchronization on social bonding have been well documented (Hove & Risen, 2009; Tarr et al., 2014). Indeed, the effects of group music making on social cohesion may have promoted the evolution of musicality in early humans (Savage et al., 2020). Recent research has begun to investigate how shared perceptions of artistic success and absorption may further strengthen interpersonal relationships and performance quality (Gaggioli et al., 2017; Himberg et al., 2018; Lee et al., 2020; Noy et al., 2015).

In the following sections, we will discuss, first, the cognitive mechanisms involved in coordinating ensemble performance, and second, how communication and interaction at the level of expressive body motion arise, helping ensembles create a unified presentation. Next, we describe the process of rehearsal and how ensembles go about establishing a performance script over time that will allow for flexibility in later performances. Finally, we discuss how creative collaboration unfolds in real-time during ensemble playing, supported by exchanges in leader/follower roles.

13.2 Real-Time Synchronization Mechanisms: Anticipation, Adaptation, and Attention

Maintaining tight synchronization despite large intentional tempo fluctuations requires the ensemble members to anticipate their co-performers' future actions and, at the same time, to flexibly adapt their own actions to those of the others (Keller et al., 2014). Adaptation processes have been studied extensively in sensorimotor synchronization research involving individual humans tapping to a metronome emitting completely regular or experimentally manipulated pulse sequences (Repp,

2005; Repp & Su, 2013). Musical experts are able to successfully synchronize from rates as slow as a tap every 2 s up to rates as fast as about 8 taps per second (corresponding to a 125-ms intertap interval, Repp, 2005). To maintain synchronization, timing differences between the stimulus and one's own actions are compensated through error correction processes involving adjusting for the time differences of the last event ('phase correction') and updating one's own notion of the musical tempo over time ('period correction', see Repp, 2005). The former process is largely unconscious (Repp, 2002) and operates automatically when timing information is transmitted through the auditory modality despite conflicting instructions (Goebl & Palmer, 2009). The latter, by contrast, is under deliberate control of the performers and contributes to the flexibility in timekeeping found in ensemble performance. When two or more musicians synchronize simultaneously, as in music ensemble performance, these processes operate simultaneously (Keller, 2008).

The extent to which these adaptation processes function jointly may depend on the individual ability to adapt, the cooperativity of the partner, or the rhythmic complexity of the stimulus (Repp et al., 2012). For example, when humans synchronized with uncooperative (compared to cooperative) virtual tapping partners, higher levels of phase and period correction were found (Keller, 2008) corresponding to higher levels of cognitive load (Fairhurst et al., 2013). By quantifying a 'correction gain', the extent one ensemble member adapts to the others, Wing et al. (2014) contrasted group adaptation behaviour in two professional string quartets: while in one quartet the ensemble members were adjusting more to the principal violin, the other quartet showed more equal gains across all four members (Wing et al., 2014).

As these error correction processes correspond to a human's capacity to track and maintain synchrony with the other musicians, the ability to anticipate the timing of the others is an integral aspect in ensemble music performance. The familiarity with the others' expressive intentions modulates the ability to predict upcoming events and, thus, the synchronization success of the joint performance. In a four-hand piano performance paradigm, for example, pianists synchronized better with recordings that they had played themselves earlier than with those by others, suggesting that differences in playing style and understanding of the piece affected the quality of the joint performance (Keller et al., 2007). Expert pianists were more successful in synchronizing with novice pianists when they were familiar with their idiosyncratic timing (Wolf et al., 2018), suggesting that previous knowledge of the others' understanding of the music substantially facilitates anticipation processes (van der Steen et al., 2015).

Alongside adaptation and anticipation, careful regulation of attention is needed to achieve and maintain coordination with ensemble partners. Musicians must attend to their own playing, to the collective output of the ensemble, and to the relationships between parts. 'Prioritized integrative attending' describes a particular form of divided attention in which a musician prioritizes attention towards their own playing while assigning a lower priority to others' playing (Keller, 2008). This process is cognitively demanding and effortful, so is not sustainable throughout an entire performance. Instead, it might be used in select circumstances to achieve expressive goals. Performers otherwise use a combination of selective attention, where they focus on a specific part or voice, and non-prioritized integrative attention, where they focus on the collective output as a whole. Performers' mode of attention can change from moment to moment, depending on the demands of the music.

13.3 Visual Communication

Beyond the auditory modality, the range of information potentially communicated within the visual domain is vast, ranging from the rich expressive loading of performers' body movements to explicit gestures to signal timing information such as conducting gestures or cueing-in gestures, from subtle gestures like raising an eye brow to overt eye-gazing behaviour among ensemble members.

Musicians' physical actions embody their cognitive states and mental representations of the music during their performance (Leman & Maes, 2014; see Maes & Leman, this volume) and are loaded with communicative information for audiences and fellow musicians alike. Actions are cognitively coded in terms of their action goals; in the case of music performance this means that actions are represented by the specific sound they will produce (perceptual– motor coupling; see, e.g. Prinz & Hommel, 2002; Schütz-Bosbach & Prinz, 2007). Action–perception associations become stronger with training and run in both directions: observing a specific sound-producing action will activate the pertinent sound expectation, whereas hearing a specific sound will activate the required action, more so for motor experts such as professional musicians (Bishop & Goebl, 2018c).

Human movements during music performance may serve different functions: they are immediately necessary to produce the intended sounds on a musical instrument, but they also may facilitate coordination in ensemble performance, balance the performer's own experience in music making, and communicate emotional states to the audience or ensemble members (Dahl et al., 2010). Musicians' visual expressivity during performance is sometimes even more important than the sounding information. In a successful replication of a classical experiment (Behne & Wöllner, 2011), musicians rated the expressive content of video recordings differently when seeing different visual performances matched with the same audio. Similar results were found testing the emotional impact of performances with different expressive intentions, the visual and sounding information of which was systematically recombined; taken together, these findings confirm the strong influence of visual information (Vuoskoski et al., 2016). One singular study even revealed that visual information of expert performances, alone, is more conducive to predicting the winners of international competitions than combined audio visual or sounding information alone (Tsay, 2013).

To coordinate their performances, musicians are generally very effective in performing together through only the auditory domain without exchanging much visual information. However, in situations with reduced auditory reliability, musicians use visual cues to maintain high levels of synchrony (Bishop & Goebl, 2015; Kawase, 2014), such as when members of a string section in an orchestra observe their principal players' bowing gestures. Visual information is deliberately used in situations of uncertainty, such as at piece beginnings or after long pauses, at sudden tempo changes, or when the tempo is free and unspecified (Bishop & Goebl, 2018a, see also Figure 13.1, top panel). The cueing gestures that are used in these situations have been found to display characteristic kinematic patterns involving a steep acceleration peak that usually occurs one beat ahead of the mutual starting note (Bishop & Goebl, 2018a). They are often related to breathing-in gestures and may contain information about the upcoming tempo (Coorevits & Moelants, 2015).

Musicians viewing professional cueing-in gestures could synchronize better with them when their kinematics were low in jerk and featured large movement amplitudes (Bishop & Goebl, 2018b). This coincides with evidence from conducting studies where smoothness and prototypicality in the conducting gestures facilitated synchronization through the visual domain (Wöllner et al., 2012). In the broader joint action literature, people also commonly modify their body motion when performing joint tasks so that their motion is more predictable (Vesper et al., 2016).

Also, eye gaze behaviour is an important vehicle for communication among performing musicians. Musicians watch each other more at moments of uncertainty in a musical piece (see the introduction section, blue, and free section, purple, in Figure 13.1, bottom panel). However, against the expectation that musicians would look at each other more when they are unfamiliar with other performer's intentions, gaze frequency was found to increase over ensemble rehearsal (Bishop et al., 2019a), suggesting that watching each other is something musicians do when they have established a common understanding of a piece and concentrate on bringing the timing synchronization to perfection, as this belongs to the main challenges of ensemble synchronization.

Eye gaze, directed at another person, is a strong social cue that commonly communicates an intention to interact (Khalid et al., 2016). Gaze more broadly reflects a person's focus of attention, with changes in gaze direction subject to both top-down and bottom-up influences (Frischen et al., 2007). In addition, gaze can be a means of securing joint attention to a particular stimulus (Bristow et al., 2007). Even infants are receptive to gaze cues and follow the gaze of others to focus on a shared object (Tomasello et al., 2007). During ensemble playing, gaze that is directed at a co-performer is not only a means of acquiring information, it is also a cue to the gazer's attention. A case study of a string quartet showed gaze patterns that were highly skewed, in line with the traditional leader/follower roles of a classical quartet: the first violinist was watched more than any other player, but almost never looked at their co-performers (Bishop et al., 2021). Such a finding suggests that the first violinist was frequently a focus of the other musicians' attention. Eye gaze between ensemble members may contribute to the feelings of togetherness that arise during

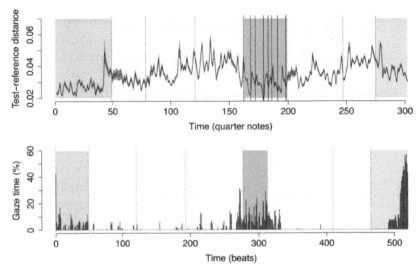

Figure 13.1 Dissimilarity to typical cueing gestures (lower values denote greater similarity to cueing gestures, top panel) and unidirectional partner-directed eye gaze time (bottom panel) over multiple performances of the same piece. Score time was either evaluated per quarter note (top panel) or per beat (bottom panel) which results in different time axes depending on the changing time signatures in the score. Vertical lines indicate section boundaries. The introduction section (blue) and middle section (purple) have to be performed freely; the final section (yellow) requires tight synchronization in a 2 + 3 + 3 metre. In the middle section of the top panel, vertical lines indicate the position of expected cueing gestures. IBI, interbeat interval. Figure adapted from Bishop et al., 2019a (top panel) and Bishop et al. 2019b (bottom panel).

creative music making by providing confirmation, both of musicians' attention as well as of their intention to interact.

Beyond communication goals of visual signalling, body motion among ensemble members is often similar. For example, body sway of ensemble members often appears to be synchronized during performance (Keller et al., 2010)—more so when auditory communication is reduced (Goebl & Palmer, 2009) but, then, only for cases in which visual contact among musicians remains possible (Colley et al., 2020). Performers' movement amplitude has also been shown to increase over rehearsal, and was larger when the musicians could see each other compared to when visual contact was prevented (Bishop et al., 2019b), suggesting that ensemble musicians are prompted to move in a more communicative and interactive way once they have a shared understanding of the music and are able to see each other. Interestingly, this kind of interactive body motion does not seem to affect the quality of an ensemble's synchronization outside of isolated moments where clear visual signals are needed (e.g. at piece entrances or following pauses; Bishop et al., 2019b).

Coordination of expressive body motion may partly arise as musicians respond similarly to the structure of the music, for which they share an interpretation, and may communicate which aspects of the music they are attending to or emphasizing (Chang et al., 2019). In this way, body motion, like gaze, may inform ensemble musicians about each other's attention. In addition to synchronization of body sway and coordinated changes in movement amplitude, interactive body motion can take other forms, like coordinated changes in posture or a collective reduction in the space between musicians. The latter effect has been observed among string quartets under conditions that are meant to disrupt normal ensemble dynamics (Glowinski et al., 2013), and may reflect musicians' heightened attention towards each other. Coordination in body motion might also be driven by our natural tendency to imitate aspects of each other's expressive behaviour during interactive tasks, which has been observed, for example, during conversation (Richardson et al., 2008).

By moving together, ensemble musicians may facilitate shared attention towards aspects of their collective interpretation. Coordinated motion may also strengthen the relationships between performers, thereby enhancing experiences of togetherness. Some recent research has shown that coordination in body motion increases audiences' perceptions of group strength and synchronization; it may therefore affect an ensemble's presentation of themselves as a unified entity (Jakubowski et al., 2020; Lee et al., 2020).

13.4 Establishing Artistic Goals Through Rehearsal

For ensembles in the Western classical tradition, different forms of musical collaboration occur in rehearsal as opposed to live concert or studio recording settings. During rehearsal, ensemble members work together to decide on artistic goals and establish a joint interpretation of the music (a 'performance script'), which they will loosely follow during subsequent performances. In contrast to concert or studio settings, rehearsals typically involve verbal discussion, demonstration of ideas through playing, deliberate practice of specific sections, and 'experimenting-while-playing', or trying out different expressive or interpretive ideas while playing through the piece (Ginsborg et al., 2006; Seddon & Biasutti, 2009).

Key decisions relating to interpretation are made during rehearsal, but players ideally maintain some flexibility around these agreed-upon points. This flexibility enables the ensemble to keep their performances fresh and engaging, gives them room to introduce new ideas, and prepares them to compensate for disruptions or errors during later performances (Glowinski et al., 2016). Flexibility in practised performance is a marker of high-level musicianship (Chaffin et al., 2007). Developing musicians, who have less musical knowledge and technical skill, may have to prepare more detailed performance scripts.

Longitudinal studies of rehearsal with high-level solo musicians have shown that musicians' focus on different technical or expressive aspects of a piece changes over the weeks, months, or years that they spend preparing for public performance. Long-term strategies for establishing a performance script vary from person to person. Some musicians practise technical aspects of the music before expressive and interpretive aspects (Chaffin & Logan, 2006) while others develop an expressive understanding of the music first, before addressing technical issues (Chaffin et al., 2010).

Both strategies involve segmenting the music based on structural features and identifying landmarks where attention should be directed towards specific musical features, be they structural, technical, interpretive, or expressive. Music is normally segmented hierarchically, with large-scale works dividing into movements, sections, subsections, phrases, bars, and, finally, individual notes. Landmarks may redirect attention on different timescales. For example, the start of a new section or subsection might signal a change in musical character, prompting attention towards certain expressive features for a period of some tens of seconds; alternatively, the start of a technically demanding bar might draw attention towards technique for a period of a couple of seconds.

During ensemble rehearsals, musicians also establish common landmarks where their attention should be directed towards group-level musical features (Williamon & Davidson, 2002). These may include instances where temporal coordination must be managed carefully, or instances where musicians attend to the same interpretive or expressive feature to achieve a coherent effect (King & Ginsburg, 2011). As discussed earlier in the section on real-time synchronization mechanisms, ensemble musicians distribute their attention between their own part and those of others, their focus may change from moment to moment depending on the demands of the performance (Keller, 2008). One goal of rehearsal is to identify points in a piece where attention should be managed in a certain way.

A case study of a singer–violist duo considered the annotations that the musicians made in their scores as indicative of attention landmarks (Ginsborg & Bennett, 2021). It was notable that the musicians differed in the types of annotations that they made. In particular, the violist often made annotations relating to coordination with the singer; the singer, by contrast, made very few annotations relating to coordination with the violist, and many annotations relating to when she needed to prepare for entries. The musicians also differed as to which hierarchical level of the music they tended to focus on, with the singer attending to subsections and the violist attending to complete sections. Overall, it seems that the way musicians prepare to distribute their attention during rehearsal depends both upon the physical demands of their instrument (e.g. the singer's need to prepare in time for entries) and upon individual roles in the ensemble.

In the previous section on visual communication, we discussed a study of rehearsal behaviour carried out in our laboratory with piano duos and clarinet duos (Bishop et al., 2019a). Performers' body motion and eye gaze were analysed to show how interaction between performers changed during a rehearsal session and varied in relation to musical structure. We found that instances of partner-directed gaze tended to occur consistently around certain points in the piece (Bishop et al., 2019a). For example, many performers looked at their partner just before piece onset, just before transitioning from a section with 7/8 metre to a section without a notated metre, and during the final few beats of the piece (Figure 13.1, bottom panel). These points correspond to the moments in the piece with high temporal ambiguity, for which timing must be more deliberately controlled, and coordination between partners demands increased cognitive effort. The pattern of partner-directed gaze became increasingly clear across the course of the rehearsal period, suggesting that the duos integrated these moments of partner-directed attention into their performance script.

Some studies have considered how the process of negotiating a shared interpretation unfolds in the earliest stages of joint rehearsal, when fluency and basic synchronization tend to be the primary goals. Often, when an ensemble plays a piece together for the first time, the performers have studied the music already and have individual preferences for how the music should be interpreted. Pianists who have practised both parts of a duet prior to their first joint rehearsal synchronize less precisely during their first performances than do pianists who have practised only their own part (Ragert et al., 2013). This is likely because the pianists who have practised both parts already have an individualized interpretation of a piece and introduce expressive variability into their playing that their duet partners cannot accurately predict. This effect of prior practise can, however, disappear quickly after a couple of runs through the piece, showing that those pianists quickly readjusted their expectations for how the music should sound.

A study of rehearsals carried out by a singing quintet showed that synchronization continued to improve across five rehearsal sessions for a complex polyphonic piece but improved only between the first and second rehearsal for a simpler homophonic piece (D'Amario et al., 2020). Thus, the rate at which an ensemble can achieve optimal levels of synchronization seems to depend on the complexity of the music.

A study of ours examined how advanced piano students adapt their expressive timing and dynamics when playing a duet together for the first time, following individual practice (Bishop & Goebl, 2020). We compared pianists' solo (recorded first) and duet (recorded second) performances of the same piece and found that duets were played with less temporal and dynamic variability than solo performances. This reduced variability suggests that the pianists played more predictably when coordinating their first duet performances together than when playing alone. Figure 13.2 shows tempo curves for solo and duet performances by some of the pianists in this study (those who played the primo part during the duets). 'Prototypical' solo and duet tempo curves, calculated by averaging across all performers, are also shown. The prototypical tempo curve for the duet condition was smoother than the prototypical tempo curve for the solo condition, indicating less variability. Prototypicality (i.e. similarity to the prototypical curve) was similar for solo and duet performances, increasing in relation to pianists' musical experience.

High prototypicality in the timing of advanced students' solo piano performances following a short rehearsal was similarly observed by Repp (1997), who found

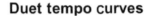

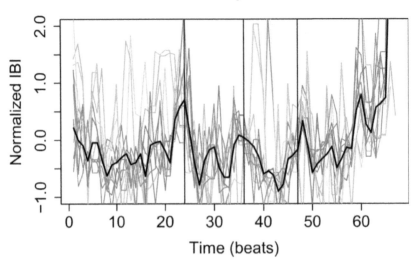

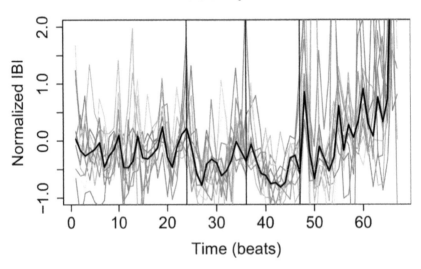

Figure 13.2 Individual (thin lines) and prototypical (thick lines) tempo curves for joint duet (top) and individual solo (bottom) performances of the *Minuet in C-sharp minor* by Maurice Ravel. Tempo curves represent the performances of the performers assigned the 'primo' role. Tempo curves are smoother in the duet performances than in the solo performances of the same piece. Figure adapted from Bishop and Goebl (2020).

timing in professional pianists' performances of the same piece to be more distinctive. These findings are notable because creativity and individuality are widely valued among musicians in the Western classical tradition (Clarke, 2012), and advanced students are generally already expected to perform with an individualized expressive style. The convergence towards prototypicality observed in these studies suggests that students require more time to study a new piece of music before they can play in an individualized way. Ensemble musicians also need time to exchange ideas in an offline context, as normally happens during ensemble rehearsals.

The conditions surrounding musicians' rehearsal and performance may also either encourage or discourage creativity in interpretation. Creativity is defined partially in terms of how original an interpretation is relative to others' performances of the same piece, and partially in terms of how stylistically appropriate the interpretation is. Highly creative performances are not necessarily more variable in features like timing than less creative performances are, but they may use microtiming or tempo changes in a more individualized manner. In some cases, the way that a performance task is framed and the instructions that musicians are given may prompt them to adopt a cautious playing style that minimizes errors instead of a playing style that prioritizes expressivity and creative risk-taking.

In the broader psychological literature on creativity, the effects of regulatory focus on creative processing have been discussed. A promotion-oriented focus is associated with striving towards an 'ideal' self and behaviours that aim to promote positive outcomes, while a prevention-oriented focus is associated with striving towards an 'ought' self and behaviours that aim to prevent negative outcomes (Lam & Chiu, 2002). In studies of individual creativity, additive effects of regulatory focus and cooperative versus competitive goals on creativity have also been observed (Bittner et al., 2016). Cooperative goals combined with a promotion-oriented focus lead to more creative performance than competitive goals combined with a prevention-oriented focus.

Music ensemble playing is, inherently, both cooperative and competitive, so performers' immediate goals and regulatory focus may vary from one situation to another. Because development of an individualized interpretation usually requires some time and study, performers' goals and changes in focus may have variable effects at different points throughout the process.

13.5 Emergent Creative Behaviour

Coordination and creativity are closely linked in the domain of ensemble playing. The relationship is perhaps most obvious in the case of improvising ensembles, who must generate new musical material that is collectively meaningful (Aucouturier & Canonne, 2017; Canonne & Aucouturier, 2016; Schober & Spiro, 2016). Coordination is needed at different musical levels during ensemble improvisation: in the timing of individual utterances, such as phrases lasting several seconds; the development of harmonies; the creation of larger-scale musical structures, such as groups of phrases lasting several minutes; and expressive nuances.

For classical ensembles, the relationship between coordination and creativity is less obvious because creativity centres exclusively on interpretation and unfolds within a different set of constraints. Still, even if the relationship is less obvious for classical ensembles than for improvising ensembles, it is no less important. Professional musicians' careers depend on their ability to distinguish themselves from their contemporaries through creative interpretation of a relatively limited repertoire.

In the previous section on rehearsal, we discussed how ensembles collaboratively interpret music during rehearsal using a combination of offline and online techniques. In this section, we will consider how the creative process of real-time interpretation unfolds as an ensemble plays together.

Real-time interpretation, like coordination, is an emergent process that cannot be attributed to the actions of any one contributor. Rather, it results from interactions between components of the dynamic system that comprises a music ensemble: the performers, their instruments, the physical performance space, the social environment, and other social-cognitive factors contributing to the performance ecology (e.g. the musicians' goals and the significance of the performance; van der Schyff et al., 2018).

Real-time interpretation involves a process of listening-while-playing that occurs in parallel for members of an ensemble (Linson & Clarke, 2017). This process requires players to listen to the ensemble's collective musical output while simultaneously responding to it. Throughout a performance, each unfolding musical utterance affords the players a range of responses (Gibson, 1979; Knoblich et al., 2011; Windsor & de Bézenac, 2012). The breadth of this range of affordances depends on many factors, including how familiar the players are with the musical style, how well the players' technical abilities match the demands of the music, and how the players have distributed their attention across the different components of the musical structure. Interaction between other components of the ensemble system (e.g. room acoustics, audience expectations, etc.) may help to shape the affordances that arise during performance, as well. A notable feature of ensemble performance is its emergent set of affordances that would not have been available to individual performers, because the ensemble can collectively produce music that individuals cannot.

A particular musical utterance may afford congruent responses from collaborating players, facilitating coordination, or it may afford incongruent responses, disrupting coordination. If coordination is disrupted, the ensemble may be able to recover, provided the players can adapt to each other and align more predictably. In some cases, depending on the music, performance may even benefit from some divergence in response between players (Schiavio & Høffding, 2015).

Leader/follower relationships often emerge during classical ensemble playing and can facilitate coordination during real-time interpretation, reducing the risk of divergent interpretations. Leader/follower roles may change throughout a performance as the musical structure changes. In cases where ensemble performers expect to receive information from a leader and fail to receive that information, their performance approach may change as they try to compensate by increasing regulation of their own playing. In a recent study, violinists performed in a normal condition where the group was led by a conductor that everyone could see, and in a perturbed condition where half the violinists turned away from the conductor and instead faced the other half of the group (Laroche et al., 2021; see Laroche et al., this volume). In the perturbed condition, coupling between violinists' head and bow motion increased, suggesting that head motion might have been used to help regulate the timing of bowing motion.

Some empirical studies have investigated how ensembles respond to unexpected changes or conflicts in interpretation. A common method has been to prompt individual players to introduce unexpected or contrasting expressive nuances. In a study by Glowinski et al. (2013), body motion among members of a string quartet was more interactive during 'perturbed' performances (in which the first violinist introduced unexpected expressive features) than it was during control performances without perturbations. The influence that the first violinist had on the others' body motion also decreased during the perturbed performances. The increase in interactivity suggests that ensemble musicians communicate more through their bodies when they are uncertain about how their performance will unfold. The first violinist's reduced influence over the others might reflect a more restricted playing style while their attention was directed towards performing perturbations.

In another study, piano duos were given conflicting tempo or dynamics instructions when performing a piece together (MacRitchie et al., 2018). Pianists prioritized their own playing during the conditions with incongruent dynamics instructions, but prioritized the joint coordination task in the conditions with incongruent tempo instructions. This tendency to adapt to each other's unexpected tempo changes likely reflects the automatic and difficult-to-override nature of error correction that occurs during synchronization tasks, as well as the centrality of temporal coordination to classical music performance.

13.6 Conclusion

The cognitive-motor processes and interpersonal skills required for an ensemble to jointly shape musical time are complex and manifold. Music ensemble performance usually involves comprehensive preparatory planning in rehearsal as well as real-time communication and interaction during performance. Body motion, eye gaze behaviour, and acoustic performance parameters are important measures that allow detailed experimental insight in this highly skilled—often professionalized—domain of ensemble music performance.

Under optimal performance conditions, music ensembles may enter a stage of group flow, when ensemble members are completely absorbed in the music, forget about time and their performances, play seemingly effortlessly, and ultimately experience a feeling of intense togetherness (Cochrane, 2017). This togetherness may be experienced by performers and audiences alike, and describes the feeling of a shared cognitive-emotional state (D'Amario et al., 2021). The behavioural and cognitive correlates of this experience are still being investigated, but they may include balanced levels of empathy (Gaggioli et al., 2017) and optimally matched skill levels among group members.

Joint music making seems to have played an important role at different stages of human evolution (Merker, 2000; Savage et al., 2020) because it promotes social bonding and affiliation among members of the synchronizing group (Hove & Risen, 2009). This evolutionary view on the experience of togetherness may (in part) explain why we humans do not shy away from effort and cost to make music together or attend events in order to experience collective togetherness in music.

References

Aucouturier, J.-J., & Canonne, C. (2017). Musical friends and foes: The social cognition of affiliation and control in improvised interactions. *Cognition*, *161*, 94–108. http://doi.org/10.1016/j.cognition.2017.01.019

Behne, K.-E., & Wöllner, C. (2011). Seeing or hearing the pianists? A synopsis of an early audiovisual perception experiment and a replication. *Musicae Scientiae*, *15*(3), 324–342. http://doi.org/10.1177/1029864911410955

Bishop, L., Cancino-Chacón, C. E., & Goebl, W. (2019a). Eye gaze as a means of giving and seeking information during musical interaction. *Consciousness and Cognition*, *68*(1), 73–96. http://doi.org/10.1016/j.concog.2019.01.002

Bishop, L., Cancino-Chacón, C. E., & Goebl, W. (2019b). Moving to communicate, moving to interact: Patterns of body motion in musical duo performance. *Music Perception*, *37*(1), 1–25. http://doi.org/10.1525/mp.2019.37.1.1

Bishop, L., & Goebl, W. (2015). When they listen and when they watch: Pianists' use of nonverbal audio and visual cues during duet performance. *Musicae Scientiae*, *19*(1), 84–110. http://doi.org/10.1177/1029864915570355

Bishop, L., & Goebl, W. (2018a). Beating time: How ensemble musicians' cueing gestures communicate beat position and tempo. *Psychology of Music*, *46*(1), 84–106. http://doi.org/10.1177/0305735617702971

Bishop, L., & Goebl, W. (2018b). Communication for coordination: Gesture kinematics and conventionality affect synchronization success in piano duos. *Psychological Research*, *82*(6), 1177–1194. http://doi.org/10.1007/s00426-017-0893-3

Bishop, L., & Goebl, W. (2018c). Performers and an active audience: Movement in music production and perception. *Jahrbuch Musikpsychologie*, *28*, e19. http://doi.org/10.5964/jbdgm.2018v28.19

Bishop, L., & Goebl, W. (2020). Negotiating a shared interpretation during piano duo performance. *Music & Science*, *3*, 2059204319896152. http://doi.org/10.1177/2059204319896152

Bishop, L., Gonzalez Sanchez, V., Laeng, B., Jensenius, A. R., & Høffding, S. (2021). Move like everyone is watching: Social context affects head motion and gaze in string quartet performance. *Journal of New Music Research*, *50*(4), 392–412. https://doi.org/10.1080/09298215.2021.1977338

Bittner, J. V., Bruena, M., & Rietzschel, E. F. (2016). Cooperation goals, regulatory focus, and their combined effects on creativity. *Thinking Skills and Creativity*, *19*, 260–268. http://doi.org/10.1016/j.tsc.2015.12.002

Bristow, D., Rees, G., & Frith, C. D. (2007). Social interaction modifies neural response to gaze shifts. *Social Cognitive and Affective Neuroscience*, *2*(1), 52–61. http://doi.org/10.1093/scan/nsl036

Canonne, C., & Aucouturier, J.-J. (2016). Play together, think alike: Shared mental models in expert music improvisers. *Psychology of Music*, *44*(3), 544–558. http://doi.org/10.1177/0305735615577406

Chaffin, R., Lemieux, A. F., & Chen, C. (2007). 'It is different each time I play': Variability in highly prepared musical performance. *Music Perception*, *24*(5), 455–472. http://doi.org/10.1525/mp.2007.24.5.455

Chaffin, R., Lisboa, T., Logan, T., & Begosh, K. T. (2010). Preparing for memorized cello performance: The role of performance cues. *Psychology of Music*, *38*(1), 3–30. http://doi.org/10.1177/0305735608100377

Chaffin, R., & Logan, T. (2006). Practicing perfection: How concert soloists prepare for performance. *Advances in Cognitive Psychology*, 2(2), 113–130. http://doi.org/10.2478/v10053-008-0050-z

Chang, A., Kragness, H. E., Livingstone, S. R., Bosnyak, D. J., & Trainor, L. J. (2019). Body sway reflects joint emotional expression in music ensemble performance. *Scientific Reports*, 9(1), 205. http://doi.org/10.1038/s41598-018-36358-4

Chang, A., Livingstone, S. R., Bosnyak, D. J., & Trainor, L. J. (2017). Body sway reflects leadership in joint music performance. *Proceedings of the National Academy of Sciences of the United States of America*, 114(21), E4134–E4141. http://doi.org/10.1073/pnas.1617657114

Clarke, E. F. (2012). Creativity in performance. In D. J. Hargreaves, D. Miell, & R. MacDonald (Eds.), *Musical imaginations: Multidisciplinary perspectives on creativity, performance, and perception* (pp. 17–30). Oxford University Press.

Cochrane, T. (2017). Group flow. In M. Lesaffre, P.-J. Maes, & M. Leman (Eds.), *The Routledge companion to embodied music interaction* (pp. 133–140). Taylor & Francis. http://doi.org/10.4324/9781315621364

Colley, I. D., Varlet, M., & Keller, P. E. (2020). The influence of a conductor and co-performer on auditory-motor synchronisation, temporal prediction, and ancillary entrainment in a musical drumming task. *Human Movement Science*, 72, 102653. http://doi.org/10.1016/j.humov.2020.102653

Coorevits, E., & Moelants, D. (2015). Synchronization in ensemble performance: The sniff as a temporal cue. *Proceedings of the 8th International Conference of Students of Systematic Musicology (SysMus 2015)* [Paper presentation] (p. 44). University of Leipzig.

Dahl, S., Bevilacqua, F., Bresin, R., Clayton, M., Leante, L., Poggi, I., & Rasamimanana, N. (2010). Gestures in performance. In R. I. Godøy & M. Leman (Eds.), *Musical gestures: Sound, movement, and meaning* (pp. 36–68). Routledge.

D'Amario, S., Bishop, L., Goebl, W., & Niemand, A. (2021). *Judging togetherness in point-light displays of professional duo performances.* [Presentation]. 16th International Conference on Music Perception and Cognition, Sheffield, UK.

D'Amario, S., Daffern, H., and Bailes, F. (2020). A longitudinal study investigating synchronization in a singing quartet. *Journal of Voice*, 34(1), 159.e1-159.e12.

Fairhurst, M. T., Janata, P., & Keller, P. E. (2013). Being and feeling in sync with an adaptive virtual partner: Brain mechanisms underlying dynamic cooperativity. *Cerebral Cortex*, 23(11), 2592–2600. http://doi.org/10.1093/cercor/bhs243

Frischen, A., Bayliss, A. P., & Tipper, S. P. (2007). Gaze cueing of attention: Visual attention, social cognition, and individual differences. *Psychological Bulletin*, 133(4), 694–724. http://doi.org/10.1037/0033-2909.133.4.694

Gaggioli, A., Chirico, A., Mazzoni, E., Milani, L., & Riva, G. (2017). Networked flow in musical bands. *Psychology of Music*, 45(2), 283–297. http://doi.org/10.1177/0305735616665003

Gibson, J. J. (1979). *The ecological approach to visual perception*. Houghton Mifflin.

Ginsborg, J., & Bennett, D. (2021). Developing familiarity in a new duo: Rehearsal talk and performance cues. *Frontiers in Psychology*, 12, 222. http://doi.org/10.3389/fpsyg.2021.590987

Ginsborg, J., Chaffin, R., & Nicholson, G. (2006). Shared performance cues in singing and conducting: A content analysis of talk during practice. *Psychology of Music*, 34(2), 167–194. http://doi.org/10.1177/0305735606061851

Glowinski, D., Bracco, F., Chiorri, C., & Grandjean, D. (2016). Music ensemble as a resilient system. Managing the unexpected through group interaction. *Frontiers in Psychology*, 7, 1548. http://doi.org/10.3389/fpsyg.2016.01548

Glowinski, D., Gnecco, G., Piana, S., & Camurri, A. (2013). Expressive non-verbal interaction in string quartet. In *Proceedings of the Humaine Association Conference on Affective Computing and Intelligent Interaction (ACII 2013)* (pp. 233–238). IEEE. http://doi.org/10.1109/ACII.2013.45

Goebl, W., & Palmer, C. (2009). Synchronization of timing and motion among performing musicians. *Music Perception*, 26(5), 427–438. http://doi.org/10.1525/mp.2009.26.5.427

Himberg, T., Laroche, J., Bigé, R., Buchkowski, M., & Bachrach, A. (2018). Coordinated interpersonal behaviour in collective dance improvisation: The aesthetics of kinaesthetic togetherness. *Behavioral Sciences*, 8(2), 23. http://doi.org/10.3390/bs8020023

Hove, M. J., & Risen, J. L. (2009). It's all in the timing: Interpersonal synchrony increases affiliation. *Social Cognition, 27*(6), 949–961. http://doi.org/10.1521/soco.2009.27.6.949

Jakubowski, K., Eerola, T., Blackwood Ximenes, A., Ma, W. K., Clayton, M., & Keller, P. E. (2020). Multimodal perception of interpersonal synchrony: Evidence from global and continuous ratings of improvised musical duo performances. *Psychomusicology: Music, Mind, and Brain, 30*(4), 159–177. http://doi.org/10.1037/pmu0000264

Kawase, S. (2014). Gazing behavior and coordination during piano duo performance. *Attention, Perception and Psychophysics, 76*(2), 527–540. http://doi.org/10.3758/s13414-013-0568-0

Keller, P. E. (2008). Joint action in music performance. In F. Morganti, A. Carassa, & G. Riva (Eds.), *Enacting intersubjectivity: A cognitive and social perspective to the study of interactions* (pp. 205–221). IOS Press.

Keller, P. E., Dalla Bella, S., & Koch, I. (2010). Auditory imagery shapes movement timing and kinematics: Evidence from a musical task. *Journal of Experimental Psychology: Human Perception and Performance, 36*(2), 508–513. http://doi.org/10.1037/a0017604

Keller, P. E., Knoblich, G., & Repp, B. H. (2007). Pianists duet better when they play with themselves: On the possible role of action simulation in synchronization. *Consciousness and Cognition, 16*(1), 102–111. http://doi.org/10.1016/j.concog.2005.12.004

Keller, P. E., Novembre, G., & Hove, M. J. (2014). Rhythm in joint action: Psychological and neurophysiological mechanisms for real-time interpersonal coordination. *Philosophical Transactions of the Royal Society of London. Series B, Biological Sciences, 369*(1658), 20130394. http://doi.org/10.1098/rstb.2013.0394

Khalid, S., Deska, J. C., & Hugenberg, K. (2016). The eyes are the windows to the mind: Direct eye gaze triggers the ascription of others' minds. *Personality and Social Psychology Bulletin, 42*(12), 1666–1677. http://doi.org/10.1177/0146167216669124

King, E., & Ginsburg, J. (2011). Gestures and glances: Interactions in ensemble rehearsal. In A. Gritten and E. King (Eds.), *New perspectives on music and gesture* (pp. 177–201). Ashgate.

Knoblich, G., Butterfill, S., & Sebanz, N. (2011). Psychological research on joint action: Theory and data. In B. Ross (Ed.), *The psychology of learning and motivation* (Vol. 54, pp. 59–101). Academic Press/Elsevier.

Lam, T. W. H., & Chiu, C. Y. (2002). The motivational function of regulatory focus in creativity. *Journal of Creative Behavior, 36*(2), 138–150. http://doi.org/10.1002/j.2162-6057.2002.tb01061.x

Laroche, J., Tomassini, A., Fadiga, L., Camurri, A., Volpe, G., & d'Ausilio, A. (2021). *Intrapersonal coupling within the orchestra and the 'head department' of rhythm*. [Presentation]. In 16th International Conference on Music Perception and Cognition, Sheffield, UK.

Lee, H., Launay, J., & Stewart, L. (2020). Signals through music and dance: Perceived social bonds and formidability on collective movement. *Acta Psychologica, 208*, 103093. http://doi.org/10.1016/j.actpsy.2020.103093

Leman, M., & Maes, P.-J. (2014). The role of embodiment in the perception of music. *Empirical Musicology Review, 9*(3), 236–246. http://doi.org/10.18061/emr.v9i3-4.4498

Linson, A., & Clarke, E. F. (2017). Distributed cognition, ecological theory and group improvisation. In E. F. Clarke & M. Doffman (Eds.), *Distributed creativity: Collaboration and improvisation in contemporary music* (pp. 52–69). Oxford University Press.

MacRitchie, J., Herff, S. A., Procopio, A., & Keller, P. E. (2018). Negotiating between individual and joint goals in ensemble musical performance. *Quarterly Journal of Experimental Psychology, 71*(7), 1535–1551. http://doi.org/10.1080/17470218.2017.1339098

Merker, B. (2000). Synchronous chorusing and human origins. In N. L. Wallin, B. Merker, & S. Brown (Eds.), *The origins of music* (pp. 315–327). MIT Press.

Noy, L., Levit-Binun, N., & Golland, Y. (2015). Being in the zone: Physiological markers of togetherness in joint improvisation. *Frontiers in Human Neuroscience, 9*, 187. http://doi.org/10.3389/fnhum.2015.00187

Prinz, W., & Hommel, B. (2002). *Common mechanisms in perception and action: Attention and Performance* (Vol. 19). Oxford University Press.

Ragert, M., Schroeder, T., & Keller, P. E. (2013). Knowing too little or too much: The effects of familiarity with a co-performer's part on interpersonal coordination in musical ensembles. *Frontiers in Psychology, 4*, 368. http://doi.org/10.3389/fpsyg.2013.00368

Repp, B. H. (1997). Expressive timing in a Debussy Prelude: A comparison of student and expert pianists. *Musicae Scientiae, 1*, 257–268. http://doi.org/10.1177/102986499700100206

Repp, B. H. (2002). The embodiment of musical structure: Effects of musical context on sensorimotor synchronization with complex timing patterns. In W. Prinz & B. Hommel (Eds.), *Common mechanisms in perception and action: Attention and performance* (Vol. XIX, pp. 245–265). Oxford University Press.

Repp, B. H. (2005). Sensorimotor synchronization: A review of the tapping literature. *Psychonomic Bulletin and Review, 12*(6), 969–992. http://doi.org/10.3758/bf03206433

Repp, B. H., Keller, P. E., & Jacoby, N. (2012). Quantifying phase correction in sensorimotor synchronization: Empirical comparison of three paradigms. *Acta Psychologica, 139*(2), 281–290. http://doi.org/10.1016/j.actpsy.2011.11.002

Repp, B. H., & Su, Y.-H. (2013). Sensorimotor synchronization: A review of recent research (2006–2012). *Psychological Bulletin and Review, 20*(3), 403–452. http://doi.org/10.3758/s13423-012-0371-2

Richardson, D. C., Dale, R., & Shockley, K. (2008). Synchrony and swing in conversation: Coordination, temporal dynamics, and communication. In I. Wachsmuth, M. Lenzen, & G. Knoblich (Eds.), *Embodied communication in humans and machines* (pp. 75–94). Oxford University.

Savage, P. E., Loui, P., Tarr, B., Schachner, A., Glowacki, L., Mithen, S., & Fitch, W. T. (2020). Music as a coevolved system for social bonding. *Behavioral and Brain Sciences, 44*, e59. http://doi.org/10.1017/S0140525X20000333

Schiavio, A., & Høffding, S. (2015). Playing together without communicating? A pre-reflective and enactive account of joint musical performance. *Musicae Scientiae, 19*(4), 366–388. http://doi.org/10.1177/1029864915593333

Schober, M. F., & Spiro, N. (2016). Listeners' and performers' shared understanding of jazz improvisations. *Frontiers in Psychology, 7*, 1629. http://doi.org/10.3389/fpsyg.2016.01629

Schütz-Bosbach, S., & Prinz, W. (2007). Perceptual resonance: Action-induced modulation of perception. *Trends in Cognitive Sciences, 11*(8), 349–355. http://doi.org/10.1016/j.tics.2007.06.005

Seddon, F. A., & Biasutti, M. (2009). A comparison of modes of communication between members of a string quartet and a jazz sextet. *Psychology of Music, 37*(4), 395–415. http://doi.org/10.1177/0305735608100375

Tarr, B., Launay, J., & Dunbar, R. I. (2014). Music and social bonding: 'Self-other' merging and neurohormonal mechanisms. *Frontiers in Psychology, 5*, 1096. http://doi.org/10.3389/fpsyg.2014.01096

Tomasello, M., Hare, B., Lehmann, H., & Call, J. (2007). Reliance on head versus eyes in the gaze following of great apes and human infants: the cooperative eye hypothesis. *Journal of Human Evolution, 52*(3), 314–320. http://doi.org/10.1016/j.jhevol.2006.10.001

Tsay, C.-J. (2013). Sight over sound in the judgment of music performance. *Proceedings of the National Academy of Sciences of the United States of America, 110*(36), 14580–14585. http://doi.org/10.1073/pnas.1221454110

van der Schyff, D., Schiavio, A., Walton, A. E., Velardo, V., & Chemero, A. (2018). Musical creativity and the embodied mind: Exploring the possibilities of 4E cognition and dynamical systems theory. *Music & Science, 1*, 1–18. http://doi.org/10.1177/2059204318792319

van der Steen, M. M., Jacoby, N., Fairhurst, M. T., & Keller, P. E. (2015). Sensorimotor synchronization with tempo-changing auditory sequences: Modeling temporal adaptation and anticipation. *Brain Research, 1626*, 66–87. http://doi.org/10.1016/j.brainres.2015.01.053

Vesper, C., Schmitz, L., Safra, L., Sebanz, N., & Knoblich, G. (2016). The role of shared visual information for joint action coordination. *Cognition, 153*, 118–123. http://doi.org/10.1016/j.cognition.2016.05.002

Vuoskoski, J. K., Thompson, M. R., Spence, C., & Clarke, E. F. (2016). Interaction of sight and sound in the perception and experience of musical performance. *Music Perception, 33*(4), 457–471. http://doi.org/10.1525/mp.2016.33.4.457

Williamon, A., & Davidson, J. W. (2002). Exploring co-performer communication. *Musicae Scientiae, 6*(1), 53–72. http://doi.org/10.1177/102986490200600103

Windsor, W. L., & de Bézenac, C. (2012). Music and affordances. *Musicae Scientiae, 16*(1), 102–120. http://doi.org/10.1177/1029864911435734

Wing, A., Endo, S., Bradbury, A., & Vorberg, D. (2014). Optimal feedback correction in string quartet synchronization. *Journal of the Royal Society Interface, 11*(93), 20131125. http://doi.org/10.1098/rsif.2013.1125

Wolf, T., Sebanz, N., & Knoblich, G. (2018). Joint action coordination in expert-novice pairs: Can experts predict novices' suboptimal timing? *Cognition, 178*, 103–108. http://doi.org/10.1016/j.cognition.2018.05.012

Wöllner, C., Deconinck, F. J. A., Parkinson, J., Hove, M. J., & Keller, P. E. (2012). The perception of prototypical motion: Synchronization is enhanced with quantitatively morphed gestures of musical conductors. *Journal of Experimental Psychology: Human Perception and Performance, 38*(6), 1390–1403. http://doi.org/10.1037/a0028130

14

Making Time Together

An Exploration of Participatory Time-Making Through
Collective Dance Improvisation

Julien Laroche, Tommi Himberg, and Asaf Bachrach

14.1 The Dynamical, Multiscale, and Participatory Nature of Time-Making

If dancing and playing music together require a timely coordination of behaviours, what is the nature of this shared time? In this chapter, we take a step back from the traditional acceptance of time as either an objective phenomenon that is independent of us or as a purely subjective intra-individual experience, and we reconsider its phenomenology from an intersubjective and enactive point of view (something our collective bodily activities make together), for which collective improvisation offers a privileged window.

14.1.1 From Dualistic to Autonomous-Relational Multiscale Time

Time is often taken for granted as a pre-existing category or an objective dimension of our world. By flowing uninterruptedly, time seems to be permanently there, preceding both the phenomena that occur in its course and our own experience. We thus tend to assimilate time to its measurement, as classical physics does: a linear and regular unfolding of successive units that can be universally captured in terms of duration (Varela, 1999). Cognitive scientists have generally tended to take objective properties of the world as a reliable starting point and then wonder how minds consequently form inner representations of this outer reality (Varela, 1989). From this perspective, it is tempting to assume that we experience time by reconstituting temporal lengths as if they were a separable trait of external events—for instance, by having recourse to some internal clocks or counters (Treisman et al., 1990; Wing & Kristofferson, 1973). More recently, the predictive coding theory has hypothesized the presence of mechanisms that generate (and test) predictions about upcoming sensory states based on prior experiences (e.g. Vuust & Witek, 2014). This account shifts the view of time perception from a reactive to an anticipatory one, but the

Julien Laroche, Tommi Himberg, and Asaf Bachrach, *Making Time Together* In: *Performing Time*. Edited by: Clemens Wöllner and Justin London, Oxford University Press. © Oxford University Press 2023. DOI: 10.1093/oso/9780192896254.003.0015 idea that internal models represent and adapt to the temporality defined by external events remains intact.

Such duality between the outer time of the world-as-objects and the inner time of the subject was noticed by Husserl (1928): we perceive outer events as having a duration, and our inner, felt experience of those events is, itself, enduring. Yet, he pointed out that we do not experience these aspects separately; rather, they present themselves in a unified fashion. This is because temporality is the most irreducible, fundamental level of lived experience. No experience happens outside time, and all experiences possess a similar temporal structure, where the present moment exists in the interplay between retention and protention. Retention designates the context formed by past experiences in light of which the present is experienced (e.g. a single note in the context of a melody). Protention designates the soft anticipation of upcoming experiences that gives the present experience a horizon towards which it tends (the implicit sensation that the melody is going to continue in a certain direction—which is not necessarily predicted yet not fully indeterminate, either). As retention holds previous experiences, it holds previous retentions as well, forming a nesting of contexts formed by past experiences (the current note heard in the light of not only its intervallic relationship to the previous note, but also of the whole melody; or the rhythmic pattern experienced in the context of a metrical hierarchy, and not merely as a succession of events separated by various lengths of time). This gives the present experience a thick, complex, and even fractal structure (Gallagher & Zahavi, 2014; Laroche et al., 2014). Past protentions are retained as well, and the ways in which they are confirmed or superseded by the unfolding of external events allows us to experience their temporal organization within the lived flow of experience itself (rather than dualistically, as a representation that seeks to duplicate reality).

Enactive and dynamical approaches can jointly account for the endogeny of temporal experiences described by Husserl and their relation to external temporalities such as those found in music and dance (Laroche et al., 2014). In effect, our behaviours and experiences emerge from a biological background where different parts of our body interact with each other. Each internal process therefore has causes in and consequences for other internal processes (Varela, 1979), giving rise to a closed network of interactions that has self-organizing properties. As such, coherent patterns of activity can emerge as a result of the reciprocal influences between the processes that compose them. In other words, coordinated patterns of activity exist dynamically as the outcomes of interaction processes. Thus two improvising musicians influenced by and adjusting to each other's temporal fluctuations can give rise to a coherent tempo without any external timekeeper (i.e. a metronome or a conductor).

Emergent patterns tend to operate at their own timescale: they display slower dynamics of change than their components do, as we observe in the oscillations involved in neural assemblies or in the phase relationships between coordinated limbs (Kelso, 1995). In return, emergent patterns constrain the activity of their component processes and, thereby, modulate their dynamics. As a result, dynamics at faster timescales (i.e. activity of component processes at lower levels of organization) both bring forth and are nested within dynamics at slower timescales (i.e. patterns of interaction at higher levels of organization; see Ihlen & Vereijken, 2010). In the example of our two interacting improvisers, the long-term stability of the common tempo they bring forth, or the slow trend of acceleration that sometimes results from a long build-up that rises in intensity, become constraining influences over the short-term timing of each musician.

This circular principle of organization recurs at many timescales, giving rise to a complex mesh of temporalities that influence each other across timescales. This mesh provides biological agents with a background of endogenous dynamics through which their behaviours and experiences can emerge. Therefore, the temporal 'grid' to which they refer is essentially non-linear and multiscale. In other words, time as measured by a linear clock does not constitute a valid baseline for gauging the temporalities we enact. On the contrary, viewing the temporal dynamics that underlie our behaviours and experiences as the nesting of multiple timescales allows us to understand the present as emerging from a retentional context that is heading towards a protentional horizon (Varela, 1999). This also allows us to better grasp the temporal foundations of our behaviours and experiences through the prism of collectively improvised activities.

In effect, while the closure of the network that enables these endogenous dynamics marks the autonomy of a living agent, it does not isolate us from the external reality, nor does it trap us within a temporality that is purely subjective. On the contrary, to sustain its autonomy, a living agent must interact with the outer world in adaptive ways (Di Paolo, 2005). The condition of our continued existence is thus an active and meaningful exploration of our world, a process of sense-making that is therefore fundamentally temporal (Di Paolo, 2005). As external events act as perturbations of our own ongoing dynamics, their temporal structure modulates the dynamical background of our behaviours and experiences. Our intrinsic temporality can thus be informed by the temporality of external events (Doelling et al., 2019). As such, the way we attend to the outer world over time is shaped by the temporal structure of external events we interact with (Large & Jones, 1999). This explains how we can feel the underlying pulse of music even when no acoustic events coincide with those pulses (Large & Snyder, 2009; Nozaradan et al., 2012), and why our behaviours can unintentionally entrain to external rhythms (Varlet et al., 2017).

As inherently autonomous yet relational agents, we thus 'sense' temporal events, but in our own terms—that is, in the flow of our own background dynamics. However, our experiences do not stem from passive processes whereby we merely submit to the influence of external temporalities. Rather, we enact our experiences in the course of our sensorimotor interactions with the world: what we do affects how we sense our environment (Varela et al., 1991). By regulating our sensorimotor coupling with the world, we thus actively create the temporal structure of our own experiences. As such, body movements contribute to frame the temporality with which we attend to, process, and experience sensory events (Hammerschmidt & Wöllner, 2020; Morillon et al., 2014; Tichko et al., 2021; Wöllner & Hammerschmidt, 2021). For instance, head movements during music listening do not just express our perceptual experiences but they actively contribute to our perception of the beat and the metre of rhythmical patterns (Phillips-Silver & Trainor, 2005, 2008). By actively interacting with external temporal events, and thereby affecting our own dynamical background, our behaviour comes to embed both the complex structuration (Stephen & Dixon, 2011) and the multiscale nature (Toiviainen et al., 2010) of sensory events.

In sum, sense-making (making the world a meaningful place by actively sensing through our movements) is a temporal process. The origins of this temporality are simultaneously endogenous (it stems from the constitutive dynamics of our embodiment) and relational (it is modulated by the temporality of external events and takes form within a process of sensorimotor interactions). As we interact with the world (modifying our intrinsic dynamics by regulating our relational dynamics and vice versa), we thus make up our own—autonomous yet relational—temporality (Laroche et al., 2014).

14.1.2 The Intersubjective Embodiment of Time

What we come to call our world, however, is first and foremost constituted by the relations we have with others, that is, other autonomous and relational sense-makers that can directly react to our own sense-making activities. The reciprocity of our interactions opens up a properly collective level of organization. Indeed, when two or more agents interact, their respective sensorimotor coupling become coupled, themselves (McGann & De Jaegher, 2009): what I do factors in what you sense, and therefore in what you do next, which factors in my own sensorimotor coupling in return (Hari et al., 2009). We thus become part of each other's sensorimotor coupling and, subsequently, of each other's resulting experiences (Fuchs & De Jaegher, 2009). Because these experiences are temporal in nature, we participate interactively in each other's temporal dynamics (Laroche et al., 2014).

The intersubjective aspect of the temporalities subtending our behaviours and experiences stems from the dynamical nature of both ourselves and our interactions with others. By scaling this dynamical perspective up to the interpersonal domain, we can think of individual behaviours as the component processes of collective patterns of coordination. Indeed, although patterns of coordination formed by the self or across individuals have most often been studied separately, they can exhibit similar dynamical laws (e.g. two persons moving one of their arms rhythmically vs one person moving both of her arms rhythmically; Amazeen et al., 1995; Fine & Amazeen, 2011; Schmidt et al., 1998; Schmidt & Richardson, 2008). Because they primarily rely on the interactions between component processes (and not their specific isolated structure), principles of coordination can therefore apply across intra- and interpersonal levels of organization (Kelso & Engstrom, 2006).

As we have already pointed to earlier, in complex dynamical systems, the formation of collective dynamics constrains the lower-level processes that participate in their emergence (Kelso, 1995). In other words, the temporal dynamics that subtend individual behaviours can nest within the collective dynamics their interactions give rise to (Ramenzoni et al., 2011). As such, the very process of interaction (how the interplay of reciprocal influences between persons unfolds) influences the coordination of individual behaviours. For instance, sensorimotor interactions can stabilize individual rhythmic behaviours (Miyata et al., 2018) and help partners to compensate for each other's fluctuations (Miyata et al., 2017). Interaction can improve habitual patterns, such as an individual's gait coordination when walking synchronously with another person (Nessler et al., 2015); or it can aid the performance of more complex patterns than we normally could on our own (Wolf et al., 2020). On the other hand, interpersonal coupling constraints can sometimes impede the timely regulation of behaviours at the intrapersonal level (Finkel et al., 2006; Galbusera et al., 2019; Lorås et al., 2019; Miyata et al., 2021). In summary, sensorimotor interactions with others change, willingly or not, how we move ourselves in time (Fine et al., 2013).

The constraints of the interaction process, nonetheless, do not simply affect individual behaviours as if they were isolated from each other. Rather, as they become constrained by their very own relations, interacting behaviours tend to coordinate synergistically (Riley et al., 2011). In effect, interpersonal coordination spontaneously emerges with mere visual coupling, and it can do so at different timescales, for instance, by swinging a pendulum with the arm (Schmidt & O'Brien, 1997), rocking a chair with the whole body (Richardson et al., 2007), or during postural oscillations (Athreya et al., 2014; Gueugnon et al., 2016; Varlet et al., 2011, 2014). Participants thus converge in tapping tempo when they see each other (Oullier et al., 2008), and even when they tap together to a metronome, the product of their interaction structures their timing more than the regular external beat does (Himberg, 2014), an effect that is observed in ancillary movements as well (Colley, 2020). Interacting individuals also spontaneously align the rhythm of their words (Himberg et al., 2015), showing that interpersonal coordination does not only happen when participants' activities are similar and synchronized (Hari et al., 2013). In fact, interpersonal temporal coordination of behaviours emerges even when participants are asked to ignore each other (Rosso et al., 2021) or to explicitly avoid coordination (Issartel et al., 2007), as well as when they are simply unaware of their mutual interactions (Auvray et al., 2009). The strength with which interactions modulate our own temporality and coordinate it with others is such that we retain a trace of others' movement dynamics after an encounter (Nordham et al., 2018; Oullier et al., 2008), even a purely spectatorial one (Bachrach et al., 2015).

Individual temporality is thus constituted by collective social dynamics. However, we described temporality at the individual level as emerging from a multiscale network of interactions. Therefore, when people interact, the entirety of their underlying dynamics influence and are influenced by each other (Laroche et al., 2014). The coordinative outcomes of the interaction process thus go beyond mere synchronized entrainment at one timescale (Tomassini et al., 2022). Rather, the very multiscale complexity of movements aligns when persons walk (Almurad et al., 2017), talk

(Abney et al., 2014), or tap beats together (Coey et al., 2016). Interacting persons thus coordinate at multiple timescales simultaneously during many activities, whether it is problem-solving (Wiltshire et al., 2019), music playing (Walton et al., 2015), or dancing (Washburn et al., 2014).

Coherent coordination at multiple and distinctly functional timescales has been observed from infancy onwards. When a mother and child interact, their vocalizations not only coordinate to a common pulse, they also coordinate at the level of proto-phrases, taking turns to form a larger coherent narrative structure at even slower timescales of interaction (Malloch & Trevarthen, 2009). By actively regulating the dynamics of our interactions, we create a properly intersubjective timescale (Gratier, 2007). Importantly, the temporal structuring of our interactive behaviours is not a simple mechanical or motor epiphenomenon. Rather, the subtle temporality of our interactions makes sense to us. Indeed, the quality of coordination across scales during mother–infant interactions is deeply associated with affective and cognitive outcomes (Gratier & Apter-Danon, 2009). Interaction dynamics thus constitute an intersubjectively lived temporality whose coordination is at the source of common meaning making (Gratier & Magnier, 2012). This has been observed in adult conversation as well (De Jaegher & Di Paolo, 2007; Fusaroli et al., 2014); it impacts affective outcomes of psychotherapeutic interventions (Ramseyer & Tschacher, 2011), and many laboratory experiments have shown the pro-social and affiliative effects of temporal coordination of movements (Marsh et al., 2009).

In short, coordinated timing induced by sensorimotor interactions does not just happen to us: we actively and sensitively make time together by regulating our interactions. Unfortunately, most current experimental set-ups related to temporal coordination use sensorimotor laboratory tasks that do not reflect the complex temporal organizations of ecological social interactions and are not affectively involving or meaningful to participants (e.g. dyadic synchronization tasks); crucially, they also do not let participants actively shape the temporal form of their interactions (but see Dell'Anna et al., 2021, for instance, where experimental designs lean towards more realistic situations that rely on a joint sense of agency). Yet it is in those complex real-world situations, such as collective music and dance performances, that our joint temporal interactions make the most sense and require the most pristine regulation (D'Ausilio et al., 2012; Gratier et al., 2018). How, then, to better study the key mechanisms of interaction that subtend what we call 'participatory time-making'—in reference to 'participatory sense-making' (De Jaegher & Di Paolo, 2007) and to 'participatory (time) discrepancies' described in jazz improvisation (Keil, 1987)?

14.2 Collective Improvisation as a Study of Participatory Time-Making

We hold that improvisational activities constitute a relevant tool to explore how we bodily make and experience time together. It is often taken for granted that, as our activities are generally poorly scripted, improvisation reflects the ecological condition of daily behaviours. However, improvising because rules or scripts are missing versus improvising for its own sake are different in nature (Krueger & Salice, 2021). In the latter case (e.g. artistic collective improvisation in dance or music), the intersubjective negotiations of temporality become the focus of interactions and a source of meaningfulness (Butterfield, 2010; Chauvigné et al., 2018; Noy et al. 2011; Vicary et al. 2017; Walton et al., 2018). Indeed, the temporal organization of interaction in collective improvisation, being underspecified (Goupil et al., 2021), has to be co-enacted and co-regulated by the performers. Furthermore, the way temporality takes form in the course of the performance incites further regulation of the group coordination. Thus, the sharing and regulating of temporalities (especially when they collapse) are among the most—if not the most—critical elements that motivate and inspire the organization of improvised interaction (Laroche & Kaddouch, 2014; Walton et al., 2018). Making time together in artistic collective improvisation is therefore both a means (coordinating the group's activity) and an end (producing aesthetically interesting temporal shapes or structures).

14.2.1 Experiencing and Experimenting Participatory Time-Making

To understand participatory time-making in collective improvisation, we thus need to understand the articulation between emergent temporal coordination and the resulting experiences that motivate strategic decisions about its co-regulation (Saint-Germier & Canonne, 2020). In other words, third-person observations and first-person experiences of interaction dynamics should be explored hand in hand (Dumas et al., 2014). Since collective improvisation consists in the very practice (and at the same time the study) of 'participatory time-making', improvisers do have a rich first-person perspective on the active sharing and making of temporality: they are proper researchers within that field. To explore participatory time-making by crossing the first- and third-person perspectives of experiential reflections and observational knowledge, a strong collaboration with practitioners is therefore necessary.

Since the multiple timescales that characterize collective improvisation are complex and intertwined, the study of their emergence and their participatory negotiation in a repeatable and trackable manner requires one to design tasks where this complexity is reduced. Yet, the temporal structure of such tasks should neither be given extrinsically, nor should they operate as canonical forms, and movement choices and timing should be free enough to let the coordination of the collective be driven by the dynamics of the members of the group and their interaction. To that effect, and by bringing scientific and artistic worlds together, we designed 'Group Improvisation Games' (GIGs; see Himberg et al., 2018, for more details): 'scores' (i.e. sets of constraints) that keep instructions sufficiently open-ended to allow for spontaneous and creative interactions while keeping a format that is amenable to empirical studies and which do not require any specific expertise for participation.

In the previous literature (e.g. Noy et al., 2011), a practice of this kind has already been repeatedly used by researchers to study the free on-line temporal negotiation of movements by reducing the degrees of freedom allowed to participants: the mirror game (MG). The MG used by researchers is based on a movement and theatre-pedagogical tool that consists of full-body mirroring exercises. It has been simplified and brought to behavioural laboratories, where dyads synchronize freely impro-vised movements along one dimension without verbal communication (Noy et al., 2011). This paradigm revealed correlations between intersubjective affects and kin-ematic dynamics (Noy et al., 2015), highlighting how individual kinematic proper-ties blend during interactions to form an emergent intersubjective behavioural space (Słowiński et al., 2016). While this practice affords rich interactions and a variety of modes of coordination, the dyadic setting reduces the space of interactional choices to a somewhat trivial level (participants can either lead or follow the partner), at the risk of masking key aspects of group coordination dynamics (Bourbousson & Fortes-Bourbousson, 2016).

To study the multiscale negotiation and emergence of intersubjective temporality, we introduce a GIG that expands the MG to a four-person setting. This configu-ration creates conflicts among possible choices, both in terms of how to negotiate common movements and in terms of who to follow. This constitutes an ecological case of joint improvisation that reflects the main 'coordination problems' identified in music improvisation: the consolidation of an idea and the articulation between different ideas (Goupil et al., 2021). Below, we present previously published results, and a new exploratory analysis of the same data in order to illustrate the intersubjec-tive and multiscale nature of time discussed above.

14.2.2 The Four-Person Mirror Game

In a small-scale study published previously (see Himberg et al., 2018, for details), we recruited four groups of four participants (with no to moderate prior experience in dance) to participate in a MG. Twelve reflective markers were placed on the parti-cipants' bodies to capture their motion (using an OptiTrack system with a 100-Hz sampling frequency). They stood in a circle, extended one arm towards the centre, and were instructed to mirror each other's movements without an assigned role and without verbal communication. Each group performed the task twice. We collected their first-person experience after the experiment and they completed personality questionnaires as well. To gauge interpersonal coordination, quantity of motion, and cross-correlations between the acceleration time series of index fingers were com-puted. To understand how partners organized their participation in the game, we qualitatively annotated the video recordings of their performances by segmenting them in terms of movement 'propositions' and 'responses'.

A striking feature of this game was pointed out by the participants in their reports: they felt that shared leadership was difficult to envisage and that they needed a leader to make collective movement possible. This was illustrated by the turn-taking structure revealed by qualitative annotations: participants spontaneously took turns in proposing movements and responding to the movements of others. Interestingly, the promptness to respond to others' propositions correlated with (self-reported) cognitive empathy, highlighting the link between relational kinematic patterns and the socio-affiliative meaningfulness of making time together.

A limitation of these analyses is that propositions and responses, despite referring to socially complementary acts, still take the structure of individual actions as a point of departure. What lacks is a collective characterization of the temporality of the whole group. Another limitation is that, as with most published research on the topic, analyses of interpersonal coordination (cross-correlation) were performed by referring to a linear scale and took moment-to-moment synchronicity as a ground truth. Missing from this analysis is an exploration of the multiscale nature of the temporal dynamics involved in the task and of the characteristic timescales at which the group evolves as a collective (i.e. the possibility of higher-level group co-ordination wherein performance is structured at slower timescales). To address the theoretical perspective of this chapter and provide an empirical illustration of the multiple scales at which participatory time-making occurs, we present below new methods and an exploratory analysis of the above kinematic data. In particular, we expected to find temporal signatures of collective organization of behaviour that are distinct from the temporal structure of individual behaviours.

14.2.3 The Mirror Game From a Multiscale Perspective: Analysis

In the MG data discussed above, the mere visualization of the finger velocity time series suffices to suggest a collective organization at a slower timescale: we can notice several episodes during which kinematic features such as movement velocity, amplitude, frequency, or shape were rather stable (collective sequences separated by smaller movements, as if participants were waiting for an impulse to enter a new sequence; see Figure 14.1a). To quantify interpersonal coordination from a multiscale perspective, we measured cross-wavelet coherence between the velocity time series of the index finger of each pair of partners. Next, we averaged the amount of coherence observed across each trial for each pair. Then, we averaged the resulting spectra across each group. We thus obtain, for each game, a measure of group coherence, which estimates the overall coordination of each group at each frequency band. To evaluate the significance of the results, we computed the group coherence of 100 randomly created surrogate ensembles of four participants who each originally belonged to a different group. At each frequency band, the coherence value observed at the 95th percentile was taken as the chance level.

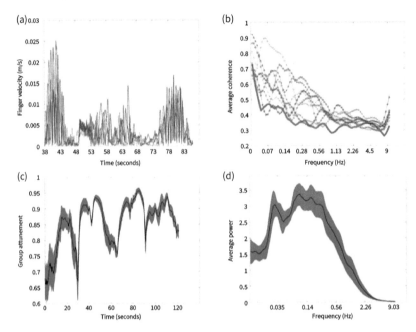

Figure 14.1 (a) Excerpt of finger velocity time series of the four participants (each represented by a different colour) of a group where collective sequences can be observed. (b) Group coherence for the two trials of the four groups. The continuous red line indicates the chance level for every frequency band. Group coherence was above chance in all trials for almost the entire spectrum. (c) Time series of group attunement (same group and trial as in (a); shaded areas represent standard error). Peaks and plateaus of high attunement of about a dozen of seconds on average followed each other, separated by abrupt drops of coordination. (d) Frequency composition of group attunement evolution. The spectrum was dominated by frequency components that correspond to a few seconds, reflecting episodical attunement spanning several individual movement propositions. Another peak was observed and corresponded to periods of 30 s approximately, reflecting the long-lasting plateaus of high group attunement observed in many trials that were separated by abrupt drops in frequency attunement.

To probe the presence of an intersubjective timescale of organization, we then quantified the evolution of the attunement of the group in the frequency domain. To do so, we first performed wavelet transforms on each participant's finger velocity to track the temporal evolution of their respective kinematics. For each 1-s window, we computed real-time cross-correlations between the power spectra of each pair of partners. We then averaged the resulting cross-correlations time series across each trial of each group. We thus obtained a time series of the evolution of frequency attunement within each trial of each group—group attunement, for short.

To capture the timescales at which group dynamics evolved, we analysed the fluctuations of group attunement in the frequency domain. We first differentiated the time series to represent how group attunement changed over time, and then submitted the resulting time series to wavelet transforms. Finally, we averaged power across time to reveal the frequency bands at which group attunement was evolving.

14.2.4 The Mirror Game: Results

Group coherence obtained with wavelet transforms spanned many frequency bands in all trials (Figure 14.1b). In fact, in nearly all trials coherence was superior to the surrogate baseline for almost the entire spectrum, between roughly 0.04 and 9.00 Hz, and especially below 2.25 Hz. This simple game thus affords the exploration of movement coordination across a wide range of frequency bands, and more particularly so in low-frequency areas.

Time series of group attunement generally displayed plateaus of high coordination during which the frequency compositions of the partners' movements converge. These plateaus are often separated by drops that reflect unstable transitions towards a novel phase of collective coordination (Figure 14.1c). The clarity of collectively structured sequences can vary between groups: the stability of segments of attunement and the drops in coordination were more or less clear depending on the trial, which possibly marks different strategies (and perhaps success) in managing coordination collectively. Interestingly, the shape of these collective dynamics is strikingly similar to the 'segmental form' observed in musical collective improvisation (Goupil et al., 2021) and reflects well the alternation between 'phases of synchrony' and 'phases of diachrony' described in musical collective improvisation as the core dialectic of group creativity (Laroche & Kaddouch, 2015; see also Dahan et al., 2016, in the context of the MG).

Group attunement was observed at several timescales (Figure 14.1d). In particular, the spectrum was dominated by frequency components roughly situated between 0.075 and 0.28 Hz, reflecting cycles of episodical attunement of about 4–12 s. Another salient peak was present around 0.03 Hz. It reflects the aforementioned long plateaus of attunement that last for about 30 s. This peak thus captures the slowly evolving dynamics of the intersubjective organization of movement. Importantly, these timescales of fluctuations encompass several individual movement propositions, which, according to our qualitative segmentation, occur every 2 s on average. During spontaneous, unscripted, and non-verbal interactions between multiple agents, stable collective sequences can thus emerge at their own timescale, beyond the temporal windows of individual actions. This structure is similar to the segmental form observed in musical collective improvisation: without any prescription, structuration emerges as a succession of collective sequences that contain a plurality of individual actions but are yet shaped by stable features (Canonne & Garnier, 2015; Goupil et al., 2021). Here, the coordinated interactions between partners' movement brought forth this form at a properly intersubjective timescale. Unlike the case of music improvisation, our task invited simple movement gestures that participants were not familiar with, and it didn't require any expertise.

Overall, the MG appears well suited to study how we make and share time to-gether through sensorimotor interactions. Whereas earlier results pointed to the importance of integrating quantitative and qualitative analysis to understand affective and motor processes of group coordination (Himberg et al., 2018), these new results show that this phenomenon takes place at multiple timescales. Importantly, the collectively improvised movements it elicits have a temporal organization that goes beyond individual action propositions and reactions. Rather, the very dynamics of sensorimotor interactions seem to bring forth temporal structures that exist at noticeably slower timescales, reflecting a properly intersubjective organization of time—a time whose shape we make and experience together. Future research should gauge if these different timescales of coordination are linked with distinct experiential profiles and degrees of intersubjective connection.

14.3 Conclusion

In this chapter, we define time as a complex and multiscale phenomenon that is inherent to our bodily dynamics, but that is yet lived relationally in our active coupling with the world. During our encounters with others, sense-making becomes participatory: by coupling through bodily interactions, we play a role in each other's experiences. As such, we make time together: the way we shape the temporality of our interactions is meaningful to us personally and to our interpersonal relationship(s). Indeed, the intersubjective organization constitutes a source of lived experience and can become the very object of the regulation of our sensorimotor interactions (Gratier, 2007). The dynamics of interaction, as they affect us mutually, form a pool of shared retention and protention, their temporality becoming part of our own present experience. To fully understand our capacity of not only performing *in* time but also of enacting time itself (i.e. bringing forth temporal qualities that we experience aesthetically, in music or dance), we should thus study time as a participatory phenomenon. In particular, time-making activities such as music and dance aim at shaping temporal forms that are, by nature, collective.

Collective improvisation stands out as the very practice of participatory time-making and, therefore, it offers a privileged window into this phenomenon. Such a practice, even in reduced forms like those found in our GIGs (Himberg et al., 2018), can reveal the complexity and the multiscale nature that is inherent to our interactions, as well as the link between such coordination and socio-affective and semiotic/meaning-making processes. Beyond a mere alignment of lived and acted temporalities, the study of interactional time reveals the emergence of temporalities that are proper to the interaction, such as the structuration of collective sequences we observed in the MG and whose organization spans slower timescales than those of individual actions.

This kind of research should help us better grasp how we develop capacities involved in multiscale coordination, and how we use it, even in solitary situations

(Dumas et al., 2014). It should also highlight phenomena and mechanisms that might escape us if we solely look for synchronized behaviours in laboratory settings. Such studies can open perspectives in other domains of human or animal behaviour where the temporality of collective organization is key. In particular, making time together plays a tremendous role in social cohesion (McNeill, 1995) and the subtleties of participatory time-making participate in the cognitive and affective development of infants (Gratier & Apter-Danon, 2009). Potential applications in social interventions extend to the domain of health, where practices such as dancing in a group can benefit individuals in rehabilitation contexts (Bégel et al., 2022). Taken together, these studies demonstrate how crucial it is to investigate the underpinnings of participatory time-making.

References

Abney, D. H., Paxton, A., Dale, R., & Kello, C. T. (2014). Complexity matching in dyadic conversation. *Journal of Experimental Psychology: General, 143*(6), 2304–2315.

Almurad, Z. M., Roume, C., & Delignières, D. (2017). Complexity matching in side-by-side walking. *Human Movement Science, 54*, 125–136.

Amazeen, P. G., Schmidt, R. C., & Turvey, M. T. (1995). Frequency-detuning of the phase entrainment dynamics of visually coupled rhythmic movements. *Biological Cybernetics, 72*, 511–518.

Athreya, D. N., Riley, M. A., & Davis, T. J. (2014). Visual influences on postural and manual interpersonal coordination during a joint precision task. *Experimental Brain Research, 232*(9), 2741–2751.

Auvray, M., Lenay, C., & Stewart, J. (2009). Perceptual interactions in a minimalist virtual environment. *New Ideas in Psychology, 27*(1), 32–47.

Bachrach, A., Fontbonne, Y., Joufflineau, C., & Ulloa, J. L. (2015). Audience entrainment during live contemporary dance performance: Physiological and cognitive measures. *Frontiers in Human Neuroscience, 9*, 179.

Bégel, V., Bachrach, A., Dalla Bella, S., Laroche, J., Clément, S., Riquet, A., & Dellacherie, D. (2022). Dance improves motor, cognitive, and social skills in children with developmental cerebellar anomalies. *Cerebellum, 21*(2), 264–279.

Butterfield, M. (2010). Participatory discrepancies and the perception of beats in jazz. *Music Perception, 27*(3), 157–176.

Bourbousson, J., & Fortes-Bourbousson, M. (2016). How do co-agents actively regulate their collective behavior states? *Frontiers in Psychology, 7*, 1732.

Canonne, C., & Garnier, N. (2015). Individual decisions and perceived form in collective free improvisation. *Journal of New Music Research, 44*(2), 145–167.

Chauvigné, L. A., Belyk, M., & Brown, S. (2018). Taking two to tango: fMRI analysis of improvised joint action with physical contact. *PLoS One, 13*(1), e0191098.

Coey, C. A., Washburn, A., Hassebrock, J., & Richardson, M. J. (2016). Complexity matching effects in bimanual and interpersonal syncopated finger tapping. *Neuroscience Letters, 616*, 204–210.

Colley, I., Varlet, M., MacRitchie, J., & Keller, P. E. (2020). The influence of a conductor and co-performer on auditory-motor synchronisation, temporal prediction, and ancillary entrainment in a musical drumming task. *Human Movement Science, 72*, 102653.

Dahan, A., Noy, L., Hart, Y., Mayo, A., & Alon, U. (2016). Exit from synchrony in joint improvised motion. *PLoS One, 11*(10), e0160747.

D'Ausilio, A., Badino, L., Li, Y., Tokay, S., Craighero, L., Canto, R., Aloimonos, Y., & Fadiga, L. (2012). Leadership in orchestra emerges from the causal relationships of movement kinematics. *PLoS One, 7*(5), e35757.

De Jaegher, H., & Di Paolo, E.A. (2007). Participatory sense-making: An enactive approach to social cognition. *Phenomenology and the Cognitive Sciences, 6*(4), 485–507.

Dell'Anna, A., Leman, M., & Berti, A. (2021). Musical interaction reveals music as embodied language. *Frontiers in Neuroscience*, *15*, 667838.

Di Paolo, E. A. (2005). Autopoiesis, adaptivity, teleology, agency. *Phenomenology and the Cognitive Sciences*, *4*(4), 429–452.

Doelling, K. B., Assaneo, M. F., Bevilacqua, D., Pesaran, B., & Poeppel, D. (2019). An oscillator model better predicts cortical entrainment to music. *Proceedings of the National Academy of Sciences of the United States of America*, *116*(20), 10113–10121.

Dumas, G., Laroche, J., & Lehmann, A. (2014). Your body, my body, our coupling moves our bodies. *Frontiers in Human Neuroscience*, *8*, 1004.

Fine, J. M., & Amazeen, E. L. (2011). Interpersonal Fitts' law: When two perform as one. *Experimental Brain Research*, *211*(3), 459–469.

Fine, J. M., Gibbons, C. T., & Amazeen, E. L. (2013). Congruency effects in interpersonal coordination. *Journal of Experimental Psychology: Human Perception and Performance*, *39*(6), 1541.

Finkel, E. J., Campbell, W. K., Brunell, A. B., Dalton, A. N., Scarbeck, S. J., & Chartrand, T. L. (2006). High-maintenance interaction: Inefficient social coordination impairs self-regulation. *Journal of Personality and Social Psychology*, *91*(3), 456.

Galbusera, L., Finn, M. T., Tschacher, W., & Kyselo, M. (2019). Interpersonal synchrony feels good but impedes self-regulation of affect. *Scientific Reports*, *9*(1), 1–12.

Fuchs, T., & De Jaegher, H. (2009). Enactive intersubjectivity: Participatory sense-making and mutual incorporation. *Phenomenology and the Cognitive Sciences*, *8*(4), 465–486.

Fusaroli, R., Rączaszek-Leonardi, J., & Tylén, K. (2014). Dialog as interpersonal synergy. *New Ideas in Psychology*, *32*, 147–157.

Gallagher, S., & Zahavi, D. (2014). Primal impression and enactive perception. In V. Arstila & D. Lloyd (Eds.), *Subjective time: The philosophy, psychology, and neuroscience of temporality* (pp. 83–99). MIT Press.

Goupil, L., Wolf, T., Saint-Germier, P., Aucouturier, J. J., & Canonne, C. (2021). Emergent shared intentions support coordination during collective musical improvisations. *Cognitive Science*, *45*(1), e12932.

Gratier, M. (2007). Les rythmes de l'intersubjectivité. *Spirale*, *44*(47), 10–3917.

Gratier, M., & Apter-Danon, G. (2009). The musicality of belonging: Repetition and variation in mother–infant vocal interaction. In S. Malloch & C. Trevarthen (Eds.), *Communicative musicality: Narratives of expressive gesture and being human* (pp. 301–327). Oxford University Press.

Gratier, M., & Magnier, J. (2012). Sense and synchrony: Infant communication and musical improvisation. *Intermédialités: Histoire et théorie des arts, des lettres et des techniques*, *19*, 45–64.

Gratier, M., Ksenija, S., & Evans, R. (2018). Negotiations: Sound and speech in the making of a studio recording. In E. Clarke & M. Doffman (Eds.), *Distributed creativity: Collaboration and improvisation in contemporary music* (pp. 163–180). Oxford University Press.

Gueugnon, M., Salesse, R. N., Coste, A., Zhao, Z., Bardy, B. G., & Marin, L. (2016). Postural coordination during socio-motor improvisation. *Frontiers in Psychology*, *7*, 1168.

Hammerschmidt, D., & Wöllner, C. (2020). Sensorimotor synchronization with higher metrical levels in music shortens perceived time. *Music Perception*, *37*(4), 263–277.

Hari, R., & Kujala, M. V. (2009). Brain basis of human social interaction: From concepts to brain imaging. *Physiological Reviews*, *89*(2), 453–479.

Hari, R., Himberg, T., Nummenmaa, L., Hämäläinen, M., & Parkkonen, L. (2013). Synchrony of brains and bodies during implicit interpersonal interaction. *Trends in Cognitive Sciences*, *17*(3), 105–106.

Himberg, T. (2014). *Interaction in musical time* [Doctoral dissertation, University of Cambridge].

Himberg, T., Hirvenkari, L., Mandel, A., & Hari, R. (2015). Word-by-word entrainment of speech rhythm during joint story building. *Frontiers in Psychology*, *6*, 797.

Himberg, T., Laroche, J., Bigé, R., Buchkowski, M., & Bachrach, A. (2018). Coordinated interpersonal behaviour in collective dance improvisation: The aesthetics of kinaesthetic togetherness. *Behavioral Sciences*, *8*(2), 23.

Husserl, E. (1928). *The phenomenology of internal time-consciousness* (J. S. Churchill, Trans.). Indiana University Press.

Ihlen, E. A., & Vereijken, B. (2010). Interaction-dominant dynamics in human cognition: Beyond $1/f\alpha$ fluctuation. *Journal of Experimental Psychology: General, 139*(3), 436–463.

Issartel, J., Marin, L., & Cadopi, M. (2007). Unintended interpersonal coordination: 'Can we march to the beat of our own drum?' *Neurosciences Letters, 411*, 174–179.

Keil, C. (1987). Participatory discrepancies and the power of music. *Cultural Anthropology, 2*(3), 275–283.

Kelso, J. S. (1995). *Dynamic patterns: The self-organization of brain and behavior.* MIT Press.

Kelso, J. S., & Engstrom, D. (2006). *The complementary nature.* MIT Press.

Krueger, J., & Salice, A. (2021). Towards a wide approach to improvisation. In J. McGuirk, S. Ravn, & S. Høffding (Eds.), *Improvisation: The competence(s) of not being in control* (pp. 50–69). Routledge.

Large, E. W., & Jones, M. R. (1999). The dynamics of attending: How people track time-varying events. *Psychological Review, 106*(1), 119–159.

Large, E., & Snyder, J. (2009). Pulse and meter as neural resonance. *Annals of the New York Academy of Sciences, 1169*(1), 46–57.

Laroche, J., Berardi, A. M., & Brangier, E. (2014). Embodiment of intersubjective time: Relational dynamics as attractors in the temporal coordination of interpersonal behaviors and experiences. *Frontiers in Psychology, 5*, 1180.

Laroche, J., & Kaddouch, I. (2014). Enacting teaching and learning in the interaction process: Keys' for developing skills in piano lessons through four-hand improvisations. *Journal of Pedagogy, 5*(1), 24.

Laroche, J., & Kaddouch, I. (2015). Spontaneous preferences and core tastes: Embodied musical personality and dynamics of interaction in a pedagogical method of improvisation. *Frontiers in Psychology, 6*, 522.

Lorås, H., Aune, T. K., Ingvaldsen, R., & Pedersen, A. V. (2019). Interpersonal and intrapersonal entrainment of self-paced tapping rate. *Plos One, 14*(7), e0220505.

Malloch, S., & Trevarthen, C. (2009). Musicality: Communicating the vitality and interests of life. In S. Malloch & C. Trevarthen (Eds.), *Communicative musicality: Exploring the basis of human companionship* (pp. 1–15). Oxford University Press.

Marsh, K. L., Richardson, M. J., & Schmidt, R. C. (2009). Social connection through joint action and interpersonal coordination. *Topics in Cognitive Science, 1*(2), 320–339.

McGann, M., & De Jaegher, H. (2009). Self-other contingencies: Enacting social perception. *Phenomenology and the Cognitive Sciences, 8*(4), 417–437.

McNeill, W. H. (1995). *Keeping together in time.* Harvard University Press.

Miyata, K., Varlet, M., Miura, A., Kudo, K., & Keller, P. E. (2017). Modulation of individual auditory-motor coordination dynamics through interpersonal visual coupling. *Scientific Reports, 7*(1), 1–11.

Miyata, K., Varlet, M., Miura, A., Kudo, K., & Keller, P. E. (2018). Interpersonal visual interaction induces local and global stabilisation of rhythmic coordination. *Neuroscience Letters, 682*, 132–136.

Miyata, K., Varlet, M., Miura, A., Kudo, K., & Keller, P. E. (2021). Vocal interaction during rhythmic joint action stabilizes interpersonal coordination and individual movement timing. *Journal of Experimental Psychology: General, 150*(2), 385–394.

Morillon, B., Schroeder, C. E., & Wyart, V. (2014). Motor contributions to the temporal precision of auditory attention. *Nature Communications, 5*(1), 1–9.

Nessler, J. A., Gutierrez, V., Werner, J., & Punsalan, A. (2015). Side by side treadmill walking reduces gait asymmetry induced by unilateral ankle weight. *Human Movement Science, 41*, 32–45.

Nordham, C. A., Tognoli, E., Fuchs, A., & Kelso, J. S. (2018). How interpersonal coordination affects individual behavior (and vice versa): Experimental analysis and adaptive HKB model of social memory. *Ecological Psychology, 30*(3), 224–249.

Noy, L., Dekel, E., & Alon, U. (2011). The mirror game as a paradigm for studying the dynamics of two people improvising motion together. *Proceedings of the National Academy of Sciences of the United States of America, 108*(52), 20947–20952.

Noy, L., Levit-Binun, N., & Golland, Y. (2015). Being in the zone: Physiological markers of togetherness in joint improvisation. *Frontiers in Human Neuroscience, 9*, 187.

Nozaradan, S., Peretz, I., & Mouraux, A. (2012). Selective neuronal entrainment to the beat and meter embedded in a musical rhythm. *Journal of Neuroscience, 32*(49), 17572–17581.

Oullier, O., De Guzman, G. C., Jantzen, K. J., Lagarde, J., & Kelso, J. A. S. (2008). Social coordination dynamics: Measuring human bonding. *Social Neuroscience*, *3*(2), 178–192.

Phillips-Silver, J., & Trainor, L. J. (2005). Feeling the beat: Movement influences infant rhythm perception. *Science*, *308*(5727), 1430–1430.

Phillips-Silver, J., & Trainor, L. J. (2008). Vestibular influence on auditory metrical interpretation. *Brain and Cognition*, *67*(1), 94–102.

Ramenzoni, V. C., Davis, T. J., Riley, M. A., Shockley, K., & Baker, A. A. (2011). Joint action in a cooperative precision task: Nested processes of intrapersonal and interpersonal coordination. *Experimental Brain Research*, *211*(3), 447–457.

Ramseyer, F., & Tschacher, W. (2011). Nonverbal synchrony in psychotherapy: Coordinated body movement reflects relationship quality and outcome. *Journal of Consulting and Clinical Psychology*, *79*(3), 284–295.

Richardson, M. J., Marsh, K. L., Isenhower, R. W., Goodman, J. R., & Schmidt, R. C. (2007). Rocking together: Dynamics of intentional and unintentional interpersonal coordination. *Human Movement Science*, *26*(6), 867–891.

Riley, M. A., Richardson, M., Shockley, K., & Ramenzoni, V. C. (2011). Interpersonal synergies. *Frontiers in Psychology*, *2*, 38.

Rosso, M., Maes, P. J., & Leman, M. (2021). Modality-specific attractor dynamics in dyadic entrainment. *Scientific Reports*, *11*(1), 1–13.

Saint-Germier, P., & Canonne, C. (2020). Coordinating free improvisation: An integrative framework for the study of collective improvisation. *Musicae Scientiae*, *26*(3), 1029864920976182.

Schmidt, R. C., & O'Brien, B. (1997). Evaluating the dynamics of unintended interpersonal coordination. *Ecological Psychology*, *9*(3), 189–206.

Schmidt, R. C., Bienvenu, M., Fitzpatrick, P. A., & Amazeen, P. G. (1998). A comparison of intra-and interpersonal interlimb coordination: Coordination breakdowns and coupling strength. *Journal of Experimental Psychology: Human Perception and Performance*, *24*(3), 884–900.

Schmidt, R. C., & Richardson, M. J. (2008). Dynamics of interpersonal coordination. In A. Fuchs & V. K. Jirsa (Eds.), *Coordination: Neural, behavioral and social dynamics* (pp. 281–308). Springer.

Słowiński, P., Zhai, C., Alderisio, F., Salesse, R., Gueugnon, M., Marin, L., Bardy, B., Di Bernardo, M., & Tsaneva-Atanasova, K. (2016). Dynamic similarity promotes interpersonal coordination in joint action. *Journal of the Royal Society Interface*, *13*(116), 20151093.

Stephen, D. G., & Dixon, J. A. (2011). Strong anticipation: Multifractal cascade dynamics modulate scaling in synchronization behaviors. *Chaos, Solitons & Fractals*, *44*(1–3), 160–168.

Tichko, P., Kim, J. C., & Large, E. W. (2021). Bouncing the network: A dynamical systems model of auditory–vestibular interactions underlying infants' perception of musical rhythm. *Developmental Science*, *24*(5), e13103.

Toiviainen, P., Luck, G., & Thompson, M. R. (2010). Embodied meter: Hierarchical eigenmodes in music-induced movement. *Music Perception*, *28*(1), 59–70.

Tomassini, A., Laroche, J., Emanuele, M., Nazzaro, G., Petrone, N., Fadiga, L., & D'Ausilio, A. (2022). Interpersonal synchronization of movement intermittency. *Iscience*, *25*(4), 104096.

Treisman, M., Faulkner, A., Naish, P. L. & Brogan, D. (1990). The internal clock: Evidence for a temporal oscillator underlying time perception with some estimates of its characteristic frequency. *Perception*, *19*(6), 705–743.

Varela, F. J. (1979). *Principles of biological autonomy*. Elsevier.

Varela, F. J. (1989). *Invitation aux sciences cognitives*. Éd. du Seuil.

Varela, F. J. (1999). The specious present: A neurophenomenology of time consciousness. In J. Petitot, F. J. Varela, B. Pachoud, & J.-M. Roy (Eds.), *Naturalizing phenomenology* (pp. 266–314). Stanford University Press.

Varela, F. J., Thompson, E., & Rosch, E. (1991). *The embodied mind: Cognitive science and human experience*. MIT Press.

Varlet, M., Marin, L., Lagarde, J., & Bardy, B. G. (2011). Social postural coordination. *Journal of Experimental Psychology: Human Perception and Performance*, *37*(2), 473–483.

Varlet, M., Schmidt, R. C., & Richardson, M. J. (2017). Influence of stimulus velocity profile on unintentional visuomotor entrainment depends on eye movements. *Experimental Brain Research*, 235(11), 3279–3286.

Varlet, M., Stoffregen, T. A., Chen, F. C., Alcantara, C., Marin, L., & Bardy, B. G. (2014). Just the sight of you: Postural effects of interpersonal visual contact at sea. *Journal of Experimental Psychology: Human Perception and Performance*, 40(6), 2310–2318.

Vicary, S., Sperling, M., von Zimmermann, J., Richardson, D. C., & Orgs, G. (2017). Joint action aesthetics. *PLoS One*, 12(7), e0180101.

Vuust, P., & Witek, M. A. (2014). Rhythmic complexity and predictive coding: A novel approach to modeling rhythm and meter perception in music. *Frontiers in Psychology*, 5, 1111.

Walton, A. E., Richardson, M. J., Langland-Hassan, P., & Chemero, A. (2015). Improvisation and the self-organization of multiple musical bodies. *Frontiers in Psychology*, 6, 313.

Walton, A. E., Washburn, A., Langland-Hassan, P., Chemero, A., Kloos, H., & Richardson, M. J. (2018). Creating time: Social collaboration in music improvisation. *Topics in Cognitive Science*, 10(1), 95–119.

Washburn, A., DeMarco, M., de Vries, S., Ariyabuddhiphongs, K., Schmidt, R. C., Richardson, M. J., & Riley, M. A. (2014). Dancers entrain more effectively than non-dancers to another actor's movements. *Frontiers in Human Neuroscience*, 8, 800.

Wiltshire, T. J., Steffensen, S. V., & Fiore, S. M. (2019). Multiscale movement coordination dynamics in collaborative team problem solving. *Applied Ergonomics*, 79, 143–151.

Wing, A. M. & Kristofferson, A. B. (1973). Response delays and the timing of discrete motor responses. *Perception and Psychophysics*, 14(1), 5–12.

Wolf, T., Sebanz, N., & Knoblich, G. (2020). Adaptation to unstable coordination patterns in individual and joint actions. *PloS One*, 15(5), e0232667.

Wöllner, C., & Hammerschmidt, D. (2021). Tapping to hip-hop: Effects of cognitive load, arousal, and musical meter on time experiences. *Attention, Perception, & Psychophysics*, 83(4), 1552–1561.

Focus Chapters

15

Time and Synchronization in Dance Movement

Birgitta Burger and Petri Toiviainen

15.1 Introduction

Music has the capacity to induce movements in humans (Keller & Rieger, 2009), particularly movements that bear a temporal, periodic relationship with the musical structure. Such temporal alignment of two or more independent processes is generally referred to as synchronization or entrainment (Clayton, 2012) which can allude to period locking, that is, processes have the same or similar periodicity, or phase locking, that is, processes are also aligned in their phase relationship (phase locking always implies period locking, but not vice versa). Periodic beat structures in music enable listeners to establish and maintain a stable periodic pattern of synchronized movement, such as nodding their head or tapping their foot. Humans tend to easily perceive and process such periodic beat patterns and spontaneously synchronize with them (for reviews on human spontaneous motor synchronization abilities, see Repp, 2005; Repp & Su, 2013). Moreover, most cultures have developed (temporally) coordinated movements to rhythmically predictable music (Brown et al., 2000).

The human capability to spontaneously synchronize with musical beats has been extensively studied using finger-tapping paradigms (Repp, 2005; Repp & Su, 2013). Various studies ranging from tapping with metronomes to complex music (e.g. Keller & Repp, 2004; Toiviainen & Snyder, 2003) suggest that humans are able to spontaneous and accurately find and entrain to (musical) beats for periods between 300 and 900 ms (e.g. Fraisse, 1982). In a tapping experiment, Janata and colleagues (2012) discovered that participants not only tapped their finger, but also moved other body parts when being asked to synchronize. Su and Pöppel (2012) found that non-musicians, in particular, tapped more synchronously with a musical stimulus when moving compared to sitting still, strongly suggesting a bodily component to the human ability to synchronize to music. This is commonly assumed to result from the coupling of the motor and auditory timing loops (Chen et al., 2008) and possibly also from the vestibular system's response to movement (Todd & Lee, 2015). For related information, see Dalla Bella (this volume).

Analysing whole-body movement induced by rhythmic stimuli or music allows one to study synchronization with tasks that are ecologically more valid than tapping,

Birgitta Burger and Petri Toiviainen, *Time and Synchronization in Dance Movement* In: *Performing Time*. Edited by: Clemens Wöllner and Justin London, Oxford University Press. © Oxford University Press 2023. DOI: 10.1093/oso/9780192896254.003.0016 as they take into account the embodied nature of music perception. Zentner and Eerola's (2010) findings regarding the ability of infants to bodily synchronize with periodic musical stimuli imply a predisposition for rhythmic movement identifiable at a young age. Furthermore, whole-body movement facilitates the identification of the complex hierarchical nature of beat perception. For instance, Toiviainen et al. (2010) showed that participants entrained to different metrical levels present in the music using different body parts and movement directions: mediolateral sway was prevalently synchronized to the whole-note level, while mediolateral and vertical arm movement was frequently synchronized to the quarter-note level. Burger et al. (2013) found that beat- and rhythm-related musical characteristics affected participants' movement responses such that torso speed increased with stronger pulse clarity, speed of head increased with stronger low-frequency spectral flux, while enhanced hand movement related to high-frequency spectral flux. These results could further suggest tighter synchronization with stronger beat structures. In the following, we will outline three studies tackling how synchronization in full-body music-induced movement is related to different musical, in particular rhythmic, characteristics and social context.

15.2 Three Studies on Human Synchronization

Experiment 1 (Burger et al., 2014) aimed to investigate relationships between periodic movement and musical, in particular beat- and rhythm-related, characteristics. Sixty participants moved individually to 30 randomly ordered stimuli of different popular music styles. All stimuli were 30 s long, non-vocal, and in 4/4 time, but differed in their musical characteristics. Participants' movement was recorded using an optical motion capture system with 28 reflective markers attached to each person (Figure 15.1a,b). Using the MATLAB Motion Capture Toolbox (Burger & Toiviainen,

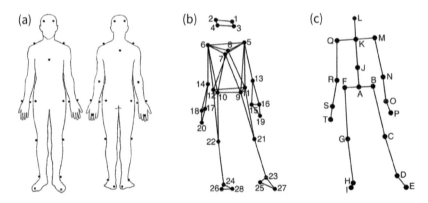

Figure 15.1 Marker and joint locations. (a) Anterior and posterior view of marker placement. (b) Anterior view of marker locations as stick figure illustration. (c) Anterior view of secondary markers/joints after a marker-to-joint transformation.

2013), acceleration of nine body parts (joints B, D, F, H, K, M, O, Q, and S, see Figure 15.1c) was calculated and subjected to periodicity estimation using autocorrelation. Each estimation was then compared to four different metrical levels—eighth-, quarter-, half-, and whole-note level—resulting in either being period locked to one of the four or not being period locked. A period-locking index per metrical level was then calculated by averaging the period occurrences. Furthermore, pulse clarity, low- and high-frequency spectral flux, and tempo from the musical stimuli were extracted and correlated with the period-locking index per metrical level and movement direction.

Results (Figure 15.2) showed significant positive correlations of quarter-note level synchronization with both pulse clarity and low-frequency flux in all directions, as well as of whole-note level synchronization with low-frequency flux in the horizontal

Study 1

Correlations (r(30))

	Eighth-note level		**Quarter-note level**		**Whole-note level**	
	sideways	**vertical**	**sideways**	**vertical**	**sideways**	**vertical**
Pulse clarity	−0.05	−0.04	**0.42***	**0.57***	0.18	−0.19
Low freq. flux	−0.10	−0.25	**0.63***	**0.54***	**0.55***	−0.08
Tempo	**−0.53***	**−0.76***	0.06	−0.17	**0.86***	**0.58***

* $p < .05$

Study 2

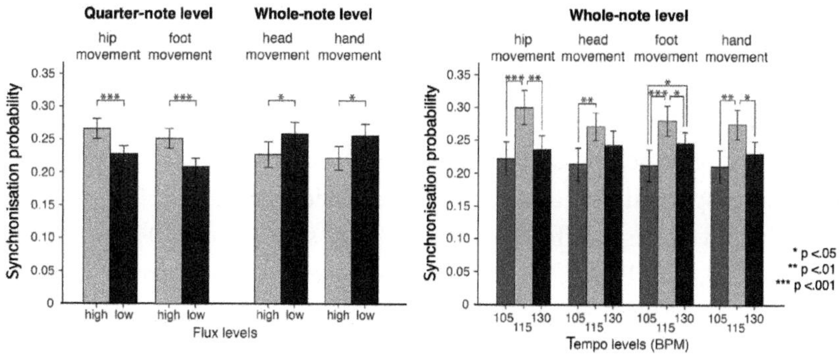

Study 3

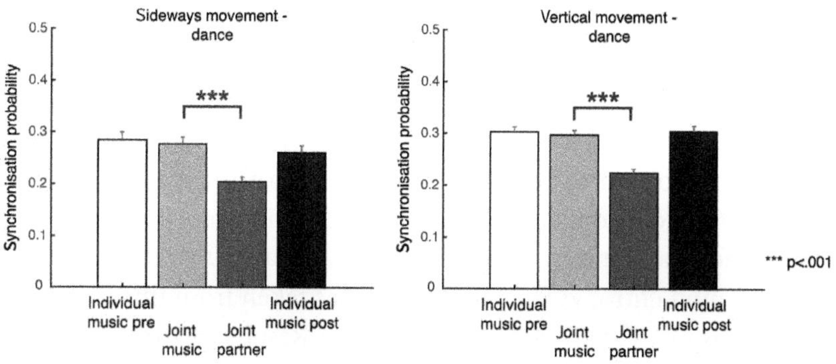

Figure 15.2 Selected results for each study.

directions, suggesting distinct relationships between low-frequency beat-related musical characteristics and periodic movement and confirming previous results by Toiviainen et al. (2010) and Burger et al. (2013). Thus, participants were strongly period locked with beat- and rhythm-related features of the music, as such features give structure and possibility for beat prediction, affording quick and spontaneous entrainment. Furthermore, tempo showed significant negative correlations with eighth-note level synchronization in mediolateral and vertical directions and positive correlations with whole-note level synchronization in all directions, suggesting that period locking to the eighth-note level was more likely for slow stimuli, while period locking to the whole-note level was more often occurring for fast stimuli. Thus, at slower tempi participants tended to synchronize more often with faster metrical levels, while at faster tempi the opposite happened, possibly due to biomechanical constraints of the human body (i.e. not being able to move too slow or too fast). These results can also be related to perceptual factors, such as the metrical level detected when listening to the stimuli, and thus seen in light of the *Dynamic Attending Theory*, according to which humans are able to switch between metrical levels, and attune to the one that seems the best fit (e.g. Jones, 1976). Furthermore, the concept of the preferred beat period of around 500 ms could play a role, in that participants adapted their movements to be as close as possible to the tempo range of around 110/120 beats per minute (BPM; e.g. Fraisse, 1982). Moreover (what this study, however, did not look into), such period-locking behaviour could be mediated by individual differences in synchronization ability, such that a person who has difficulties extracting the beat in music would display less synchronized and periodic movement than someone for whom beat extraction is easier (see also Dalla Bella, this volume).

The second study (Burger et al., 2018) aimed to extend the previous findings by investigating phase locking and its relationship to musical characteristics, namely low-frequency spectral flux and tempo. We motion-captured 30 participants who individually moved to six different Motown/R&B songs (each 30 s) at three different tempi (105, 115, 130 BPM). At each tempo, one song had strong low-frequency spectral flux, while the other exhibited weak flux. In order to quantify synchronization between music and movement, phase locking of the movement was calculated by first taking the acceleration of head, hands, hip, and feet for vertical movement at quarter-note level and mediolateral movement at whole-note level, followed by bandpass-filtering the data, and subsequently applying Hilbert transform, yielding the movement phase relative to the respective metrical level. The beat timepoints were manually annotated using SonicVisualiser (http://www.sonicvisualiser.org) and linearly interpolated to match the sample size of the movement phase data. Subsequently, to allow comparison between music and movement, the difference between the music and movement phases was calculated, and the neg-entropy (the inverse of Shannon entropy; Shannon, 1948) was taken from this difference distribution as a measure of phase-locking probability. Results (Figure 15.2) suggest that participants differed in their synchronization with respect to metrical levels, flux, and tempo. Vertical movement of hip and feet at quarter-note level was more tightly synchronized to stimuli containing strong low-frequency flux, whereas sideways movement of head and hands was better synchronized to the weak flux stimuli at whole-note level. Moreover, at whole-note level the medium tempo exhibited tighter synchronization than the other two tempi, which could relate to the concept of pre-ferred tempo around 110/120 BPM (Fraisse, 1982). These outcomes imply beat-related synchronization being embodied with particularly vertical feet and torso movement when the music showed strong beat-related characteristics. This is in line with the above presented study as well as with previous research (e.g. Toiviainen et al., 2010). Furthermore, results suggest that participants used more extensive and complex horizontal movement to entrain to stimuli containing less clear rhythmic structures, particularly with respect to longer time spans and higher metrical levels (cf. Burger et al., 2013). In addition, the results support the Dynamic Attending Theory (e.g. Jones, 1976) that participants perceived and attuned to the different metrical levels simultaneously or shifted in between to match the most-fitting level based on musical characteristics and body constraints (and certainly preferences and personality features).

The third study aimed to investigate synchronization precision in a social setting. Sixteen pairs (both familiar and unfamiliar pairs, occasional dancers) were asked to sway sideways, bounce up and down, and freely dance to six different music stimuli of popular music (30 s each), first individually, then together, and then individually again, while being recorded with optical motion capture. Speed of the hip marker was calculated, followed by phase analysis using Hilbert transform and manual phase an-notation of the music. To quantify the phase-locking probability between movement and music, the neg-entropy of the difference between movement and music phases was taken, while the neg-entropy of the difference between the movement phases of both participants was taken to quantify the phase-locking probability between the two partners. There was neither a difference in the music synchronization for any con-dition nor in the partner synchronization for sway and bounce. However, synchroni-zation probability differed significantly between music and partner synchronization in the joint dance condition for both sideways and vertical synchronization (Figure 15.2): participants were more tightly synchronized to the music than to their partner when moving together, suggesting that synchronization to music seems rather stable. Music could give flexibility to express one's own individuality, thus precise synchro-nization with each other could be diminished, while still being interactive. However, this could be mediated by the stimulus lengths (as they were rather short), the musical genre, participants' preference and familiarity, or instructions. These preliminary, but interesting results would therefore warrant further investigation.

15.3 Conclusion

Humans are able to synchronize with music; however, the highlighted studies indicate that synchronization with music and with others comprises complex relationships.

Results indicate commonalities and differences in synchronization behaviours that involve the whole body, affect body parts and movement directions differently and distinctively, occur at several metrical levels, and depend on musical characteristics that particularly relate to rhythmic and temporal structures. Furthermore, the social context could play a role in shaping synchronization responses, as well as possibly other factors, such as participants' background, individual differences, or (musical) training (see also Dalla Bella, this volume).

Real music presents a complex and rich set of affordances for rhythmic synchronization. Appropriate analysis of human movement to such musical stimuli helps to disclose these affordances. Besides attempts to generalize results of movement behaviour, neuroscientific approaches (e.g. combining motion capture with electroencephalography) could provide further insights into the underlying mechanisms of human synchronization with complex musical stimuli.

There is a need to study interaction, synchronization in particular, in social settings, in which there are two potentially competing influences occurring simultaneously: the music and other dancers (including individual differences, such as personality traits or individual synchronization abilities). Furthermore, the question whether synchronization implies interaction as well as whether a subjectively experienced 'successful interaction' even requires temporally precise synchronization or broader interactive behaviours instead, such as movement similarity, remains to be studied in the future.

References

Brown, S., Merker, B., & Wallin, N. L. (2000). An introduction to evolutionary musicology. In N. L. Wallin, B. Merker, & S. Brown (Eds.), *The origins of music* (pp. 3–24). MIT Press.

Burger, B., London, J., Thompson, M. R., & Toiviainen, P. (2018). Synchronization to metrical levels in music depends on low-frequency spectral components and tempo. *Psychological Research, 82*(6), 1195–1211.

Burger, B., Thompson, M. R., Luck, G., Saarikallio, S., & Toiviainen, P. (2014). Hunting for the beat in the body: On period and phase locking in music-induced movement. *Frontiers in Human Neuroscience, 8*, 903.

Burger, B., Thompson, M. R., Saarikallio, S., Luck, G., & Toiviainen, P. (2013). Influences of rhythm- and timbre-related musical features on characteristics of music-induced movement. *Frontiers in Psychology, 4*, 183.

Burger, B., & Toiviainen, P. (2013). MoCap Toolbox—A Matlab toolbox for computational analysis of movement data. In *Proceedings of the 10th Sound and Music Computing Conference* (pp. 172–178). KTH Royal Institute of Technology.

Chen, J. L., Penhune, V. B., & Zatorre, R. J. (2008). Listening to musical rhythms recruits motor regions of the brain. *Cerebral Cortex, 18*(12), 2844–2854.

Clayton, M. (2012). What is entrainment? Definition and applications in musical research. *Empirical Musicology Review, 7*, 49–56.

Fraisse, P. (1982). Rhythm and tempo. In D. Deutsch (Ed.), *The psychology of music* (pp. 149–180). Academic Press.

Janata, P., Tomic, S. T., & Haberman, J. M. (2012). Sensorimotor coupling in music and the psychology of the groove. *Experimental Psychology, 141*(1), 54–75.

Jones, M. C. (1976). Time, our lost dimension: Toward a new theory of perception, attention, and memory. *Psychological Review, 83*(5), 323–355.

Keller, P., & Repp, B. H. (2004). When two limbs are weaker than one: Sensorimotor syncopation with alternating hands. *Quarterly Journal of Experimental Psychology, 57*(6), 1085–1101.

Keller, P., & Rieger, M. (2009). Special issue—musical movement and synchronization. *Music Perception, 26*(5), 397–400.

Repp, B. H. (2005). Sensorimotor synchronization: A review of the tapping literature. *Psychonomic Bulletin and Review, 12*(6), 969–992.

Repp, B. H., & Su, Y.-H. (2013). Sensorimotor synchronization: A review of recent research (2006–2012). *Psychonomic Bulletin and Review, 20*(3), 403–452.

Shannon, C. E. (1948). A mathematical theory of communication. *Bell System Technical Journal, 27*(3), 379–423.

Su, Y.-H., & Pöppel, E. (2012). Body movement enhances the extraction of temporal structures in auditory sequences. *Psychological Research, 76*(3), 373–382.

Todd, N., & Lee, C. (2015). The sensory-motor theory of rhythm and beat induction 20 years on: A new synthesis and future perspectives. *Frontiers in Human Neuroscience, 9*, 444.

Toiviainen, P., Luck, G., & Thompson, M. R. (2010). Embodied meter: Hierarchical eigenmodes in music-induced movement. *Music Perception, 28*(1), 59–70.

Toiviainen, P., & Snyder, J. S. (2003). Tapping to Bach: Resonance-based modeling of pulse. *Music Perception, 21*(1), 43–80.

Zentner, M., & Eerola, T. (2010). Rhythmic engagement with music in infancy. *Proceedings of the National Academy of Sciences of the United States of America, 107*(13), 5768–5773.

16

Unravelling Individual Differences in Synchronizing to the Beat of Music

Simone Dalla Bella

16.1 Moving to a Musical Beat

When we speak, walk, or play a musical instrument we naturally and mostly automatically coordinate our actions with what we perceive. Music in particular is an excellent model for studying auditory–motor skills. This power of music to prompt a motor response is associated with features such as its rhythmic complexity, syncopation, and harmonic complexity, among others (Matthews et al., 2019; Witek et al., 2014). Humans can easily extract the regular pulse of music (i.e. its beat) from a complex auditory sequence, and align their movements to this pulse by foot tapping, dancing, or walking (beat perception and synchronization - BPS). These abilities are typically hindered by degenerative and neurodevelopmental disorders in patient populations (e.g. those with Parkinson's disease, attention deficit hyperactivity disorder, or developmental dyslexia; Bégel et al., 2022; Dalla Bella, 2020; Grahn & Brett, 2009; Puyjarinet et al.; 2017).

Music, because of its temporal regularity and the predictability of its beat, is perfectly suited to entrain our movements (Damm et al., 2020; Patel & Iversen, 2014). Motor entrainment to the beat is mediated by mechanisms whereby attention is dynamically allocated to the most rhythmically prominent elements in an auditory stimulus (e.g. the beat; Large & Jones, 1999). This process can be successfully modelled by internal neurocognitive self-sustained oscillations (Fujioka et al., 2012; Nozaradan et al., 2011). Even in the absence of motor movement, listening to a rhythmic sequence engages motor regions of the brain, such as the basal ganglia and motor cortical areas (Chen et al., 2008; Grahn & Brett, 2007).

16.2 Individual Differences in Beat Perception and Synchronization

BPS skills are widespread in the general population (Sowiński & Dalla Bella, 2013; Tranchant et al., 2016). Yet, single-case evidence suggests that individuals vary significantly in their ability to perceive the underlying pulse when listening to music,

Simone Dalla Bella, *Unravelling Individual Differences in Synchronizing to the Beat of Music* In: *Performing Time*. Edited by: Clemens Wöllner and Justin London, Oxford University Press. © Oxford University Press 2023. DOI: 10.1093/oso/9780192896254.003.0017 and in synchronizing to its beat. Rhythmic abilities can be considered on a continuum in the general population, from the most proficient (e.g. drummers, dancers) to the least proficient ones.

The latter, referred to as 'beat-deaf' or 'poor synchronizers', display poor perception of the beat and/or poor synchronization, in a variety of profiles. Rhythm perception and production are often both impaired in beat-deaf individuals (Palmer et al., 2014; Phillips-Silver et al., 2011). However, synchronization to the beat can be selectively impaired in the presence of spared beat perception (Sowiński & Dalla Bella, 2013). The reverse—poor perception with unimpaired synchronization to the beat—is also observed (Bégel et al., 2017). Also, among rhythmic stimuli, synchronization to a musical beat can be selectively impaired, while moving to a simple metronome is spared (Launay et al., 2014). Dissociations between rhythm perception and production point to partial separability of the mechanisms underpinning BPS. These individual differences are further exacerbated by disease, such as neurodegenerative and neurodevelopmental disorders, such as Parkinson's disease (Benoit et al., 2014; Grahn & Brett, 2009), attention deficit hyperactivity disorder (Puyjarinet et al., 2017), and speech and language impairments (Bégel et al., 2022; Corriveau & Goswami, 2009).

16.3 Limitations of Current Research

While single-case evidence pointing to different profiles of BPS is informative and suggestive, its generalization to the general population is not warranted. A systematic investigation in large cohorts is still lacking. In addition, the sources of this variability are still elusive. It is still unclear whether these individual profiles can account for variability in cognitive functions not related to rhythm per se. For example, recent evidence indicates a separation between the performance of beat-based and memory-based tasks (Bouwer et al., 2020; Fiveash et al., 2022; Tierney & Kraus, 2015). Yet, evidence showing links between cognitive functions such as working memory or executive functions and the performance in rhythm tasks (Puyjarinet et al., 2017; Tierney & Kraus, 2013; Woodruff Carr et al., 2014) suggests that BPS and cognitive functions may be intermingled. Another limitation of previous work is that the tasks used for testing BPS (synchronized tapping or beat perception), by requiring either voluntary rhythm production or a judgement of stimulus timing, target primarily explicit timing mechanisms. However, BPS can also engage implicit timing mechanisms, visible in the effects of temporal regularity on a non-rhythmic judgement (Nobre & Coull, 2010). Interestingly, individual differences found using explicit timing tasks may not be apparent when testing implicit timing. For example, in a recent study we contrasted the performance on explicit perceptual and auditory–motor tasks (tapping to a beat, detecting whether a metronome is aligned or not to the beat), to the performance on an implicit task in beat-deaf individuals (Bégel et al., 2017). The implicit task consisted in detecting a pitch difference following a temporally regular or irregular tone sequence (Cutanda et al., 2015). Two cases with beat-deafness displayed poor beat perception in explicit timing tasks, but spared processing of temporal regularity in an implicit timing task (Bégel et al., 2017). Thus, individual profiles for BPS skills may vary depending on the explicit or implicit nature of the tested timing mechanisms, which are known to recruit different neuronal circuitries (Coull et al., 2011).

16.4 Future Research Perspectives

Single-case evidence and studies of BPS in patient populations reveal intriguing dissociations between perception and production, and between beat-based and memory-based processes. These differences may translate into profiles characterizing individual differences in the general population, and potentially markers of impairment. Detecting individual profiles of rhythmic abilities in patient populations may play a pivotal role in devising personalized rhythm-based interventions (e.g. Dalla Bella, 2020, 2022; Dalla Bella, Benoit, et al., 2017). This possibility is appealing. However, owing to the complexity of these profiles, the task of identifying them and pinpointing the underlying mechanisms may be daunting. This difficulty can be tackled by systematic assessment of BPS using multiple tests, coupled with testing of non-rhythmic cognitive abilities.

Widespread examples of tasks testing BPS are based on finger tapping (Repp, 2005), or perceptual judgements (e.g. the Beat Alignment Test; Iversen & Patel, 2008). Fully capturing individual differences in BPS can be arduous on the basis of a single rhythm task, though. Performance in perceptual and production tasks are not always correlated (Dalla Bella, Farrugia, et al., 2017; Fujii & Schlaug, 2013). This points to the existence of potentially separable rhythmic abilities that may be underpinned by distinct neural mechanisms. To systematically probe BPS abilities, batteries of perception and production tests have been recently devised such as the Battery for the Assessment of Auditory Sensorimotor and Timing Abilities (BAASTA; Dalla Bella, Farrugia, et al., 2017), and the Harvard Beat Alignment Test (H-BAT; Fuji & Schlaug, 2013). Owing to the portability of these testing tools on mobile devices (e.g. Zagala et al., 2021), they can afford reliable data collection from large samples of participants. Data collection using an extensive set of tests (rhythmic and non-rhythmic), in large samples, is conducive to applying data mining techniques and machine learning, such as clustering and supervised learning (e.g. Hastie et al., 2009). This approach can serve for identifying the minimal set of measures for characterizing individual profiles based on BPS measures in the general population and in patients, and to determine whether these profiles are influenced by more general cognitive functions. In addition, knowledge of individual profiles in BPS can be used to guide music-based interventions based on auditory–motor synchronization. Along this line, recent examples show that the individual performance in BPS allows prediction of the success of a rhythm-based intervention on motor performance (i.e. gait) in patients with movement disorders (Dalla Bella et al., 2018). Moreover this information can be integrated in applications capable of providing individualized rhythmic stimulation to patients in real time (for an example with Parkinson's disease, see Dotov et al., 2019).

16.5 Conclusion

Individuals vary significantly in their capacity to track the beat of music and move along with it. These differences may reveal the complex cognitive and neuronal architecture underpinning BPS skills. Methods relying on multivariate measures coupled with advanced data mining techniques can unravel this complexity, while paving the way to personalized music-based interventions (e.g. Agres et al., 2021).

References

Agres, K. R., Schaefer, R. S., Volk, A., van Hooren, S., Holzapfel, A., Dalla Bella, S., Müller, M., de Witte, M., Herremans, D., Ramirez Melendez, R., Neerincx, M., Ruiz, S., Meredith, D., Dimitriadis, T., & Magee, W. L. (2021). Music, computing, and health: A roadmap for the current and future roles of music technology for healthcare and well-being. *Music & Science, 4*, 1–32.

Bégel, V., Benoit, C. E., Correa, A., Cutanda, D., Kotz, S. A., & Dalla Bella, S. (2017). 'Lost in time' but still moving to the beat. *Neuropsychologia, 94*, 129–138.

Bégel, V., Dalla Bella, S., Devignes, A., Vanderbergue, M., Lemaître, M. P., & Dellacherie, D. (2022). Rhythm as an independent determinant of developmental dyslexia. *Developmental Psychology, 58*(2), 339–358.

Benoit, C.E., Dalla Bella, S., Farrugia, N., Obrig, H., Mainka, S., & Kotz, S. A. (2014). Musically cued gait-training improves both perceptual and motor timing in Parkinson's disease. *Frontiers in Human Neuroscience, 8*, 494.

Bouwer, F. L., Honing, H., & Slagter, H. A. (2020). Beat-based and memory-based temporal expectations in rhythm: Similar perceptual effects, different underlying mechanisms. *Journal of Cognitive Neuroscience, 32*(7), 1221–1241.

Chen, J. L., Penhune, V. B., & Zatorre, R. J. (2008). Listening to musical rhythms recruits motor regions of the brain. *Cerebral Cortex, 18*(12), 2844–2854.

Corriveau, K. H., & Goswami, U. (2009). Rhythmic motor entrainment in children with speech and language impairments: Tapping to the beat. *Cortex, 45*(1), 119–130.

Coull, J. T., Cheng, R.-K., & Meck, W. H. (2011). Neuroanatomical and neurochemical substrates of timing. *Neuropsychopharmacology, 36*(1), 3–25.

Cutanda, D., Correa, A., & Sanabria, D. (2015). Auditory temporal preparation induced by rhythmic cues during concurrent auditory working memory tasks. *Journal of Experimental Psychology: Human Perception and Performance, 41*(3), 790–797.

Dalla Bella, S. (2020). The use of rhythm in rehabilitation for patients with movement disorders. In L. Cuddy, S. Belleville, & A. Moussard (Eds.), *Music and the aging brain* (pp. 383–406). Elsevier.

Dalla Bella, S. (2022). Rhythmic serious games as an inclusive tool for music-based interventions. *Annals of the New York Academy of Sciences, 1517*(1), 15–24.

Dalla Bella, S., Benoit, C.-E., Farrugia, N., Keller, P. E., Obrig, H., Mainka, S., & Kotz, S. A. (2017). Gait improvement via rhythmic stimulation in Parkinson's disease is linked to rhythmic skills. *Scientific Reports, 7*, 42005.

Dalla Bella, S., Dotov, D. G., Bardy, B., & Cochen de Cock, V. (2018). Individualization of music-based rhythmic auditory cueing in Parkinson's disease. *Annals of the New York Academy of Sciences, 1423*(1), 308–317.

Dalla Bella, S., Farrugia, N., Benoit, C. E., Bégel, V., Verga, L., Harding, E., & Kotz, S. A. (2017). BAASTA: Battery for the Assessment of Auditory Sensorimotor and Timing Abilities. *Behavior Research Methods, 49*(3), 1128–1145.

Damm, L., Varoqui, D., Cochen De Cock, V., et al. (2020). A multi-scale approach, from physical principles to brain dynamics. *Neuroscience & Biobehavioral Reviews, 112*, 553–584.

Dotov, D. G., Cochen de Cock, V., Geny, C., Ihalainen, P., Moens, B., Leman, M., Bardy, B., & Dalla Bella, S. (2019). The role of mutual synchronization and predictability in entraining walking to an auditory stimulus. *Journal of Experimental Psychology: General, 148*(6), 1041–1057.

Fiveash, A., Dalla Bella, S., Bigand, E., Gordon, R., & Tillmann, B. (2022). You got rhythm, or more: The multidimensionality of rhythmic abilities. *Attention, Perception & Psychophysics, 84*, 1370–1392.

Fujii, S., & Schlaug, G. (2013). The Harvard Beat Assessment Test (H-BAT): A battery for assessing beat perception and production and their dissociation. *Frontiers in Human Neuroscience, 7*, 771.

Fujioka, T., Trainor, L. J., Large, E. W., & Ross, B. (2012). Internalized timing of isochronous sounds is represented in neuromagnetic β oscillations. *Journal of Neuroscience, 32*(5), 1791–1802.

Grahn, J. A., & Brett, M. (2007). Rhythm and beat perception in motor areas of the brain. *Journal of Cognitive Neuroscience, 19*(5), 893–906.

Grahn, J. A., & Brett, M. (2009). Impairment of beat-based rhythm discrimination in Parkinson's disease. *Cortex, 45*(1), 54–61.

Hastie, T., Tibshirani, R., & Friedman, J. (2009). *The elements of statistical learning.* Springer.

Iversen, J. R., & Patel, A. D. (2008). The Beat Alignment Test (BAT): Surveying beat processing abilities in the general population. In K. Miyazaki, Y. Hiraga, M. Adachi, Y. Nakajima, and M. Tsuzaki (Eds.), *Proceedings of the 10th International Conference on Music Perception and Cognition (ICMPC10) Sapporo, Japan* (pp. 465–468). Causal Productions.

Large, E. W., & Jones, M. R. (1999). The dynamics of attending: How people track time-varying events. *Psychological Review, 106*(1), 119–159.

Launay, J., Grube, M., & Stewart, L. (2014). Dysrhythmia: A specific congenital rhythm perception deficit. *Frontiers in Psychology, 5*, 18.

Matthews, T. E., Witek, M. A. G., Heggli, O. A., Penhune, V. B., & Vuust, P. (2019). The sensation of groove is affected by the interaction of rhythmic and harmonic complexity. *PLoS One, 14*(1), e0204539.

Nobre, K., & Coull, J. T. (2010). *Attention and time.* Oxford University Press.

Nozaradan, S., Peretz, I., Missal, M., & Mouraux, A. (2011). Tagging the neuronal entrainment to beat and meter. *Journal of Neuroscience, 31*(28), 10234–10240.

Palmer, C., Lidji, P., & Peretz, I. (2014). Losing the beat: Deficits in temporal coordination. *Philosophical Transactions of the Royal Society of London. Series B, Biological Sciences, 369*(1658), 20130405.

Patel, A. E., & Iversen, J. R. (2014). The evolutionary neuroscience of musical beat perception: The Action Simulation for Auditory Prediction (ASAP) hypothesis. *Frontiers in Systems Neuroscience, 8*, 57.

Phillips-Silver, J., Toiviainen, P., Gosselin, N., Piche, O., Nozaradan, S., Palmer, C., & Peretz, I. (2011). Born to dance but beat deaf: A new form of congenital amusia. *Neuropsychologia, 49*(5), 961–969.

Puyjarinet, F., Bégel, V., Lopez, R., Dellacherie, D., & Dalla Bella, S. (2017). Children and adults with attention-deficit/hyperactivity disorders cannot move to the beat. *Scientific Reports, 7*(1), 11550.

Repp, B. H. (2005). Sensorimotor synchronization: A review of the tapping literature. *Psychonomic Bulletin & Review, 12*(6), 969–992.

Sowiński, J., & Dalla Bella, S. (2013). Poor synchronization to the beat may result from deficient auditory-motor mapping. *Neuropsychologia, 51*(10), 1952–1963.

Tierney, A. T., & Kraus, N. (2013). The ability to tap to a beat relates to cognitive, linguistic, and perceptual skills. *Brain and Language, 124*(3), 225–231.

Tierney, A., & Kraus, N. (2015). Evidence for multiple rhythmic skills. *PLoS One, 10*(9), e0136645.

Tranchant, P., Vuvan, D.T., & Peretz, I. (2016). Keeping the beat: A large sample study of bouncing and clapping to music. *PLoS One, 11*(7), e0160178.

Witek, M. A., Clarke, E. F., Wallentin, M., Kringelbach, M. L, & Vuust, P. (2014). Syncopation, body-movement and pleasure in groove music. *PLoS One, 9*(4), e94446.

Woodruff Carr, K., White-Schwoch, T., Tierney, A. T., Strait, D. L., & Kraus, N. (2014). Beat synchronization predicts neural speech encoding and reading readiness in preschoolers. *Proceedings of the National Academy of Sciences of the United States of America, 111*(40), 14559–14564.

Zagala, A., Foster, N. E. V., & Dalla Bella, S. (2021). Commentary: A tablet-based assessment of rhythmic ability. *Frontiers in Psychology, 12,* 607676.

17

Shaping the Beat Bin in Computer-Based Grooves

Anne Danielsen

17.1 Introduction

Catching the correct or intended basic pulse is fundamental to the production and perception of all musical rhythms with a metre. This pulse can be more or less articulated in sound and is vital to understanding a groove. That the pulse is not always clear, or even present (see London, this volume), in the sound points to the fact that the feeling of pulse emerges in the meeting of sound and listener. Importantly, the beats in such a pulse are not simply a stream of points in time but have a distinct shape: they can be narrow or wide, have a more or less clear peak, be skewed to one side, and so on. The shape of this internal pulse is important for the overall feel of the rhythm.

The rhythmic events evoking the internal pulse in the listener may be shaped in different ways. Sometimes they are clear and sharp, inducing an unambiguous point-like pulse in the perceiver. However, they may also have a temporal shape that makes their location in time difficult to locate relative to a single point in time, inducing a pulse with a wider, more saddle-like shape in the listener. Often this comes as a consequence of multiple, but slightly asynchronous events marking the beat or digital sound processing obscuring the beat's exact location.

In the following, I present the beat bin theory and discuss its implications for synchronizing with a musical rhythm. The theory states that the precision with which we process beats in a groove-based context varies systematically with the width and shape of the beat-related rhythmic events in the sounding rhythm. The beat bin is defined as the *perceptual* counterpart to the sound(s) that are located at beat-related metrical positions. I will focus on how various acoustic factors influence the beat bin and present some examples of beat-related events in computer-based musical grooves. Ultimately, I discuss how different beat bins might affect the feel of a rhythmic groove and provide different affordances for synchronization.

Anne Danielsen, *Shaping the Beat Bin in Computer-Based Grooves* In: *Performing Time*. Edited by: Clemens Wöllner and Justin London, Oxford University Press. © Oxford University Press 2023. DOI: 10.1093/oso/9780192896254.003.0018

17.2 What Is the Beat Bin and What Acoustic Factors Influence It?

The beat bin theory grew out of musical analyses of African American groove-based music of the last three decades. In hip-hop and related musical styles, one often finds that beat-related sound events are 'muddy' (i.e. have no clear attack) or that several, asynchronous events (with or without clear attacks) refer to the same metrical position. Both make the exact location of beats unclear and work to extend the perceptual beat bin. In neo-soul, for example, rhythmic layers are often deliberately displaced from 50 ms to as much as 100 ms in relation to each other, producing multiple locations of the same beat at the microrhythmic level (Figure 17.1).

The beat bin theory states that in response to such 'multiple' beats, the *perceptual* beat, or tactus, will normally take the shape of a wider 'bin' that encompasses *all* beat-related events, merging them into one compound sound. The width and shape of the beat bin is influenced by the acoustic features of the beat-related events. However, the stylistic expectations of the listener also play a role here. If 'muddy' or 'multiple' beats are typical of the style, an enculturated listener will probably immediately apply a wide beat bin to the processing of rhythmic events, and vice versa: if the listener has been trained in a 'tight' timing tradition, that is, where rhythmic events are produced and perceived with high temporal resolution, the beat bin will probably be narrow from the outset.

The probability distribution of perceived synchronization points within the beat bin is not flat. As has been shown in perception experiments (Danielsen et al., 2019; Wright, 2008), there is usually a peak (sometimes also more than one) in the probability distribution. Depending on the shape of the sound, this peak can be flat or sharp. It has been labelled the perceptual centre (P-centre) of the sound (Morton et al., 1976) or the perceptual attack time (Gordon, 1987), and various methods of adjustment and tapping tasks have been used to identify its location and variability (London et al., 2019; Villing, 2010).

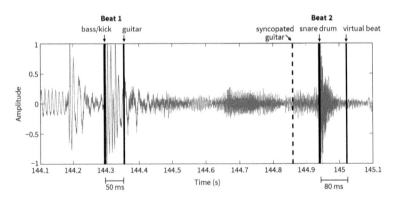

Figure 17.1 Asynchronies between bass drum/bass and guitar stroke at beat 1, and snare drum and virtual beat position projected by the syncopated guitar at beat 2 in D'Angelo's 'Left & Right'. Reproduced from Danielsen et al. (2015).

Some acoustic factors have repeatedly been found to have a systematic effect on the location of the P-centre and shape of the beat bin. The perception of varying *attack rise times* (from now on 'attack') has been tested for both music and speech sounds (for a review, see Villing, 2010). If the rise time of the sound is slow/ gradual, the peak is later and the distribution of synchronization points wider compared to sound with a fast/sharp attack (Danielsen et al., 2019; Gordon, 1987; London et al., 2019; Vos & Rasch, 1981; Wright, 2008). As to duration, longer durations produce wider beat bins than short durations. However, there is a strong interaction with attack since the effect of duration is by and large limited to sounds with a slow attack (Danielsen et al., 2019). Frequency range has also been tested, but the results are mixed (Danielsen et al., 2019; Hove et al., 2007; Seton, 1989). Relative intensity also seems to influence the perceptual location of a sound, such that higher relative intensity leads the listener to perceive the beat earlier (Bechtold & Senn, 2018; Gordon, 1987). Contextual factors are also likely to influence the perceived location and width of beat bins, but little research into this has been conducted so far.

17.3 Extending the Beat Bin by Multiple or Muddy Beats

There are many production and performance techniques for manipulating beat shapes. One is to introduce multiple, slightly asynchronous events at beat-related positions, either by relative microtiming between rhythmic layers in performed grooves or by stacking sounds atop of each other in a digital audio workstation. A classic example is D'Angelo's and other neo-soul artists' preference for inserting 'glitches' between rhythmic layers in an otherwise organic-sounding rhythmic context. D'Angelo's song 'Left & Right' (from the album *Voodoo*, 2000), for example, begins with just guitar and percussion. All sounds in this part are sharp, percussive sounds with fast attack and short duration, which is likely to yield a narrow beat bin and tight phase and period synchronization. Next follows the entrance of the combined drum kit and bass layer. This introduces a discrepancy between the two pulse-carrying layers of around 50 (beats 1 and 3) to 80 (beats 2 and 4) ms, that is, between 8% and 12% of a quarter note at the song's tempo of 92 beats per minute (Danielsen, 2010; see also Figure 17.1). Following this, the listener may experience a transition period where the perceptual beat bin adjusts to the glitch, that is, widens it to accommodate both beat positions. This involves a perceptual change only (i.e. there is no change in the sounding rhythm), and results in the experience of being fully synchronized with all layers in the groove. This is where the groove evolves into a more rolling feel. According to the beat bin theory, this is because the listener has adjusted to the multiple onsets: the width and shape of each pulsation in the listener's internal (perceptual) pulse reference has changed from a narrow, point-like to a wider, more saddle-shaped beat bin that encompasses the beat locations of the various rhythmic

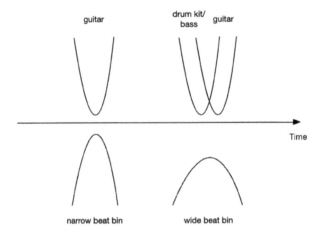

Figure 17.2 Transition from narrow to wide beat bin.

layers of the groove (Figure 17.2). This wider beat bin affords stable period synchronization but is slightly more tolerant as to phase.

Another musical aspect that may cause a widening of the beat bin is to use sounds
that in themselves are 'muddy' at beat positions in the pulse-carrying rhythmic
layers. Typically, such sounds do not display a clear attack point due to a gradual
or smooth attack. The integration of various digital music production tools in digital audio workstations has made it possible to 'muddify' sounds in new and radical ways. This has widened the sonic palette of contemporary groove-based music
considerably (Danielsen, 2019; Brøvig-Hanssen & Danielsen, 2016). A classic example of a muddy sound from hip-hop is the synth bass sound depicted in Figure
17.3, sampled from Snoop Dogg's 'Can I Get A Flicc Witchu' (from the album *R&G
[Rhythm & Gangsta]: The Masterpiece*, 2004). Due to the gradual attack, this sound
has no clear temporal location at the microlevel. When tested in a P-centre task, the
variability of click alignments to this sound was around 21 ms, which might be taken

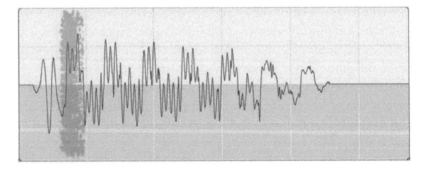

Figure 17.3 Synth bass sound from Snoop Dogg's 'Can I Get A Flicc Witchu'. Danielsen et al.
(2019) found that the P-centre of this sound was 23 ms after the onset (click alignment task),
and the variability 21 ms (location and width of beat bin illustrated in orange).

as an indication of how wide the perceptual bin produced by this sound is (Danielsen et al., 2019).

17.4 Rhythmic Feel and Affordances for Synchronization

How do these different beat bins affect the feel of the respective grooves? This is a complex question since the feel of a groove is a mix of many factors such as tempo, timing, articulation, and density of events, in combination with structural-stylistic figures (cross-rhythmic tendencies, off-beat patterns, stylistic figures, and so on). However, narrow beat bins generally mean low tolerance for timing 'deviations', that is, events that are played early and late will in such a context be heard and felt as early or late. With a wider beat bin, on the other hand, the same microtiming might be experienced as 'on the beat' since a wider bin absorbs the early/late events and make them part of the beat. Early and/or late experiences are of course also possible with wider bins, but then the microtiming needs to be more extreme.

The highly relative and contextual nature of what is actually perceived as early, on the beat, versus late (see, e.g. Danielsen et al., 2021) is an overlooked aspect in the microtiming literature, which tends to measure microtiming in relation to an isochronous grid and assume that the measured values are representative for the experience. The relative nature of experienced microtiming becomes particularly salient when comparing the very different traditions for shaping the basic pulse in different musical genres. In a grid-based genre such as electronic dance music, for example, a track delay of 5–10 ms magnitude is often characterized as late timing (Brøvig-Hanssen et al., 2022) and more extreme delays would probably be experienced as a mistake. In contrast, as demonstrated above, in neo-soul, discrepancies between layers of up to 100 ms are quite common (see also Bjerke, 2010; Carlsen & Witek, 2010; Danielsen, 2018) and will most likely be experienced as the groove having the correct 'feel'.

These differences in the ways in which microrhythmic features are perceived will, of course, affect the groove's affordances for synchronization. A wide beat bin increases the listener's overall tolerance (Johansson, 2010) for 'imprecise' location of rhythmic events. It means a greater openness to where rhythmic events can take place at the micro level and still produce a feeling of a largely isochronous pulse that invites stable synchronization. Wide beat bins also increase musicians' tolerance for where and how their respective sounds can be synchronized and still form a singular rhythmic event. Accordingly, when we have tested synchronization to a battery of sounds of different shapes (shapes were systematically varied with regard to attack and duration), slow attack sounds with long duration yielded most variability as to where the participants synchronized a click and tap with the sound (Danielsen et al., 2019, 2021). Similar results were obtained when testing with a slow attack noise sound as probe. However, when synchronizing the noise probe to a sound with a very similar shape, the variability decreased compared to results for sounds with different shapes, suggesting that the two beat bins are synchronized to create maximum overlap (London et al., 2019).

In an experiment using the groove from D'Angelo's 'Left and Right' described above (Danielsen et al., 2015), we found that beat bin width and shape also influence the shape and accuracy of synchronizing to the pulse of the music. We explained this by way of the *Dynamic Attending Theory* (Jones, 1976; Large & Jones, 1999) which claims that endogenous attending rhythms synchronize with external rhythms via a process of entrainment (Large & Jones, 1999, p. 123). Attending rhythms point to where in a repeated cycle a salient event is likely to occur and involves a process whereby attentional energy is allocated over time (Jones, 1976). Like the concept of beat bin, Dynamic Attending Theory presupposes that the distribution of attentional energy over time is flexible: depending on predictions regarding the nature of forthcoming events, it can become sharper and point-like, or conversely more extended in time. In terms of synchronization, however, the Dynamic Attending Theory claims that the beat bin/attentional peak narrows as synchronization improves and widens as synchronization degrades. However, whereas wider beat bins may result in looser phase synchronization (Danielsen et al., 2015), period synchronization does not necessarily decrease (Hove et al., 2007). Generally, overall phase error has been found to be lower between two human musicians than between a human musician and a metronome (Himberg, 2014; Repp, 2005; Repp & Su, 2013). Wider beat bins might thus be preferable in many musical contexts and engender joint action: more events are perceived as synchronous and there is less need for overt phase correction.

17.5 Conclusion

The beat bin theory suggests that the perceptual counterpart to beat asynchronies or widened beat shapes in a sounding groove is an internal reference structure of beat bins of considerable 'width' and a distinctive 'shape'. The theory aims to explain how micro-level synchronization to sound is optimized for the task at hand, taking into account the flexibility and dynamic nature of the human apparatus when it comes to perceiving, predicting, and processing rhythm. Narrow beat bins afford period synchronization with precise phase-locking. A widened beat bin still affords stable period synchronization but with a looser phase-locking. Wider beat bins might thus be beneficial for stable synchronization with auditory rhythms where micro-level features are shaped in a way that makes predicting exact beat locations irrelevant or even counterproductive.

References

Bechtold, T. A., & Senn, O. (2018). Articulation and dynamics influence the perceptual attack time of saxophone sounds. *Frontiers in Psychology*, 9, 1692–1692. https://doi.org/10.3389/fpsyg.2018.01692

Bjerke, K. (2010). Timbral relationships and microrhythmic tension: Shaping the groove experience through sound. In A. Danielsen (Ed.), *Musical rhythm in the age of digital reproduction* (pp. 85–101). Ashgate/Routledge. https://doi.org/10.4324/9781315596983-6

Brøvig-Hanssen, R., & Danielsen, A. (2016). *Digital signatures: The impact of digitization on popular music sound.* MIT Press.

Brøvig-Hanssen, R., Sandvik, B., Aareskjold, J. M., & Danielsen, A. (2022). A grid in flux: Sound and timing in electronic dance music. *Music Theory Spectrum*, 44(1), 1–16.

Carlsen, K., & Witek, M. A. G. (2010). Simultaneous rhythmic events with different schematic affiliations: Microtiming and dynamic attending in two contemporary R&B grooves. In A. Danielsen (Ed.), *Musical rhythm in the age of digital reproduction* (pp. 51–68). Ashgate/Routledge. https://doi.org/10.4324/9781315596983-4

Danielsen, A. (2010). Here, there, and everywhere. Three accounts of pulse in D'Angelo's 'Left and Right'. In A. Danielsen (Ed.), *Musical rhythm in the age of digital reproduction* (pp. 19–36). Ashgate/Routledge. https://doi.org/10.4324/9781315596983-2

Danielsen, A. (2018). Pulse as dynamic attending: Analysing beat bin metre in neo soul grooves. In C. Scotto, K. M. Smith, & J. Brackett (Eds.), *The Routledge companion to popular music analysis: Expanding approaches* (pp. 179–189). Routledge. https://doi.org/10.4324/9781315544700

Danielsen, A. (2019). Glitched and warped: Transformations of rhythm in the age of the digital audio workstation. In M. Walther-Hansen & M. Knakkergaard (Eds.), *The Oxford handbook of sound and imagination, volume 2* (pp. 595–609). Oxford University Press. https://doi.org/10.1093/oxfordhb/9780190460242.013.27

Danielsen, A., Haugen, M. R., & Jensenius. A. R. (2015). Moving to the beat: Studying entrainment to micro-rhythmic changes in pulse by motion capture. *Timing and Time Perception*, 3(12), 133–154. http://dx.doi.org/10.1163/22134468-00002043

Danielsen, A., Nymoen, K., Anderson, E., Câmara, G. S., Langerød, M. T., Thompson, M. R., & London, J. (2019). Where is the beat in that note? Effects of attack, duration, and frequency on the perceived timing of musical and quasi-musical sounds. *Journal of Experimental Psychology: Human Perception and Performance*, 45(3), 402–418. https://doi.org/10.1037/xhp0000611

Danielsen, A., Nymoen, K., Langerød, M. T., Jacobsen, E., Johansson, M., & London, J. (2022). Sounds familiar(?): Expertise with specific musical genres modulates timing perception and micro-level synchronization to auditory stimuli. *Attention, Perception and Psychophysics*, 84(2), 599–615. https://doi.org/10.3758/s13414-021-02393-z

Gordon, J. W. (1987). The perceptual attack time of musical tones. *Journal of the Acoustical Society of America*, 82(1), 88–105. https://doi.org/10.1121/1.395441

Himberg, T. (2014). *Interaction in musical time* [Doctoral dissertation]. Apollo, University of Cambridge Repository. https://doi.org/10.17863/CAM.15930

Hove, M. J., Keller, P. E., & Krumhansl, C. J. (2007). Sensorimotor synchronization with chords containing tone-onset asynchronies. *Perception & Psychophysics*, 69(5), 699–708. https://doi.org/10.3758/BF03193772

Johansson, M. (2010). The concept of rhythmic tolerance. In A. Danielsen (Ed.), *Musical rhythm in the age of digital reproduction* (pp. 69–84). Ashgate/Routledge. https://doi.org/10.4324/978131 5596983-5

Jones, M. R. (1976). Time, our lost dimension: Toward a new theory of perception, attention, and memory. *Psychological Review*, 83(5), 323–355. https://doi.org/10.1037/0033-295X.83.5.323

Large, E. W., & Jones, M. R. (1999). The dynamics of attending. *Psychological Review*, 106(1), 119–159. https://doi.org/10.1037/0033-295X.106.1.119

London, J., Nymoen, K., Langerød, M. T., Thompson, M. R., Code, D. L., & Danielsen, A. (2019). A comparison of methods for investigating the perceptual center of musical sounds. *Attention, Perception and Psychophysics*, 81(6), 2088–2101. https://doi.org/10.3758/s13414-019-01747-y

Morton, J., Marcus, S., & Frankish, C. (1976). Perceptual centers (P-centers). *Psychological Review*, 83(5), 405–408. https://doi.org/10.1037/0033-295X.83.5.405

Repp, B. H. (2005). Sensorimotor synchronization: A review of the tapping literature. *Psychonomic Bulletin & Review*, 12(6), 969–992. https://doi.org/10.3758/BF03206433

Repp, B. H., & Su, Y.-H. (2013). Sensorimotor synchronization: A review of recent research (2006–2012). *Psychonomic Bulletin & Review*, 20(3), 403–452. https://doi.org/10.3758/s13423-012-0371-2

Seton, J. C. (1989). *A psychophysical investigation of auditory rhythmic beat perception* [Doctoral dissertation]. University of York.

Villing, R. (2010). *Hearing the moment: Measures and models of the perceptual centre* [Doctoral dissertation]. National University of Ireland Maynooth.

Vos, J., & Rasch, R. (1981). The perceptual onset of musical tones. *Perception and Psychophysics, 29*(4), 323–335. https://doi.org/10.3758/BF03207341

Wright, M. (2008). *The shape of an instant: Measuring and modelling perceptual attack time with probability density functions* [Doctoral dissertation, Stanford University].

18

The 'Synchrony Effect' in Dance

How Rhythmic Scaffolding and Vision Facilitate Social Cohesion

Matthew H. Woolhouse

18.1 Introduction

The desire to watch people dance and to take part oneself, given the right conditions, appears to be universal (Hanna, 1987). From our current perspective, the mass appeal of broadcast dance shows indicates that people find it to be singularly captivating (Allen, 2010; Wood, 2010). And historically, Charles Darwin's note of the first encounter between the crew of the *Beagle* and the inhabitants of Tierra del Fuego is particularly revealing:

> When a song was struck up by our party, I thought the Fuegians would have fallen down with astonishment. With equal surprise they viewed our dancing; but one of the young men, when asked, had no objection to a little waltzing. (Darwin, 1860/1939, p. 217)

Culturally and geographically, then, dance was and continues to be a common form of entertainment and important in many human interactions. Indeed, the notion that dance is particularly able to express emotional and mental states has led some to speculate that it might have a privileged social role, a kind of *telos* of human life (LaMothe, 2015). In the meeting described by Darwin, it is difficult to imagine a more effective means of affective communication other than dance.

Between individuals, participatory dance is characterized by synchronous repetitive and rhythmic movement, a coupling process referred to as 'interpersonal entrainment' (Clayton et al., 2005; Phillips-Silver & Keller, 2012). Unsurprisingly, music—dance's ever-present counterpart—is similarly composed of repetitive and rhythmic motives and phrases, in which a hierarchy of beats and pulses (London, 2012; Large & Jones, 1999) allows dancers to plan, predict, and coordinate their movements (Himberg & Thompson, 2011). While our increasingly urban and, arguably, isolated lifestyles (Krivo et al., 2013) may currently obscure the importance of dance, recent research has sought to explore the various functions that it may play in different social settings.

Matthew H. Woolhouse, *The 'Synchrony Effect' in Dance* In: *Performing Time*. Edited by: Clemens Wöllner and Justin London, Oxford University Press. © Oxford University Press 2023. DOI: 10.1093/oso/9780192896254.003.0019

Three complementary hypotheses, relating to courtship, coalition signalling, and social bonding, are thought to account for the historic and geographic prevalence of dance. In brief, the courtship hypothesis states that dance creates a safe, power-neutral space in which people can become familiar with one another (Grammer et al., 1998; Luck et al., 2012a; Miller, 2000). In this scenario, mate-fitness selection may occur when agility and coordination are elevated in importance (Luck et al., 2012b). Proponents of the 'coalition signalling' hypothesis advance the idea that dance evolved through group coordination, principally with the aim of establishing and reinforcing alliances and/or territories (Hagen & Hammerstein, 2009; Phillips-Silver et al., 2010; Wiltermuth & Heath, 2009). The Māori haka, which is regularly performed by the New Zealand All Blacks rugby team when facing their opponents, could be considered a good exemplar (Calabrò, 2016). Lastly, theories relating to social bonding propose that dance and music co-evolved, culturally and perhaps biologically, as mechanisms for creating cohesion between non-kin individuals (Cross, 2008; Cross & Woodruff, 2009; Honing, 2013; Phillips-Silver, 2009). Experimental evidence exists to support the social bonding hypothesis (e.g. Cirelli et al., 2014; Kirschner & Tomasello, 2010; Pearce et al., 2015; Rabinowitch et al., 2013; Tarr et al., 2015) and it is this line of inquiry that was explored in the following studies, with particular reference to the role that vision may play in dance, music, and social cohesion.

18.2 Three Dance Studies

18.2.1 Group Dancing

Study 1 (Woolhouse et al., 2016) explored whether in-tempo dancing enhances interpersonal memory, a hypothesized prerequisite of social bonding—if people cannot remember aspects of one another, *ipso facto* they cannot bond. Forty participants, all of whom were unaware of the experiment's aim, were divided into four separate groups, each consisting of 10 mixed-ability dancers. Upon entry into the studio, the 10 participants of a group were photographed and provided with wireless 'silent-disco' headphones and different-coloured shoulder-to-hip sashes, some of which had cat symbols. The headphones were (surreptitiously) set to receive music on one of two channels. Depending upon the channel setting, the headphones played different music to different dancers—unbeknown to the participants, within each group, five heard music at one tempo, and five heard music at a different tempo. To ensure relatively equal overall dancer proximity, a pattern of 10 large interlocking hexagons with directional arrows was taped to the dancefloor. Using periodic auditory cues, the dancers progressed from one hexagon to the next via the arrows, resulting in each dancer being brought into a neighbour relationship with every other dancer. Immediately following the dance portion of the session, which lasted 8 minutes, the participants were visually isolated from each another and tasked with remembering the sash colours and cat-symbol status (present or absent) of the nine other members of their group; hitherto, they had been unaware of this requirement. The experiment was repeated for the remaining three groups. Results showed that participants listening to the same music (i.e. those dancing at the same tempo) had significantly increased memory for one another's sash colours and cat symbols. The recall of sash colour and cat symbol of those who danced at different tempos was relatively reduced. Woolhouse et al. (2016) conjectured that an audiovisual integration mechanism, sensitive to beat and limb movement, might account for this finding. Participants danced freely, in any manner they chose, and thus their movements were not precisely matched, as in previous synchronization research (e.g. Macrae et al., 2008). Such a mechanism might therefore require a high degree of visual acuity, which is presumably reflected in eye-movement behaviours, such as fixation durations and positions, and saccades (the path between fixations). While increased gaze between the in-tempo dancers could account for the results, the possibility also exists that audiovisual alignment of music and body leads to greater focused attention (Turino, 1999, p. 234). Alternatively, then, this could explain the observed enhanced memory effect, which, as stated above, is assumed to be a prerequisite of social bonding. The second study investigated this matter.

18.2.2 Gaze and Attentional Focus

Study 2 (see Woolhouse & Lai, 2014) examined whether audiovisual synchrony with respect to music and dance resulted in increased gaze (or 'dwell') time and/or greater attentional focus (for a related cross-cultural study, see Ponmanadiyil & Woolhouse, 2018). Twenty participants with normal or corrected-to-normal vision watched split-screen videos of two laterally positioned dancers; one dancer was synchronized with the music, the other was asynchronous. Using a bright-pupil eye-tracking camera, the dwell times, saccade lengths, and fixation durations of the participants were recoded with respect to two regions of interest: the synchronous and the asynchronous dancers, dancing either on the left or right of the screen.[1] Dwell duration was significantly greater for the synchronized dancer, indicating a preference for watching dancing in which audiovisual integration was seamless. Moreover, saccades were shorter for the synchronized dancer—relatively large scan paths occurred for the asynchronous dancer. An effect of asynchronous music and dance, therefore, is that observers' fixations are directed towards relatively distant locations of dancers' bodies, presumably in an attempt to locate and integrate perceptually non-aligned sensory inputs. There were no significant differences in fixation durations between the synchronous or asynchronous conditions. Thus, while increased dwell times may have enhanced interpersonal memorization for those who danced to the same music (and tempo) in Study 1 (Woolhouse et al., 2016), changes in fixation duration—a measure associated with attention (Rayner, 1998)—seems not to have contributed to the effect. Which is to say, at present there is little evidence

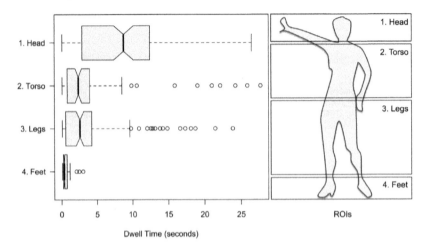

Figure 18.1 Left panel: mean dwell/gaze times for the head, torso, legs, and feet of the dancer. Right panel: corresponding regions of interest (ROIs).

that enhanced social memory within the context of music and dance results from changes in attentional focus. A subsequent, single-dancer eye-tracking experiment, conducted by Woolhouse & Lai (2014), investigated eye movements in relation to different body regions, including head, torso, legs, and feet. Significantly greater dwell times were observed for head than torso and legs. Perhaps paradoxically, the feet—arguably a dancer's greatest asset (Macaulay, 2009)—attracted significantly less dwell time than any other body region. In summary, as Figure 18.1 shows, participants' fixations were primarily drawn to the face, the primary communicative locus for intent (Trevarthen, 1979), affect (Ekman & Friesen, 1971), and empathy (Schulte-Rüther et al., 2007).

18.2.3 Aesthetic Appreciation and Attractivness

In Study 3, Tang Poy & Woolhouse (2020) investigated an evolutionary adaptive explanation for the cultural ubiquity of choreographed synchronous dance: that it evolved to increase interpersonal aesthetic appreciation and/or attractiveness. In turn, it is assumed that this may facilitate social cohesion and bonding, thereby promoting union formation and procreative opportunities. In their eye-tracking experiment, pairs of dancers were videoed performing fast- and slow-choreographed hip-hop dance moves to fast- and slow-tempo music. When laterally paired, the different combinations of dance and music gave rise to split-screen stimuli with four levels of synchrony: (level 1) synchronous dancers, synchronous music; (level 2) synchronous dancers, asynchronous music; (level 3) asynchronous dancers, one dancer synchronous with the music; and (level 4) asynchronous dancers, asynchronous music. Thirty-eight participants' pupil dilations, a proxy for for attractiveness (Murphy et al., 2011; Sepeta et al., 2012), and ratings of aesthetic appreciation were recorded for each video, with the expectation that these measures would increase with higher levels of synchronization. Increased pupil dilation allows more light to enter the eye and thus observers can collect more visual information (from synchronous dancers, for example). In theory, this allows them to process and store more social information, which may in turn lead to elevated levels of affiliation and increased prosocial behaviours.[2] Although the results were consistent with this hypothesis, the data also indicated that aesthetic appreciation depends upon a hierarchy of synchrony between dancers. Videos in which only one dancer was synchronous with the music (level 3) were rated lower than videos in which the dancers were asynchronous with each other and with the music (level 4). Thus, stimuli in which the dancers were equal with respect to the music were rated more favourably than stimuli in which the dancers were unequal, perhaps indicating that the participants were making empathetic judgements. Videos in which all elements were synchronous—dancers and music—were rated highest and, in general, elicited greater pupil dilations, that is, were most attractive to participants.

18.3 Conclusion

While the laboratory setting of the eye-tracking experiments in Studies 2 and 3 did not match the ecologically rich, group dancing experiment of Study 1, their results provide significant evidence for the role of vision in social phenomena such as increased social memorization and aesthetic appreciation/attractiveness. Dancers moving together within the rhythmic scaffolding afforded by music observe one another to a greater extent than would otherwise be the case. Whether this level of observation is greater for individuals engaged in other social interactions is unknown. A follow-up study might therefore investigate, for example, participants' memory for the attributes of actors who dance versus those who speak, or who are engaged in some other commensurate activity such as mime. Therefore, whether dance is a special category of interaction and engine of social cohesion remains to be explored.

The findings from Study 2, showing that (a) in-tempo dancing increased dwell times and (b) fixations were primarily directed towards the head, strongly suggest that synchronous movement promotes mutual eye contact. Presumably, this could create a positive feedback loop whereby dancers' bodies and limbs become increasingly synchronized, further guiding dancers to attend to one another visually. In summary, although the literature provides evidence that dance promotes prosocial behaviours and facilitates communication, the findings from Study 3 indicate that synchronized group dancing may also increase interpersonal attraction and thus the conditions under which procreation and group survival may ultimately occur. But, at this point, we stray from that which can be tested in the laboratory into the real world, where dance's multiplicity of negotiated social meanings and uses increases exponentially.

Notes

1. Dwell times represented the overall time spent gazing at a particular area of the screen; saccade lengths were measured as screen distance in mm; and fixation durations were the mean fixation lengths in seconds for a particular area of the screen.
2. For research linking pupil dilations to arousal, attention, and mental effort, see Eckstein et al. (2017) and Laeng et al. (2012).

References

Allen, N. (2010, 23 November). Strictly Come Dancing is 'world's most successful reality television format'. *The Telegraph.* http://www.telegraph.co.uk/news/worldnews/northamerica/usa/8155637/Strictly-Come-Dancing-is-worlds-most-successful-reality-television-format.html

Calabrò, D. G. (2016). Once were warriors, now are rugby players? Control and agency in the historical trajectory of the Māori formulations of masculinity in rugby. *The Asia Pacific Journal of Anthropology, 17*(3–4), 231–249.

Cirelli, L. K., Einarson, K. M., & Trainor, L. J. (2014). Interpersonal synchrony increases prosocial behavior in infants. *Developmental Science, 17*(6), 1003–1011.

Clayton, M., Sager, R., & Will, U. (2005). In time with the music: The concept of entrainment and its significance for ethnomusicology. *ESEM Counterpoint, 1*, 1–45.

Cross, I. (2008). Musicality and the human capacity for culture. *Musicae Scientiae, 12*(1 Suppl), 147–167.

Cross, I., & Woodruff, G. (2009). Music as a communicative medium. In K. Knight and C. Henshilwood (Eds.), *The prehistory of language* (Vol. 1, pp. 113–144). Oxford University Press.

Darwin, C. (1939). *A naturalist's voyage round the world: The voyage of the Beagle* (1st ed.). John Murray. (Original work published 1860)

Eckstein, M. K., Guerra-Carrillo, B., Singley, A. T. M., & Bunge, S. A. (2017). Beyond eye gaze: What else can eyetracking reveal about cognition and cognitive development? *Developmental Cognitive Neuroscience, 25*, 69–91.

Ekman, P., & Friesen, W. V. (1971). Constants across cultures in the face and emotion. *Journal of Personality and Social Psychology, 17*(2), 124.

Grammer, K., Kruck, K. B., & Magnusson, M. S. (1998). The courtship dance: Patterns of nonverbal synchronization in opposite-sex encounters. *Journal of Nonverbal Behavior, 22*(1), 3–29.

Hagen, E. H., & Hammerstein, P. (2009). Did Neanderthals and other early humans sing? Seeking the biological roots of music in the territorial advertisements of primates, lions, hyenas, and wolves. *Musicae Scientiae, 13*(2 Suppl), 291–320.

Hanna, J. L. (1987). *To dance is human: A theory of nonverbal communication.* University of Chicago Press.

Himberg, T., & Thompson, M. R. (2011). Learning and synchronising dance movements in South African songs—Cross-cultural motion-capture study. *Dance Research, 29*(Suppl), 305–328.

Honing, H. (2013). *Musical cognition: A science of listening.* Transaction Publishers.

Kirschner, S., & Tomasello, M. (2010). Joint music making promotes prosocial behavior in 4-year-old children. *Evolution and Human Behavior, 31*(5), 354–364.

Krivo, L. J., Washington, H. M., Peterson, R. D., Browning, C. R., Calder, C. A., & Kwan, M. P. (2013). Social isolation of disadvantage and advantage: The reproduction of inequality in urban space. *Social Forces, 92*(1), 141–164.

Laeng, B., Sirois, S., & Gredebäck, G. (2012). Pupillometry: A window to the preconscious? *Perspectives on Psychological Science, 7*(1), 18–27.

LaMothe, K. L. (2015). *Why we dance: A philosophy of bodily becoming.* Columbia University Press.

Large, E., & Jones, M. R. (1999). The dynamics of attending: How track time-varying events. *Psychological Review 106*(1), 119–159.

London, J. (2012). *Hearing in time: Psychological aspects of musical meter.* Oxford University Press.

Luck, G., Saarikallio, S., Thompson, M. R., Burger, B., & Toiviainen, P. (2012a). Do opposites attract? Personality and seduction on the dance floor. In E. Cambouropoulos, C. Tsougras, P. Mavromatis and K. Pastiadis (Eds.), *Proceedings of the 12th International Conference on Music Perception and Cognition* (pp. 626–629). International Conference on Music Perception and Cognition.

Luck, G., Saarikallio, S., Thompson, M. R., Burger, B., & Toiviainen, P. (2012b). Hips don't lie: Multidimensional ratings of opposite-sex dancers' perceived attractiveness. In E. Cambouropoulos, C. Tsougras, P. Mavromatis and K. Pastiadis (Eds.), *Proceedings of the 12th International Conference on Music Perception and Cognition* (pp. 630–634). International Conference on Music Perception and Cognition.

Macaulay, A. (2009, 1 August). Notice the feet in that body of work. *New York Times*. http://www.nytimes.com/2009/12/13/arts/dance/13feet.html

Macrae, C. N., Duffy, O. K., Miles, L. K., & Lawrence, J. (2008). A case of hand waving: Action synchrony and person perception. *Cognition, 109*(1), 152–156.

Miller, G. F. (2000). *The mating mind: How sexual choice shaped the evolution of human nature.* Doubleday.

Murphy, P. R., Robertson, I. H., Balsters, J. H., & O'Connell, R. G. (2011). Pupillometry and P3 index the locus coeruleus–noradrenergic arousal function in humans. *Psychophysiology, 48*(11), 1532–1543.

Pearce, E., Launay, J., & Dunbar, R. I. (2015). The ice-breaker effect: Singing mediates fast social bonding. *Royal Society Open Science, 2*(10), 150221.

Phillips-Silver, J. (2009). On the meaning of movement in music, development and the brain, *Contemporary Music Review, 28*(3), 293–314.

Phillips-Silver, J., Aktipis, C. A., & A. Bryant, G. (2010). The ecology of entrainment: Foundations of coordinated rhythmic movement. *Music Perception, 28*(1), 3–14.

Phillips-Silver, J., & Keller, P. (2012). Searching for roots of entrainment and joint action in early musical interactions. *Frontiers in Human Neuroscience, 6*, 26.

Ponmanadiyil, R., & Woolhouse, M. H. (2018). Eye movements, attention, and expert knowledge in the observation of Bharatanatyam dance. *Journal of Eye Movement Research, 11*(2), https://doi.org/10.16910/jemr.11.2.11

Rabinowitch, T. C., Cross, I., & Burnard, P. (2013). Long-term musical group interaction has a positive influence on empathy in children. *Psychology of Music, 41*(4), 484–498.

Rayner, K. (1998). Eye movements in reading and information processing: 20 years of research. *Psychological Bulletin, 124*(3), 372–422.

Schulte-Rüther, M., Markowitsch, H., Fink, G., & Piefke, M. (2007). Mirror neuron and theory of mind mechanisms involved in face-to-face interactions: A functional magnetic resonance imaging approach to empathy. *Journal of Cognitive Neuroscience, 19*(8), 1354–1372.

Sepeta, L., Tsuchiya, N., Davies, M. S., Sigman, M., Bookheimer, S. Y., & Dapretto, M. (2012). Abnormal social reward processing in autism as indexed by pupillary responses to happy faces. *Journal of Neurodevelopmental Disorders, 4*(1), 1–9.

Tang Poy, C., & Woolhouse, M. H. (2020). The attraction of synchrony: A hip-hop dance study. *Frontiers in Psychology, 11*, 588935.

Tarr, B., Launay, J., Cohen, E., & Dunbar, R. (2015). Synchrony and exertion during dance independently raise pain threshold and encourage social bonding. *Biology Letters, 11*(10), 20150767.

Trevarthen, C. (1979). Communication and cooperation in early infancy. A description of primary intersubjectivity. In M. Bullowa (Ed.), *Before speech: The beginnings of human communication* (pp. 321–348). Cambridge University Press.

Turino, T. (1999). Signs of imagination, identity, and experience: A Peircian semiotic theory for music. *Ethnomusicology, 43*(2), 221–255.

Wiltermuth, S. S., & Heath, C. (2009). Synchrony and cooperation. *Psychological Science, 20*(1), 1–5.

Wood, K. (2010). An investigation into audiences' televisual experience of Strictly Come Dancing. *Journal of Audience and Reception Studies, 7*, 1–30.

Woolhouse, M. H., Tidhar, D. & Cross, I. (2016). Effects on inter-personal memory of dancing in time with others. *Frontiers in Psychology, 7*, 167.

Woolhouse, M. H., & Lai, R. (2014). Traces across the body: Influence of music-dance synchrony on the observation of dance. *Frontiers in Human Neuroscience, 8*, 965.

SECTION 4

PERFORMANCE TIME EXPERIENCED

Attention, Expectation, and Groove

Anchor Chapters

19

Changes in Psychological Time When Attending to Different Temporal Structures in Music

Clemens Wöllner

19.1 Introduction

Music affords multiple ways of experiencing time. Listeners may focus on each note of a melody on the surface level of sound events, the underlying pulse, or on whole bars in a piece of music. These temporal levels in music provide different cues for synchronization, and in the case of dance, individuals may synchronize with various levels simultaneously. Perceiving larger temporal units such as phrases, sections, or entire pieces of music depends on working and long-term memory processes that are prone to changes in subjective time. Our temporal processing of such longer time spans involves an integration of past sound events stored in memory, perceived sounds at the present moment, and an anticipation of future musical events unfolding. This integration of past, present, and future has long been researched in the philosophy and psychology of time (for overviews, see Arstila et al., 2019; Block & Zakay, 1997; Eisler, 1976; Fraisse, 1984; Grondin, 2010; Ornstein, 1969). Curiously, while music has been called the 'temporal art' par excellence (see Kozak, this volume), there are still many open questions as to how music shapes our experience of time.

This chapter first examines the thresholds for the detection, recognition, and meaning formation of sound events at different time intervals, and asks how perceptions of coherence and large-scale forms can be achieved. Musical durations are also considered that exceed the temporal boundaries of human motor and memory processing. It is then asked which factors—be they psychophysical states of the listener or features of music, itself—lead to dilations or compression of psychological time compared to objective clock time. Long before clocks were invented, music may already have helped in shaping time and in keeping together with others in a flexible way.

Clemens Wöllner, *Changes in Psychological Time When Attending to Different Temporal Structures in Music*
In: *Performing Time*. Edited by: Clemens Wöllner and Justin London, Oxford University Press. © Oxford University Press 2023.
DOI: 10.1093/oso/9780192896254.003.0020

19.2 Perceptual, Motor, and Memory Thresholds

19.2.1 From Microseconds to the Psychological Present

The smallest temporal structures perceivable in the auditory domain have been investigated with a range of methods that permit the detection of subtle time differences. Regarding temporal resolution, trained listeners are able to perceive interaural time differences in signals when they differ by as little as 7 μs (i.e. 0.07 ms); more specifically, they can detect at which ear Gaussian white noise was presented slightly earlier (Thavam & Dietz, 2019). Gaps in continuous auditory stimuli are detectable from 2 to 20 ms, depending on intensity (detection threshold increases for low intensity) and frequency (e.g. detection threshold increases for frequencies below 200 Hz; Moore et al., 1993). For auditory temporal integration, that is, perceiving a rapid succession of stimuli as being fused into a single continuous sound event or perceptual stream, thresholds are in the range of 100 ms, with recent research tentatively suggesting that older adults might have longer integration intervals (Saija et al., 2019), as has previously been found for visual integration.

While these small temporal units in resolution experiments can be detected by attentive participants, they are usually not considered to convey meaningful information. Pöppel (1997, p. 56) called them 'pre-semantic'. Based on neural information processing, and independently of sensory modalities, he suggests a lower limit for operational time perception at 30 ms, below which before–after judgements for two stimuli are impossible, and an upper limit of 3 s, above which two or more stimuli are no longer mentally experienced as a unit. Durations up to 3 s are also termed the 'subjective present' (p. 60), since information rests in working memory only for about 3 s if there is no inner rehearsal. Correspondingly, Paul Fraisse (1984, p. 10) confined what he called the 'psychological present' between 2 and 3 s, with a maximum upper limit of 5 s, in which durations can still be perceived as a unit. Longer time intervals can only be cognitively estimated by summing up events in the range of the psychological present, or by comparing them to durations stored in long-term memory. As will be discussed below, it is particularly these longer estimations that are susceptible to a number of factors that typically lead to remarkable dilations or compressions in experienced durations. While evidence for the psychological present has been found in numerous perception and action studies, Wittmann (2011) suggests that boundaries in time processing are less fixed, and that a 'mental presence' for higher-order experiences of an acting self may exceed the 3-s time interval as previously suggested by Fraisse and by Pöppel.

Neuropsychological research on 'how and where in the brain time is processed' (Wittmann & van Wassenhove, 2009, p. 1809) has shown brain regions and neural networks for different temporal units. For instance, processing short intervals in the sub-second range involves the cerebellum (see Avanzino et al., 2015; Koch et al., 2009); timing in this range is typically beyond conscious control but crucial for 'automatic' movement production. The psychological present, in contrast, involves working memory, which is associated with the frontal lobe (Owen et al., 1990; see Grondin, 2010, for further cortical areas involved in temporal processing). Further research has highlighted the role of the basal ganglia for intervals of 2 s or more (Meck, 2005), and of the anterior insular cortex for time experiences exceeding these durations, for instance, in relation to emotional judgements and comparisons with information in long-term memory (Craig, 2009). Taken together, these studies indicate that there is no singular clock centre in the brain, and no steady, isochronously ticking timing mechanism. As a consequence, time experiences may vary inter- and intra-individually, and not having only one time system undoubtedly has the advantage that lesions in one area would not interrupt the whole system. For further discussion of the presence of an internal clock, which has been useful as a psychological metaphor for timing processes, versus state-dependent timing mechanisms, see Doelling et al. (this volume), Wang and Wöllner (2020), and Wittmann and van Wassenhove (2009).

In what ways do temporal perception and cognition thresholds come into play in music? It should be noted that temporal processing does not always result in explicitly perceived time units. For particularly small intervals, it is represented by pitch frequencies or timbre (van Wassenhove, 2009). The resolution and integration intervals (i.e. up to 100 ms) permit the perception of one or more signals and are crucial for the localization of sound sources, as they may stem from different instruments or locations. In other words, the small time intervals impel us to perceive events either as a fused, continuous stream, or as separate entities. Time intervals above 100 ms permit the recognition of meaningful qualities in musical events. Research on so-called blinks has shown that very short durations suffice for identifying the musical source they have been extracted from. For short snippets of well-known popular songs, individuals may recognize them at time intervals of only 200 ms (for a review, see Thiessen et al., 2020).

Regarding the next level, time intervals that can be processed in working memory and enable experiences of the psychological present are paramount in music. It can be argued that most musical motifs, that is, short melodic, harmonic, and rhythmic patterns, are in the range of up to 3 or 5 s. Gestalt laws come into play for those motifs that are particularly recognizable, while other motifs are perceived to be less succinct and segmented or memorized (for an overview, see Deutsch, 2013). Listeners perceive these motifs as units, typically recognize them when played again, or may find them easy to synchronize with when dancing. In this regard, Repp (2010) found that the variability in sensorimotor synchronization gets continuously larger when the metronome inter-onset intervals (IOI) increase from 1 s up to 3.25 s. Mental or physical subdivisions help participants to reduce variability, suggesting that there are upper limits for processing time intervals in sensorimotor synchronization. Lower limits, based on motor constraints, are at around 100 ms (Repp, 2003), with evidence for West African expert jembe drummers to reach IOIs as small as 80–90 ms (Polak, 2018). It should also be noted that there appear to be optimal intervals clustering around 500 ms for spontaneous motor tempo and preferred tempo (see

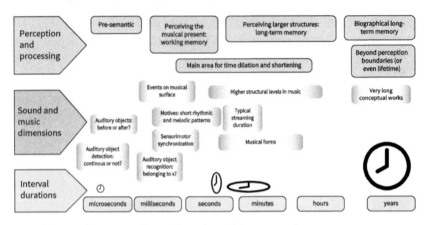

Figure 19.1 Temporal structures in music and cognitive processing.

Hammerschmidt, this volume), and longer intervals may be internally or overtly subdivided.

Figure 19.1 presents a proposed scheme of temporal structures for auditory events and music. Increasing clock-time intervals correspond with several temporal structures in music, which in turn range from preconscious processing for very short events up to compositional concepts of time that go beyond even a human lifetime. The kinds of time dilations and compressions which are thought to occur most often in musical contexts, and which have been most thoroughly investigated, typically span several seconds up to an hour.

19.2.2 Coherence

Musical-temporal structures exceeding the psychological present require long-term memory in order to be perceived as coherent and organized sounds. There is some argument as to whether larger musical structures are mainly of conceptual relevance for composers in the Western classical tradition, and hence whether violations of structural coherence can be detected by listeners at all (Karno & Konecni, 1992; McDonald & Wöllner, 2022). Composers may achieve a sense of coherence by relating different parts of a composition to each other, for instance, in terms of similarities between musical themes (Levinson, 1997). Listeners then retrieve some detail of the musical characteristics that has been stored in long-term memory when listening to music attentively. On the other hand, coherence or musical unity, as a composer may aspire to and a music theorist attempts to elucidate, can never be a sort of 'apprehension, in a single imaginative-recollective act, of all the temporal parts of a composition in all their interrelations' (Levinson, 1997, p. 59), as music unfolds as a succession of events over time. Since recognizing previous melodic–rhythmic themes or other features of the music, including orchestration and timbre, can engender a sense of coherence and enjoyment, composers and improvisers often use repetition in their works. As Huron (2013) points out, musical repetition facilitates habituation as a form of 'non-associative learning' (p. 13) as well as enhanced perceptual and processing fluency, which are supposedly related to experiences of aesthetic pleasure. On one side of the spectrum, highly repetitive music can induce a trance state by shaping attentional processes in terms of habituation; and on the other, listeners may consciously perceive a sense of unity via the return of familiar material in musical forms such as strophic songs, rondos, or theme-and-variation movements.

What are the time intervals for perceiving musical coherence, apart from the occasional long-term memory retrieval of similar musical events in attentive listening? Cook (1987) investigated the durations at which the compositional concept of tonal closure is relevant for listeners, with tonal closure referring to a piece of music beginning and ending in the same key despite modulations in between. He played original 19th-century piano compositions as well as manipulated versions that included modulations to keys other than the tonic; pieces were about 1–6 min in duration. Those pieces that were manipulated within the range of about 1 min were rated lower than the originals by music student listeners in the aesthetic dimensions of coherence, completion, pleasure, and expressiveness. For longer pieces (at, or exceeding, 2 min) listeners did not seem to have noticed the manipulations, and thus did not prefer the originals, independently of their familiarity with the music. These findings suggest that musical coherence in terms of tonal structure is less perceivable for larger time spans than commonly assumed.

19.2.3 Time Experiences Beyond Perceptual and Motor Boundaries

Human capacities for grasping coherence in temporal structures are limited in time, as are the time intervals that afford accurate synchronization with music. While the first observation points to limits in attentional span, the second limitation refers to both cognitive and sensorimotor dimensions. Composers nevertheless have been intrigued by the idea of overcoming these boundaries, in some cases striving for the essence of coherence, in that the small should be present in the large, and vice versa. This idea, frequently termed 'organicism', has been prominent particularly in 19th-century thinking and music analysis (Solie, 1980; for a recent critique, see Watkins, 2017). The idea that a longer work of Western music is built of structurally resembling material can be found, for example, in E. T. H. Hoffmann's *Kreisleriana*, in which he describes Beethoven's fifth symphony in terms of organic unity that can for the most part be traced back to 'simple' motivic material (Castein & Hoffmann, 1814/1993, Chapter 4).

Reich's composition *Proverb* (1995) is based on Wittgenstein's phrase 'How small a thought it takes to fill a whole life!' (original: 'Welch ein kleiner Gedanke doch ein ganzes Leben füllen kann!'; Wittgenstein, 1946/1998, p. 57). The composition can be heard as a form of time stretching, such that the 'small thought', first sung by one soprano, is extended to other solo voices with augmented notes, and later joined by a small instrumental ensemble. Tenor voices repeatedly perform melodic–rhythmic motives reminiscent of the *hoquetus* style of the Notre-Dame epoch (12th/13th century), and vibraphones fill the sustained sounds with notes at a rate that lie within comfortable synchronization thresholds. The fascination of this work may thus be due to the combination of small- and large-scale events at the same time. Reich has composed other conceptual works that endeavour to slow time. His 'Slow Motion Sound' (1967) consists of the single instruction, 'Very gradually slow down a recorded sound to many times its original length without changing its pitch or timbre at all'. The advent of digital music processing in recent decades has made possible the fully satisfactory realization of Reich's piece, along with other similarly conceptual works. Rehding (2015) describes the '9 Beet Stretch' project by Norwegian artist Leif Inge, in which the approximately 75 minutes of Beethoven's Ninth Symphony are stretched digitally to fill an entire day. The listening experience hardly allows for any musical orientation in the score, but instead telescopes into the timbral and tonal qualities of the recording.

Beyond Inge's transmogrification of Beethoven, the so-called Halberstadt organ project was inspired by John Cage's (1987/2002) composition *Organ²/ASLAP (As Slow as Possible)*. When it was premiered in 1987, it took the organist nearly half an hour to perform the short eight-page composition (four pages in the Edition Peters scores). Yet slower is still possible: established as an art installation in the Romanesque St. Burchadi church in the central German town of Halberstadt in 2001, the performance of Cage's composition is stretched to 639 years. Years will often pass before a new tone sounds on the organ, which is usually celebrated as a special event (see the project's webpage for what the current state of the composition sounds like: https://www.aslsp.org). At the time of the writing of this chapter, the next event will take place in February 2022 with the release of one of the two current organ sounds, to be succeeded by a single new sound 2 years later. While some listeners value primarily the concept of a creation beyond human lifetime scales, comparable perhaps to the construction of the great cathedrals, others may wish to experience a glimpse of eternity and timelessness.

19.3 Time Changes Through Music: Factors Evoking Experiences of Condensed or Expanded Durations

19.3.1 Complexity, Event Density, and Familiarity

Musical complexity is one of the factors that may cause time dilations. If the number of events to be processed is increased, as is typically the case in more complex music, then listeners should have the impression of durations lasting longer (cf. Repp & Bruttomesso, 2010, for a musical study on the filled duration illusion). Ornstein's

(1969) experiments with moving visual objects for durations from 30 s up to 9.5 min were among the first suggesting a memory storage size model of duration experiences. The greater the complexity of the visual information, the more information needs to be stored in memory, leading to subjectively longer durations than for less complex stimuli with smaller amounts of information.

A small number of studies have assessed variations in musical complexity. Clarke and Krumhansl (1990) asked musically trained listeners to rate complexity and duration of several excerpts from Stockhausen's *Klavierstück* Nr. IX and, in a separate experiment, Mozart's *Fantasie* in C minor (KV 475). Excerpt durations were in the range of 22–34 s, with an average of about 30 s. Correlations between actual excerpt durations and perceived durations were highly significant, and were not related to perceived complexity. Based on this analysis, one could assume that listeners were relatively stable in judging duration, or that the complexity differences in the excerpts taken from one composition were not sufficiently large. Nevertheless, other research had found time dilations for more complex melodies (Yeager, 1969). A further study contrasted symphonic compositions by Mahler and Bério (Bueno et al., 2002) varying in complexity. Listeners overestimated the duration of Bério's third movement from the *Sinfonia* (for eight voices and orchestra), which was supposedly higher in complexity than Mahler's third movement of the second symphony (90 s were played for both). It can be argued that time intervals in the Bério composition were filled with more events to be processed. In should be noted that in this study, white noise, perhaps by inducing boredom, resulted in even longer duration estimates than for both musical compositions. In one of our own studies, a four-voice rhythmic pattern that was typical in instrumentation for electronic dance music was also perceived to last shorter than two other, less typical patterns with the same instruments at different voices (Hammerschmidt & Wöllner, 2020), which were arguably perceived as more complex. These findings are in line with Ornstein's (1969) information processing approach for time judgements.

Complexity may to some extent be related to familiarity, such that more familiar pieces should be processed with more ease and consequently perceived as shorter. A simple analogy is walking to and fro along an unknown route, which will appear longer at first, since more events are perceived and processed. Indeed, waiting time appeared shorter for participants listening to familiar background music (Bailey & Areni, 2006). Familiarity effects were not replicated in a prospective duration estimation task with hip-hop music (Wöllner & Hammerschmidt, 2021), nor were they found for non-musical duration estimation tasks in a meta-analysis (Block et al., 2010). It may well be that attention and emotional involvement co-varied with familiarity for music in previous research, and should be systematically varied in future experiments.

It should be noted that complexity may additionally affect perceived tempo. When played at the same tempo, melodies that contained embellishments such as passing notes or arpeggios are perceived to be faster than simpler melodies (Kuhn, 1987). Melodies exhibiting higher pitch and brighter timbre are similarly perceived to be faster, as are those with ascending pitch or increasing loudness (Boltz, 2011). Hence it should be emphasized that listeners judge music and time holistically, leading to an 'overgeneralization of certain structural correlations within the natural environment' (Boltz, 2011, p. 367). Approaches by researchers that change only one dimension in music should therefore be critically reflected in comparison with the statistical likelihood of such isolated changes.

19.3.2 Tempo, Arousal, and Valence

Based on the information processing approach to time judgements (Ornstein, 1969), faster tempi in music should lead to longer duration estimations compared to slower tempo, since more events per unit of clock time are processed and stored in memory. London (2011) found that tempo perception is intrinsically linked to the density of events on the musical surface, and to a higher degree than the underlying tactus or beat rate for basic rhythmic patterns. A number of studies revealed that faster music did, indeed, lead to overestimations of time intervals and longer duration judgements in music (Droit-Volet et al., 2013; Hammerschmidt & Wöllner, 2020; Oakes, 2003). While these studies employed prospective duration estimations, a further experiment (Hammerschmidt et al., 2021) additionally asked participants to reproduce the duration of six disco songs (14.8–19.2 s) that differed in tempo (original tempi: 105–125 beats per minute). In the reproduction task, participants pressed a key on a computer keyboard at the beginning and at the end of the imagined duration immediately after hearing the stimulus. Song tempo was judged to be significantly different as expected, and duration reproduction was relatively longer for the fast-tempo songs compared to the slower-tempo songs. This finding suggests that fewer events per unit of clock time were perceived in the slower songs, which subsequently caused shorter duration reproductions. The reproductions were also more accurate than the relatively shorter duration estimations, which were not significantly influenced by the tempo of the different songs. More importantly, there was a small but significant correlation between tempo rating and duration reproduction, showing once again that the faster the tempo was perceived, the longer was the participant's reproduced time interval. A retrospective time estimation study, by contrast, varied slow and fast music in a gymnasium (North et al., 1998). Respondents underestimated the duration spent in the gymnasium in general, while there was no systematic difference according to the music. It can be speculated that other factors may have contributed to this real-world study of the perception of filled time.

Fast music is often associated with increased arousal (Ilie & Thompson, 2006; Kim et al., 2019). In psychological inner-clock models, arousal is suggested to increase the number of pulses emitted by the pacemaker (Burle & Casini, 2001; Gibbon, 1991; Noulhiane et al., 2007; Wearden, 2008). The more pulses are accumulated in an interval, the longer this interval is perceived to be. The reason for the overestimation lies in comparisons with a typical number of pulses in a reference time span that is stored in long-term memory. There is some evidence that the insula is involved in the accumulation of pulses (Wittmann et al., 2010), providing a neural basis for the theoretical model of a central clock mechanism. The higher number of pulses requires that the organism (e.g. the listener) is in a state of heightened arousal. Indeed, a study by Jakubowski and colleagues (2015) found that participants who had engaged in jogging had not only a faster heart rate, but also preferred faster song tempi in a selection task, compared to another group who stayed still. So, the first group's tempo choice reflected their higher arousal levels, and, according to the inner-clock model, the higher number of pulses emitted.

In music studies, researchers differentiate between two types of arousal. For *induced* emotional arousal, music elicits physiological responses in listeners, while for *perceived* stimulus arousal, listeners recognize different emotional arousal levels in the music without, themselves, typically experiencing corresponding physiological effects from it (Gabrielsson, 2001; Song et al., 2016). For example, emotions in music may change rapidly, and listeners may recognize these emotions but not feel them at the same rate of change. Consequently, perceived stimulus arousal should also have different effects on listeners' time experiences compared to induced physiological arousal, and it can be assumed that indeed only an altered physiological state affects the number of pulses emitted in the proposed inner-clock mechanism. While Jakubowski et al. (2015) clearly manipulated the listeners' physiological arousal, other studies aimed at varying the arousal level in musical excerpts. Droit-Volet et al. (2013) played orchestral versus piano versions of the same music at the same tempi. These differences had no impact on duration judgements. Similarly, low-arousal hip-hop songs at the same beat rates did not differ in duration estimates or passage of time judgements compared to high-arousal ones (Wöllner & Hammerschmidt, 2021; Figure 19.2, right panel). The same holds true for an unpublished study in which we presented excerpts from Beethoven's Symphony No. 7 in A Major, Op. 92, second movement. The first part of this movement, which functions as the symphony's slow movement even if the tempo and character marking (allegretto) may suggest otherwise, consists of a theme that spans eight plus 16 bars. This theme contains an omnipresent long–short–short march-like rhythm, and is repeated three times, starting with the lower strings in piano (tenuto), then including the first violins (crescendo poco a poco), and finally culminating in a tutti passage in fortissimo when occurring for the third time. We played eight- and 24-bar parts of each of the three sections to 28 participants. As expected, they judged musical arousal to be highest for the tutti and fortissimo section, and lowest for the first piano section.[1] This judgement was not associated with listeners' duration estimation or passage of time judgements. In other words, while listeners very clearly differentiated between the arousal levels in the music, they were themselves not affected by it to an extent that would have changed their inner clock and consequently their experiences of time.

In addition to arousal, effects of musical valence on time experiences have been studied by Droit-Volet and colleagues. While the mode of the music, being in major or minor, did not influence time estimations (Droit-Volet et al., 2010), playing the

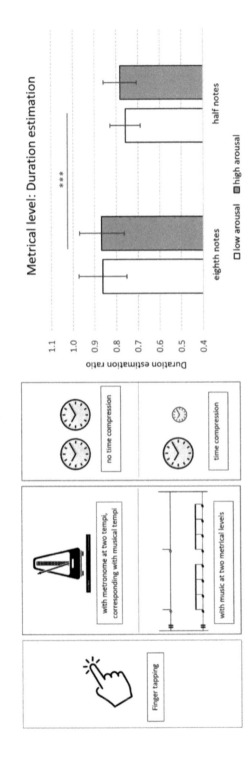

Figure 19.2 Simplified scheme of the experiment and statistical findings. When focusing on a higher metrical level (half notes), participants underestimated durations more than when they tapped at the eighth-note level of the same music. Stimulus arousal did not affect results (Wöllner & Hammerschmidt, 2021). Duration estimation ratio is calculated by dividing subjective duration estimates by clock time (both in seconds).

audio file backwards was perceived to be unpleasant in a different study (Droit-Volet et al., 2013) and resulted in longer duration estimates. Since playing music backwards violated listeners' expectations and may have increased complexity in terms of processing fluency, this finding could also be seen in light of the information processing model as discussed above. Further research has taken a back-to-front approach, in that listeners' theories about 'time flying when having fun' may influence their aesthetic appreciation. Sackett et al. (2010) asked listeners to choose a favourite song out of a selection, and manipulated the timer showing elapsed or remaining song time. If the supposedly objective elapsing time listeners saw was quicker, then they enjoyed the songs significantly more, and even more so the stronger they believed in the 'time flies' theory. When time remaining was shown, or when supposedly objective time was manipulated to last longer, no significant effect was found. These findings suggest that listeners attributed their altered time experiences to both qualities of the music and their subjective pleasure.

Taken together, faster tempo increased perceived and reproduced duration in experiments, and a plausible explanation for this effect is the higher number of events perceived per unit of clock time. Tempo may also lead to higher arousal in listeners. If this is the case, or if listeners are physiologically aroused by other means such as engaging in sports before doing the task, then their time estimations may be dilated as well, due to the higher number of pulses emitted by the putative pacemaker in the inner clock model. If listeners, by contrast, are presented with different pieces or sections of music that vary in arousal but not in tempo, then they may perceive the arousal changes, but are less likely to be affected in time perception. Hence, the information processing approach in addition to physiological arousal seems to be a more promising model to understand time dilations in music than stimulus arousal.

19.3.3 Attention to Metrical Levels

The role of attention for time estimations has been widely acknowledged. The most obvious effect is present in the difference between prospective and retrospective duration judgements. When individuals are told beforehand (prospectively) that they should judge the duration of a time interval (above 3 s), they draw their attention to judging time and are thus distracted from the stimuli or task. As a consequence, the time interval is typically judged to be shorter in comparison with retrospective, a posteriori judgements (Block et al., 2010). To make things somewhat more complicated, prospective and retrospective time estimations further depend on cognitive load, defined as attentional and working memory demands on information processing. If load is low, then the reverse is true: as Block and colleagues (2010) showed in their meta-analysis, if the task does not require active or difficult processing, and there are no particular demands on divided or selective attention, then prospective duration judgements are longer compared to retrospective judgements. Hence time tends to be more underestimated the more individuals divert their attention, and attention in turn is diverted more by difficult tasks when knowing beforehand that time should also be judged. For this reason, listening to music by focusing attention on different characteristics may lead to changes in perceived durations.

In a series of studies, we hypothesized that attending to a higher metrical level in the music, in this case by tapping a finger along with every other pulse compared to a layer of binary pulse subdivisions (half notes versus eighth notes), should result in shorter duration estimates. In other words, listeners should perceive larger structures and time should be perceived to be less filled as compared to attending to metrical levels faster than the 4/4 beat. In an experiment with different examples of hip-hop music all played at the same tempo, the duration of the music (in seconds) was underestimated in both listening conditions, but significantly more so when participants tapped along with half notes (Figure 19.2; Wöllner & Hammerschmidt, 2021). This effect was not simply due to tapping faster or slower. When asked to tap with a metronome, there was no difference between the speed of tapping at fast or slow rates that were at the same tempo as the half or eighth notes in the hip-hop music. These findings build on a previous study indicating that tapping to different metrical levels in a four-instrument drum pattern changed time estimations (Hammerschmidt & Wöllner, 2020). Our results indicate that the way listeners engage with the same music changes their judgements of the music's duration, and time is contracted more when focusing their attention on larger structures.

Furthermore, these results point to an effect of attentional demands as a measure of cognitive load. Block et al. (2010) remarked that '[d]uration judgments, especially those made under the prospective paradigm, seem to be a reliable and unobtrusive way to assess cognitive load' (p. 340). In our study (Wöllner & Hammerschmidt, 2021), the motor control task in which participants tapped to a metronome increased cognitive load, compared to listening only to the metronome. In other words, the sensorimotor synchronization of tapping increased attentional demands and resulted in shorter duration judgements. Hence, while cognitive load was higher in tapping conditions compared to non-tapping ones, the above-mentioned effect that time was shorter when attending to a higher metrical level can be attributed to the perception of larger musical structures, resulting in time intervals being subjectively less filled by musical events.

19.4 Attending to Various Temporal Structures in Music Enhances Flexibility

The wide range of musical tempi requires and may train human flexibility in synchronization and timing, that is, individuals may easily switch from one synchronization mode to another and entrain with an external source at different speeds. When listening to the same music, individuals can in some cases perceive a number of various metres (London, 2012) that may differ from what is notated in Western music. By taking into account non-Western music, it has been suggested that pulses and subdivisions do not need to be isochronous in order to establish a rhythmic period and percepts of metre, which opens the possibilities for numerous combinations (Polak et al., 2016).

If individuals move their body when finding the pulse, for instance, by tapping their feet or nodding their head, they find it easier to attune to the tempo and are more stable in synchronization, that is, they are less variable in asynchronies from the beat (Su & Pöppel, 2012). These results suggest that the body plays an important role in timing tasks (see also Stupacher et al., this volume, for feelings of groove). Extensive training has an impact on flexibility in embodied processing of music at different temporal levels. Musical training clearly improves timing at various tempi, as was shown for percussionists who were able to perform with high synchronization accuracy at tempi ranging from 60 to 200 beats per minute (Fujii et al., 2011; see also Scheurich et al., 2018, for synchronization rate flexibility of musicians compared to non-musicians). Furthermore, the synchronization accuracy of percussionists was found to be higher compared to other musicians including pianists and singers, and was extended to a cross-modal timing perception task (Krause et al., 2010), suggesting that enhanced temporal flexibility in synchronization may generalize to other domains including vision. This cross-domain temporal flexibility permits tuning in with other individuals in musical ensembles of various types (see Bishop & Goebl, 2018; Wöllner & Keller, 2017) in terms of entrainment and synchronization, and presumably extends to the coordination of movement in dance and other group contexts.

Music offers hierarchical cues for various body movements at the same time (Burger et al., 2018; Toiviainen et al., 2010; see also Burger & Toiviainen, this volume). These studies have shown that musical and acoustical characteristics such as tempo, pulse clarity, or spectral flux facilitate a dancer's synchronization with different parts of their body simultaneously at various paces. For instance, foot movements were faster than lateral hand movements, and both were thus synchronized with different metrical levels in the music. It would be interesting to investigate further which of these metrical levels are more consciously attended to, and what the effects are for perceived time (cf. Hammerschmidt & Wöllner, 2020; Wöllner & Hammerschmidt, 2021). From an information processing perspective, complex simultaneous body synchronization at various metrical levels may lead to time passing more quickly as compared to synchronizing with only one metrical level. Nevertheless, there seem to be limits to conscious multi-metre perception, and it is more likely that listeners establish an internal composite rhythmical pattern rather than perceiving two or more different metres simultaneously (Poudrier & Repp, 2013).

19.5 Conclusion and Implications for Future Research

If music can change time experiences, as discussed in this chapter, does time change music? In other words, does music reflect, for instance, the widely perceived acceleration in pace of life? Despite some controversy, musical tempo does not seem to have changed dramatically in the Western musical tradition over historical epochs (Auhagen, 1993). Rather than accelerating, in recent years the average tempo of the most widely played music on Spotify has dropped because of the popularity of hip-hop (see Wöllner & Hammerschmidt, 2021), probably due to facilitating temporal frames for rapping and breakdancing, and perhaps a certain 'laid-back' approach in some hip-hop subgenres. It can be argued that there are certain temporal boundaries for optimal musical experiences of performers, listeners, and dancers. These boundaries are grounded in perceptual, sensorimotor, and cognitive processing constraints. It thus seems unlikely that humans will come to enjoy extremely fast music with inter-onset intervals below 100 ms, or long time intervals above a few seconds for motives and repeating patterns, or minutes and hours for longer structures—simply because it is neither possible to move to fast temporal intervals nor to store very long ones in memory.

On the other hand, by engaging with music, temporal flexibility can be trained for a range of different time intervals within these boundaries. This type of flexibility leads to higher accuracy when synchronizing with a beat and coordinating actions with other individuals, both within and beyond music and dance contexts. Experienced musicians are not only able to adjust their timing to an external beat with high accuracy, but they can also retrieve timing and tempo nuances over many years for repeat performances (Clynes & Walker, 1986). Strikingly, though mastering temporal structures is at the core of the musicians' profession, their sense of time during performance has hardly been addressed. Research on contemporary dance (Stevens et al., 2009) showed stable internal clocks for the movements of an ensemble with and without music.

In this chapter it has been argued that attending to different metrical levels is one way of enhancing temporal flexibility. Less is known about how fast and how frequently individuals switch between different metrical levels (e.g. from quarter-note to half-note level), or to different metres for non-isochronous metrical structures. How consciously can listeners, musicians, and dancers attend to different metrical levels at the same time? If they can, would this lead to higher perceived event density and cognitive load, and subsequently to prolongations in perceived durations? It may be that, in this way, music helps to stretch time, offering the rather Faustian promise of a moment held in place.

Note

1. $F(1.59, 43.02) = 107.15$, $p < .001$, $\eta_p^2 = .80$, all post hoc comparisons were different at $p < .001$. Effects were not significant for duration estimation ($p = .57$, $\eta_p^2 = .05$) or passage of time judgements ($p = .33$, $\eta_p^2 = .08$).

References

Arstila, V., Bardon, A., Power, S. E., & Vatakis, A. (2019) (Eds.). *The illusions of time: Philosophical and psychological essays on timing and time perception*. Springer/Palgrave-MacMillan.

Auhagen, W. (1993). Eine wenig beachtete Quelle zur musikalischen Tempoauffassung im frühen 19. Jahrhundert [Musical tempo concepts in the early 19th century]. *Archiv Für Musikwissenschaft, 50*(4), 291. https://doi.org/10.2307/930910

Avanzino, L., Bove, M., Pelosin, E., Ogliastro, C., Lagravinese, G., & Martino, D. (2015). The cerebellum predicts the temporal consequences of observed motor acts. *PLoS One, 10*(2), e0116607. https://doi.org/10.1371/journal.pone.0116607

Bailey, N., & Areni, C. S. (2006). When a few minutes sound like a lifetime: Does atmospheric music expand or contract perceived time? *Journal of Retailing, 82*(3), 189–202. https://doi.org/10.1016/j.jretai.2006.05.003

Bishop, L., & Goebl, W. (2018). Communication for coordination: Gesture kinematics and conventionality affect synchronization success in piano duos. *Psychological Research, 82*(6), 1177–1194. https://doi.org/10.1007/s00426-017-0893-3

Block, R. A., Hancock, P. A., & Zakay, D. (2010). How cognitive load affects duration judgments: A meta-analytic review. *Acta Psychologica, 134*(3), 330–343. https://doi.org/10.1016/j.actpsy.2010.03.006

Block, R. A., & Zakay, D. (1997). Prospective and retrospective duration judgments: A meta-analytic review. *Psychonomic Bulletin & Review, 4*(2), 184–197. https://doi.org/10.3758/BF03209393

Boltz, M. G. (1989). Time judgments of musical endings: Effects of expectancies on the 'filled interval effect'. *Perception & Psychophysics, 46*(5), 409–418. https://doi.org/10.3758/BF03210855

Boltz, M. G. (2011). Illusory tempo changes due to musical characteristics. *Music Perception, 28*(4), 367–386. https://doi.org/10.1525/mp.2011.28.4.367

Bueno, J. L. O., Firmino, E. A., & Engelman, A. (2002). Influence of generalized complexity of a musical event on subjective time estimation. *Perceptual and Motor Skills, 94*(2), 541–547. https://doi.org/10.2466/pms.2002.94.2.541

Burger, B., London, J., Thompson, M. R., & Toiviainen, P. (2018). Synchronization to metrical levels in music depends on low-frequency spectral components and tempo. *Psychological Research, 82*(6), 1195–1211. https://doi.org/10.1007/s00426-017-0894-2

Burle, B., & Casini, L. (2001). Dissociation between activation and attention effects in time estimation: Implications for internal clock models. *Journal of Experimental Psychology: Human Perception & Performance, 27*, 195–205. https://doi.org/10.1037/0096-1523.27.1.195.

Cage, J. (2002). *Organ²/ASLSP*. Edition Peters. (Original work published 1987)

Castein, H., & Hoffmann, E. T. A. (1993). *Universal-Bibliothek: Nr. 5623. Kreisleriana*. Reclam. (Original work published 1814)

Clarke, E. F., & Krumhansl, C. L. (1990). Perceiving musical time. *Music Perception, 7*(3), 213–251. https://doi.org/10.2307/40285462

Clynes, M., & Walker, J. (1986). Music as time's measure. *Music Perception, 4*(1), 85–119. https://doi.org/10.2307/40285353

Cook, N. (1987). The perception of large-scale tonal closure. *Music Perception, 5*(2), 197–205. https://doi.org/10.2307/40285392

Craig, A. D. B. (2009). Emotional moments across time: A possible neural basis for time perception in the anterior insula. *Philosophical Transactions of the Royal Society of London. Series B, Biological Sciences, 364*(1525), 1933–1942. https://doi.org/10.1098/rstb.2009.0008

Deutsch, D. (2013). Grouping mechanisms in music. In D. Deutsch (Ed.), *The psychology of music* (3rd ed., pp. 183–248). Academic Press.

Droit-Volet, S., Bigand, E., Ramos, D., & Bueno, J. L. O. (2010). Time flies with music whatever its emotional valence. *Acta Psychologica, 135*(2), 226–232. https://doi.org/10.1016/j.actpsy.2010.07.003

Droit-Volet, S., Ramos, D., Bueno, J. L. O., & Bigand, E. (2013). Music, emotion, and time perception: The influence of subjective emotional valence and arousal? *Frontiers in Psychology, 4*, 417. https://doi.org/10.3389/fpsyg.2013.00417

Eisler, H. (1976). Experiments on subjective duration 1868–1975: A collection of power function exponents. *Psychological Bulletin, 83*(6), 1154–1171. https://doi.org/10.1037/0033-2909.83.6.1154

Fraisse, P. (1984). Perception and estimation of time. *Annual Review of Psychology, 35*, 1–36. https://doi.org/10.1146/annurev.ps.35.020184.000245

Fujii, S., Hirashima, M., Kudo, K., Ohtsuki, T., Nakamura, Y., & Oda, S. (2011). Synchronization error of drum kit playing with a metronome at different tempi by professional drummers. *Music Perception, 28*(5), 491–503. https://doi.org/10.1525/mp.2011.28.5.491

Gabrielsson, A. (2001). Emotion perceived and emotion felt: Same or different? *Musicae Scientiae, 5*(1 Suppl), 123–147. https://doi.org/10.1177/10298649020050S105

Gibbon, J. (1991). Origins of scalar timing. *Learning & Motivation, 22*, 3–38. https://doi.org/10.1016/0023-9690(91)90015-Z

Grondin, S. (2010). Timing and time perception: A review of recent behavioral and neuroscience findings and theoretical directions. *Attention, Perception & Psychophysics, 72*(3), 561–582. https://doi.org/10.3758/APP.72.3.561

Hammerschmidt, D., & Wöllner, C. (2020). Sensorimotor synchronization with higher metrical levels in music shortens perceived time. *Music Perception, 37*(4), 263–277. https://doi.org/10.1525/MP.2020.37.4.263

Hammerschmidt, D., Wöllner, C., London, J., & Burger, B. (2021). Disco time: The relationship between perceived duration and tempo in music. *Music & Science, 4*, 205920432098638. https://doi.org/10.1177/2059204320986384

Huron, D. (2013). A psychological approach to musical form: The habituation–fluency theory of repetition. *Current Musicology, 96*, 7–35. https://doi.org/10.7916/CM.V0I96.5312

Ilie, G., & Thompson, W. F. (2006). A comparison of acoustic cues in music and speech for three dimensions of affect. *Music Perception, 23*(4), 319–330. https://doi.org/10.1525/mp.2006.23.4.319

Jakubowski, K., Halpern, A. R., Grierson, M., & Stewart, L. (2015). The effect of exercise-induced arousal on chosen tempi for familiar melodies. *Psychonomic Bulletin & Review, 22*(2), 559–565. https://doi.org/10.3758/s13423-014-0687-1

Karno, M., & Konečni, V. J. (1992). The effects of structural interventions in the first movement of Mozart's Symphony in G Minor K. 550 on aesthetic preference. *Music Perception, 10*(1), 63–72. https://doi.org/10.2307/40285538

Kim, J., Strohbach, C. A., & Wedell, D. H. (2019). Effects of manipulating the tempo of popular songs on behavioral and physiological responses. *Psychology of Music, 47*(3), 392–406. https://doi.org/10.1177/0305735618754688

Koch, G., Oliveri, M., & Caltagirone, C. (2009). Neural networks engaged in milliseconds and seconds time processing: Evidence from transcranial magnetic stimulation and patients with cortical or subcortical dysfunction. *Philosophical Transactions of the Royal Society of London. Series B, Biological Sciences, 364*(1525), 1907–1918. https://doi.org/10.1098/rstb.2009.0018

Krause, V., Pollok, B., & Schnitzler, A. (2010). Perception in action: The impact of sensory information on sensorimotor synchronization in musicians and non-musicians. *Acta Psychologica, 133*(1), 28–37. https://doi.org/10.1016/j.actpsy.2009.08.003

Kuhn, T. L. (1987). The effect of tempo, meter, and melodic complexity on the perception of tempo. In C. K. Madsen & C. A. Prickett (eds.), *Applications of research in music behavior* (pp. 165–174). University of Alabama Press.

Levinson, J. (1997). *Music in the moment.* Cornell University Press. http://www.jstor.org/stable/10.7591/j.ctv5rdz19

London, J. (2011). Tactus ≠ tempo: Some dissociations between attentional focus, motor behavior, and tempo judgment. *Empirical Musicology Review, 6*(1), 43–55. https://doi.org/10.18061/1811/49761

London, J. (2012). *Hearing in time: Psychological aspects of musical meter* (2nd ed.). Oxford University Press.

McDonald, G. & Wöllner, C. (2022). Appreciation of form in Bach's Well-Tempered Clavier: Effects of structural interventions on perceived coherence, pleasantness and retrospective duration estimates. *Music Perception, 40*(2), 150–167. https://doi.org/10.1525/MP.2022.40.2.150

Meck, W. H. (2005). Neuropsychology of timing and time perception. *Brain and Cognition, 58*(1), 1–8. https://doi.org/10.1016/j.bandc.2004.09.004

Moore, B. C., Peters, R. W., & Glasberg, B. R. (1993). Detection of temporal gaps in sinusoids: Effects of frequency and level. *Journal of the Acoustical Society of America, 93*(3), 1563–1570. https://doi.org/10.1121/1.406815

North, A. C., Hargreaves, D. J., & Heath, S. J. (1998). Musical tempo and time perception in a gymnasium. *Psychology of Music, 26*(1), 78–88. https://doi.org/10.1177/0305735698261007

Noulhiane, M., Mella, N., Samson, S., Ragot, R., & Pouthas, V. (2007). How emotional auditory stimuli modulate time perception. *Emotion, 7*(4), 697–704. https://doi.org/10.1037/1528-3542.7.4.697

Oakes, S. (2003). Musical tempo and waiting perceptions. *Psychology & Marketing, 20*(8), 685–705. https://doi.org/10.1002/mar.10092

Ornstein, R. E. (1969). *On the experience on time* (Penguin Science of Behaviour). Penguin.

Polak, R. (2018). The lower limit for meter in dance drumming from West Africa. *Empirical Musicology Review, 12*(3–4), 205. https://doi.org/10.18061/emr.v12i3-4.4951

Polak, R., London, J., & Jacoby, N. (2016). Both isochronous and non-isochronous metrical subdivision afford precise and stable ensemble entrainment: A corpus study of Malian jembe drumming. *Frontiers in Neuroscience, 10*, 285. https://doi.org/10.3389/fnins.2016.00285

Pöppel, E. (1997). A hierarchical model of temporal perception. *Trends in Cognitive Sciences, 1*(2), 56–61. https://doi.org/10.1016/S1364-6613(97)01008-5

Poudrier, È., & Repp, B. H. (2013). Can musicians track two different beats simultaneously? *Music Perception, 30*(4), 369–390. https://doi.org/10.1525/mp.2013.30.4.369

Rehding, A. (2015). The discovery of slowness in music. In S. van Maas (ed.), *Thresholds of listening: sound, technics, space* (pp. 206–299). Fordham UP.

Reich, S. (1995). *Proverb.* Boosey & Hawkes (Hendon Music).

Repp, B. H. (2003). Rate limits in sensorimotor synchronization with auditory and visual sequences: The synchronization threshold and the benefits and costs of interval subdivision. *Journal of Motor Behavior, 35*(4), 355–370. https://doi.org/10.1080/00222890309603156

Repp, B. H. (2010). Self-generated interval subdivision reduces variability of synchronization with a very slow metronome. *Music Perception, 27*(5), 389–397. https://doi.org/10.1525/mp.2010.27.5.389

Repp, B. H., & Bruttomesso, M. (2010). A filled duration illusion in music: Effects of metrical subdivision on the perception and production of beat tempo. *Advances in Cognitive Psychology, 5*, 114–134. https://doi.org/10.2478/v10053-008-0071-7

Sackett, A. M., Meyvis, T., Nelson, L. D., Converse, B. A., & Sackett, A. L. (2010). You're having fun when time flies: The hedonic consequences of subjective time progression. *Psychological Science, 21*(1), 111–117. https://doi.org/10.1177/0956797609354832

Saija, J. D., Başkent, D., Andringa, T. C., & Akyürek, E. G. (2019). Visual and auditory temporal integration in healthy younger and older adults. *Psychological Research, 83*(5), 951–967. https://doi.org/10.1007/s00426-017-0912-4

Scheurich, R., Zamm, A., & Palmer, C. (2018). Tapping into rate flexibility: Musical training facilitates synchronization around spontaneous production rates. *Frontiers in Psychology, 9*, 458. https://doi.org/10.3389/fpsyg.2018.00458

Solie, R. A. (1980). The living work: Organicism and musical analysis. *19th-Century Music, 4*(2), 147–156. https://doi.org/10.2307/746712

Song, Y., Dixon, S., Pearce, M. T., & Halpern, A. R. (2016). Perceived and induced emotion responses to popular music. *Music Perception, 33*(4), 472–492. https://doi.org/10.1525/MP.2016.33.4.472

Stevens, C. J., Schubert, E., Wang, S., Kroos, C., & Halovic, S. (2009). Moving with and without music: Scaling and lapsing in time in the performance of contemporary dance. *Music Perception, 26*(5), 451–464. https://doi.org/10.1525/mp.2009.26.5.451

Su, Y.-H., & Pöppel, E. (2012). Body movement enhances the extraction of temporal structures in auditory sequences. *Psychological Research, 76*(3), 373–382. https://doi.org/10.1007/s00426-011-0346-3

Thavam, S., & Dietz, M. (2019). Smallest perceivable interaural time differences. *Journal of the Acoustical Society of America, 145*(1), 458. https://doi.org/10.1121/1.5087566

Thiesen, F. C., Kopiez, R., Reuter, C., & Czedik-Eysenberg, I. (2020). A snippet in a snippet: Development of the Matryoshka principle for the construction of very short musical stimuli (plinks). *Musicae Scientiae, 24*(4), 515–529. https://doi.org/10.1177/1029864918820212

Toiviainen, P., Luck, G., & Thompson, M. R. (2010). Embodied meter: Hierarchical eigenmodes in music-induced movement. *Music Perception, 28*(1), 59–70. https://doi.org/10.1525/mp.2010.28.1.59

van Wassenhove, V. (2009). Minding time in an amodal representational space. *Philosophical Transactions of the Royal Society of London. Series B, Biological Sciences, 364*(1525), 1815–1830. https://doi.org/10.1098/rstb.2009.0023

Wang, X., & Wöllner, C. (2020). Time as the ink that music is written with: A review of internal clock models and their explanatory power in audiovisual perception. *Jahrbuch Musikpsychologie, 29*, Article e67. https://doi.org/10.5964/jbdgm.2019v29.67

Watkins, H. (2017). Toward a post-humanist organicism. *Nineteenth-Century Music Review, 14*(1), 93–114. https://doi.org/10.1017/S1479409816000306

Wearden, J. H., & Lejeune, H. (2008). Scalar properties in human timing: Conformity and violations. *Quarterly Journal of Experimental Psychology, 61,* 569–587. https://doi.org/10.1080/17470210701282576

Wittgenstein, L. (1946/1998). *Culture and value* (rev. ed. by G. H. von Wright). Blackwell.

Wittmann, M. (2011). Moments in time. *Frontiers in Integrative Neuroscience, 5,* 66. https://doi.org/10.3389/fnint.2011.00066

Wittmann, M., Simmons, A. N., Aron, J. L., & Paulus, M. P. (2010). Accumulation of neural activity in the posterior insula encodes the passage of time. *Neuropsychologia, 48*(10), 3110–3120. https://doi.org/10.1016/j.neuropsychologia.2010.06.023

Wittmann, M., & van Wassenhove, V. (2009). The experience of time: Neural mechanisms and the interplay of emotion, cognition and embodiment. *Philosophical Transactions of the Royal Society of London. Series B, Biological Sciences, 364*(1525), 1809–1813. https://doi.org/10.1098/rstb.2009.0025

Wöllner, C., & Hammerschmidt, D. (2021). Tapping to hip-hop: Effects of cognitive load, arousal, and musical meter on time experiences. *Attention, Perception & Psychophysics, 83*(4), 1552–1561. https://doi.org/10.3758/s13414-020-02227-4

Wöllner, C., & Keller, P. E. (2017). Music with others: Ensembles, conductors, and interpersonal coordination. In R. Ashley & R. Timmers (Eds.), *The Routledge companion to music cognition* (pp. 313–324). Routledge.

Yeager, J. (1969). Absolute time estimates as a function of complexity and interruption of melodies. *Psychonomic Science, 15*(4), 177–178. https://doi.org/10.3758/BF03336267

20

Expressive Timing in Music and Dance Interactions

A Dynamic Perspective

Pieter-Jan Maes and Marc Leman

20.1 Introduction

In music and dance performance, timing involves the alignment of body movements with musical rhythms and temporal structures, such as tempo, metre, and phrasing. Timing may also imply *co-regulation* of this alignment among performers, based on adaptations of individual body movements to one another. In order for a performance to be successful, timing is characterized by fine-grained temporal nuances and variations that result in compelling dance grooves, typically embedded in configurations that display synchronization and counterpoint between dance and music, and exhibiting profound expressive qualities and emotional excitement. In music and dance, bodily coordination and the co-regulation of timing means walking the thin line between order and variation, between prediction and surprise, and between tension and release.

In recent decades, our scientific understanding of timing—in terms of sensorimotor coordination and co-regulation—has been growing steadily. The integration of novel technologies for recording and analysing sound and body movement within empirical research methods has greatly improved our understanding of timing, offering a fine-grained picture of specific relationships between body movement and musical signals. For example, several studies have used a frequency–time analysis of music–dance relationships; these are typically based on Fourier or wavelet analysis of movement velocity and involve subsequent correlation analysis and dimensionality reductions on frequency and/or time representations of body parts in relation to music (Amelynck et al., 2014; Hartmann et al., 2019; Toiviainen et al., 2010). However, despite overall progress in the field, two types of problems deserve our attention. The first type of problems relates to methodology and technology— when optical occlusion occurs when a body part is hidden from the view of a motion caption camera; when synchronization issues occur in contexts of multimodal data playback and recording; or simply when technology drives us to focus on kinematic parameters so that we tend to neglect other aspects of human movement, such as

Pieter-Jan Maes and Marc Leman, *Expressive Timing in Music and Dance Interactions* In: *Performing Time*. Edited by: Clemens Wöllner and Justin London, Oxford University Press. © Oxford University Press 2023. DOI: 10.1093/oso/9780192896254.003.0021 kinetic energy and muscle tension. It can be assumed that, for these problems, better measurement will move the field a step further, and issues in analysis will probably improve by applying and refining advanced analysis methods. The second type of problems, often closely related to the first type, relates to epistemology. These problems involve the gap between the artistic and the scientific approach, also known as the gap between insider and outsider knowledge, or the gap between first-person and third-person perspective (Leman, 2010). Typically, a dancer would use the term 'expressive timing' in view of an intended dance narrative, and understand timing in terms of corporeal articulations, gesturing, phrasing, communication of emotion, and storylines in relation to music. In contrast, scientists face the problem of measuring 'expressive timing', using theory to understand what measured signals mean in their context. Up to now, the scientific understanding of expressive timing is based on knowledge of short time frame sensorimotor mechanisms rather than in terms of artistic intentions. Closing this epistemological gap requires theoretical perspectives and conceptualizations from a humanities point of view, on top of the engineering challenges of measurement and analysis.

This chapter aims to provide some ingredients for understanding timing in the context of the above-mentioned epistemological problem. We show how expressive timing in music and dance can be understood in terms of ongoing sensorimotor processes and interactions within our environment. While that understanding currently focuses on short time frames, we aim to expand our understanding of expressive timing in larg(er) time frames. We suggest that the concept of embodied hierarchies and dynamical theory might help our scientific understanding of expressive timing to progress beyond the current state of the art.

At this point, most researchers tend to agree that timing is a critical issue in music and dance (Keller, 2014). Timing is typically a stabilizing factor and constancy in timing is needed to allow performers to predict the future so that collaboration and co-regulated alignments between dance and music become possible. Accordingly, the timing should be such that it entrains others to respond and that, through mutual exchanges of timing, time patterns (endowed with expression) emerge and become a new level for excitement and appeal to engagement (Leman, 2016). Key concepts in our understanding of timing are entrainment and emergence (see Madison, this volume). Entrainment occurs when patterns evolve over time towards particularly stable pattern configurations, such as when dance and music rhythms gradually reach in-phase or anti-phase synchronization. Emergence occurs when interactions between micro-patterns generate macro-pattern configurations, such as when a metre emerges from polyrhythms (both in music and body swaying).

Apart from these considerations about entrainment and emergence, we argue that a combination of two major theoretical frameworks, known as embodiment and predictive coding, can shed light on the underlying principles of timing in music and dance interactions. Embodiment theory relates to bodily realizations of timing, and to the idea that timing in humans is grounded in action repertoires shared among conspecifics (Leman, 2007; Leman et al., 2017). Predictive coding theory (Koelsch et al., 2019; Vuust & Witek, 2014) involves predictions of timing and the idea that participants in an ensemble adapt their timings based on individual assumptions about joint timing constancy. While these theories support our understanding of expressive timing in short time frames, it is of interest to investigate their potential for understanding expressive timing in large time frames such as dance narratives. A narrative occurs when entities of expressive timing (such as gestures) are sequentially ordered in particular ways, such that their contrasts and tensions tell a story. Such a (non-verbal) story offers a powerful way to create affective and emotional responses in those who perceive the narrative, even if the expressive nature of the narrative—or the responses to it—cannot be accurately described in verbal terms. At this point, it is of interest to note that expressive timing, given its non-verbal character, can be guided by a linguistic storyline such as the libretto in opera, or the lyrics of a song. For example, rather than counting a 13/12 metre, it may be easier to articulate a linguistic mantra and/or incorporate the metre in particular choreographies, which then can be cognitively *outsourced* (Maes, Giacofci, & Leman, 2015; Maes, Wanderley, & Palmer, 2015). But we should also consider facilitation of expressive timing through images that support particular postures, attitudes, and movement concepts (see also Godøy & Leman, 2010). For example, in Tchaikovsky's *Swan Lake*, the behaviour of swans (i.e. how swans move in their natural environment) provides an inspiration for a narrative of subsequent gestures endowed with expressive timing, revealing intentions related to seduction and enchantment. In short, to better understand concepts like 'expressive timing' and 'narrative of expressive timing' in terms of measured quantities, we envision an expansion of the embodied predictive coding theory in the direction of larger time frames. Given the state of the field, such an ambition cannot be anything but embryonic. Nevertheless, some ingredients are worth considering.

20.2 Outsourcing Timing to Sensorimotor Processes: The Body and Sound as Time-Keeper

At present, it is generally agreed that there is no single dedicated locus within the human brain that is solely responsible for time processing, like the central master clock operating in a computer. In contrast, there is ample support for the idea that time-keeping and -production are mediated by the intrinsic activation dynamics of a distributed network of cortical and subcortical brain regions (Buhusi & Meck, 2005; Paton & Buonomano, 2018, see Doelling et al., this volume). The specific brain regions that comprise a timing network may vary and depend on factors such as the duration of the timed intervals and the sensorimotor modalities involved (Grahn, 2012; Grondin, 2010). A better understanding of the contribution of sensorimotor mechanisms in timing is important, as timing is foundational to both music and dance.

In an earlier series of studies, we investigated in more detail how sensorimotor mechanisms, related to action-perception processing, may support timing in music performance (Maes, Giacofci, & Leman, 2015; Maes, Wanderley, & Pamer, 2015). The core idea was that time is inherently embedded in the performance of bodily gestures and in the sensory information perceived during live musical interactions (the sounds, the visual information about other's gestures, the tactile vibrations, etc.). To understand the extent to which people can rely on self-performed actions and perceived sensory patterns to regulate individual and joint time-keeping in musical performances, we designed experiments in which we studied participants' time-keeping abilities in rhythmical interval production tasks. A comparison between conditions in which, on the one hand, sensory and/or motor information was continuously available, and, on the other, conditions in which no (or only minimal) sensorimotor information was available thereby revealed underlying timing control mechanisms. For example, we hypothesized that when no continuous sensorimotor information was available, participants would need to rely more on their cognitive resources to keep track of time. This idea was grounded in earlier timing research positing a distinction between an emergent timing mechanism and an event-based timing mechanism underlying the control of rhythmic movements (Delignières et al., 2004; Robertson et al., 1999; Torre & Balasubramaniam, 2009; Zelaznik, 2005). The emergent timing mechanism is based on the idea that time-keeping is rooted in the dynamically unfolding action-perception processes going on in live embodied musical interactions. For instance, the performance of a bodily gesture, even the simplest one, necessarily implies a demarcation of a temporal interval, from the beginning of the gesture until its ending. Time thus becomes a property that is embedded in—and emerges from—the control of movement dynamics, and the body and motor system may function jointly as a timekeeper in support of rhythmical behaviour. This emergent timing mechanism assumes the presence of a continuous movement, typically periodic and oscillatory in nature, that helps to keep track of time. In many instances, however, rhythmical behaviour is performed by discrete movements, characterized by short, salient movement events that demarcate (quasi-)periodic temporal intervals in which no movement occurs. Keeping track of time during these intervals is regulated by what is called an event-based timing mechanism. It is often assumed that event-based timing relies on an explicit mental representation of time, requiring cognitive resources such as attention and working memory, such as in counting.

As a matter of fact, music and dance provide relevant contexts to study these distinct timing mechanisms. In a study on samba dance, Naveda and Leman (2010) suggested that continuous gestures mark the time points of the metre in space, with an event-based representation offering a concise representation of the dynamic continuous movement. In another study by Maes, Wanderley, and Palmer (2015), cellists were asked to perform simple melodies using two distinct types of bowing gestures, namely legato articulation and staccato articulation. Specific for legato articulation is that bowing strokes are smoothly tied to one another (cf. continuous rhythmic movement), while staccato articulation is characterized by short tone onsets separated by interspersed pauses (cf. discrete rhythmic movement). Hence, in accordance with the existing theory on emergent versus event-based timing, we hypothesized that timing of staccato articulation would rely more on cognitive resources compared to legato articulation. To test this hypothesis, we integrated a dual-task paradigm in which we crossed the primary musical timing task (production of cello tones at regular temporal intervals) with a secondary 'cognitive load' task relying on attention and working memory. Accordingly, if both tasks tapped into the same resources, it was to be expected that the tasks would mutually impair one another. In that way, it became possible to assess the relative roles of sensorimotor and cognitive resources in different musical timing contexts. The results of this experiment showed that only the timing of staccato articulation was impaired under conditions of heightened cognitive load, in particular at slower performance tempi. These findings indicated that, in line with the existing theory on emergent versus event-based timing, the temporal control of rhythmic movements may, indeed, recruit distinct neural networks depending on the performance context and modalities involved (Koch et al., 2009; Petter et al., 2016). It is also of practical interest to know that, in conditions of heightened cognitive load—frequent in music and dance contexts—body movements may support the regulation of timing.

In a follow-up study, the focus was further directed towards the possible role of sounds in support of an emergent timing mechanism (Maes, Giacofci, & Leman, 2015). As it does for bodily gestures, time may be similarly embedded in, and emerge from, the unfolding of acoustical energy and/or musical patterns. Through repeated experiences, musicians and dancers may establish an association between perceived auditory regularities in music and the duration of temporal intervals. In turn, in coupling action to perception, body movements may be aligned in time to perceived auditory regularities in order to obtain successful performance timing. Sensorimotor processing is at the core of this emergent timing mechanism. Keeping track of time becomes a matter of coupling actions to perception and of underlying sensorimotor learning processes, rather than of the purely mental act of keeping track of time. Consequently, it is to be expected that this emergent sensorimotor timing mechanism is more robust in situations of heightened cognitive load, as it relies less on cognitive resources for keeping track of time.

This idea was tested in the study by Maes, Giacofci, and Leman (2015). In this study, participants were asked to tap out a simple melody as regularly as possible by repeatedly pressing a keyboard key. This timing task was integrated into the synchronization-continuation paradigm, whereby participants were first asked to synchronize their taps to an auditory metronome (indicating the target temporal interval to be produced) and to maintain that regular pace after the metronome had stopped. The crucial aspect of the experiment resided in the manipulation of the auditory tones that were produced, in particular their amplitude envelope that captured the amplitude change of a tone over time (attack, decay, sustain, and release). Tapping the key either produced a short piano tone (discrete tone) or a long piano tone of which the amplitude envelope exactly fitted the temporal interval that needed to be produced (continuous tone). In synchronizing taps to the initial metronome ticks, participants were expected to implicitly learn the relationship between the amplitude envelope of the continuous tone, and the target temporal interval that needed to be produced; in other words, the onset of each next metronome tick (the point where a tap should be performed) occurred systematically at the point where the previous piano tone ceased to be heard. Results of the experiment showed that continuous tones contributed to regular timing production, suggesting that participants could, indeed, rely on the perceived temporal characteristics of the self-produced piano tones to regulate their timing. This conclusion was further supported by an additional temporal manipulation of the amplitude envelope of the continuous tone. While participants were tapping at a regular pace (without a metronome), we gradually shortened the duration of the continuous tone, from a duration that equalled the target temporal interval of 1,100 ms to a duration of 867 ms. Consequently, we observed that participants adapted their temporal tapping interval correspondingly in order to maintain the alignment of each tap with the ending of the piano tone produced by the previous tap. Again, this indicated that the amplitude envelope of piano tones was taken as temporal reference for participants' control of their own timing.

The studies above demonstrated that both bodily gestures and sounds can support an emergent timing mechanism, rooted in sensorimotor processing. This points to an interesting mechanism that can be of practical benefit to musicians and dancers. When relying on the alternative *event-based* timing mechanism, keeping track of time requires cognitive resources, such as attention and memory, meaning that these resources—at least to some extent—cannot be allocated anymore to other tasks in music and dance interaction that require them. In that regard, the use of sensorimotor processing skills underlying the emergent timing mechanism may be a valuable and welcome strategy to control timing in music and dance interactions in an alternative way, freeing up cognitive resources for executing additional tasks. In earlier work (Coorevits et al., 2020; Maes, Giacofci, & Leman, 2015) we have referred to this strategy as an *outsourcing* strategy. With this concept, we point to the idea that timing can be transferred, at least partly, from cognitive resources to sensorimotor processing. This idea fits within a more general tendency to use physical actions—as well as phenomena, objects, and technologies within their environment—to reduce the cognitive demands of tasks such as mental timekeeping.

In one study, we investigated how this emergent timing mechanism may not only be of relevance for regulating individual timekeeping, but also for interpersonal coregulation in music and dance performance. In Coorevits et al. (2020), we applied the framework of emergent versus event-based timing to a context of social music interaction. In particular, we were interested whether so-called ancillary movements in music performance could contribute to joint regular interval production. Unlike sound-producing movements, ancillary movements do not contribute directly to the production of musical sounds (Cadoz & Wanderley, 2000). However, they do support embodied expression and communication of musical intentions (Davidson,

1993; Wanderley, 2002). Because of the inherent spatiotemporal nature of ancillary movements, we were interested in how they might support temporal co-regulation in social music performance. In our experiment, we manipulated the type of ancillary gestures that participants were allowed to perform in a joint tapping task. The goal of this task was to perform the same musical melody together as regularly as possible by tapping their finger on tapping pads. Between conditions, we controlled for the type of tapping gestures performed. Participants were either instructed to perform prominent, continuous up/downward movements in between successive taps (continuous gestures), or were restricted to perform any movements between successive taps (discrete gestures). In line with the findings on individual timing, results showed that when participants of a dyad could see each other, continuous gestures (performed by both) led to better joint timing in terms of consistency and accuracy of synchronized tapping. In addition, we found that the type of gestures employed by musicians modulated leader–follower dynamics, in the sense that participants who performed continuous bodily gestures tended to take the leader role in the interaction.

20.3 Embodied Predictive Coding and Expressive Narratives

Until recently, sensorimotor coupling was typically studied from the viewpoint of rhythmic tapping and timekeeping (Repp & Su, 2013). For understanding the basics of music and dance interactions, this paradigm is still very relevant. Currently, however, the tapping studies are expanded in several directions, including neuroscience (Elst et al., 2021) and musicology, where limbs, full body movement, and more realistic (or artistic) movements are studied (see previous section for examples). Overall, our understanding of timekeeping and of simple (discrete, continuous) sensorimotor-based timing (both in individual and social contexts), is based on prediction, as captured by the predictive coding theory, a brain theory which holds that the brain is a prediction generating engine (Koelsch et al., 2019). In the context of timing, the engine would constantly adapt a prediction about timing based on prediction error, which is the difference between the predicted timing and the real timing (Vuust & Witek, 2014). In the context of co-regulated timing, Leman (2021) has implemented this principle in an algorithm called *BListener*, an application that solely focuses on perception (not involving any embodiment) but that clearly explicates how Bayesian inferencing about timing works. BListener could become part of an action-perception coupling mechanism in a virtual musician that could—with some further programming effort—play along with human musicians and interact with dancers. BListener perceives the duration between two consecutive onsets (so-called inter-onset intervals (IOIs)) and estimates the constancy of subsequent fluctuating IOIs. The onsets come from musical onsets of notes, hand clapping, or from dance onsets, such as feet touching the ground. The

Bayesian inference component in this approach relates to the updating mechanism for predicting timing. The Bayesian view involves a likelihood (i.e. how likely it is that a new temporal event stems from the assumed timing constancy) and a prior (the expected timing constancy in absence of observations), from which a posterior (expected timing constancy, given the new temporal event) is inferred. In view of a subsequent onset, the prior is updated by replacing the old prior with the posterior. This Bayesian inference is embedded in a system dynamic that updates the priors every sample (e.g. 100 times per second). In music and dance, the rhythms can often be conceived as a concatenation of IOIs taken from a limited set of IOI values having a simple relationship among each other, such as binary or ternary. These binary and ternary components together mark the metre. Constancy in timing is therefore typically a constancy in the fluctuation of subsequent durations that establish the metre. Repetitive dances, for example, can thus be captured in terms of metre constancy, which may even may be a marker of a qualitative performance, attracting interest and leading to excitement or empowerment.

While this theory provides a solid basis for timing (see also Vuust & Witek, 2014), it nevertheless does not incorporate the embodiment perspective, which we believe to be essential—not only for expressive timing being in line with the timing predictions, but also for generating narratives of expressive timing. Given its relation to the unfolding of a gesture over time, expression implies careful planning ahead of time, and hence careful prediction of timing. The Bayesian brain could be conceived as a controller mechanism for expressive timing necessarily connected with corporal articulations that unfold in a pattern over time (see the previous paragraphs). Looking back at finger tapping studies and extensions of the experimental paradigm of sensorimotor control in music and dance interaction studies, it can be noticed that sensorimotor mechanisms and predictions work well in the millisecond range. However, these mechanisms can typically have no awareness of larger-scale developments such as we know them in artistic performances. At that level, we often speak about patterns at larger time frames, such as expressive arcs (as in the unfolding of a gesture that starts smoothly, going to a maximum in movement speed and articulation, and then ends again smoothly) and tension bows (as in a gesture that starts in sync with the music, becomes highly de-synchronized, and ends again in sync) that may reach far beyond the 10–20 s range. Such expressive arcs and tension bows are assumed to influence the timings at the local level. Hence, for understanding this aspect, it is necessary to call upon a more global level, which is typically associated with the narrative and its associated intentionality, or goal-driven character. There is a considerable gap between sensorimotor studies, on the one hand (their underpinning by predictive coding theories and micro-embodiment), and studies about artistic expression, narratives, and intentions, on the other, and this issue is currently not well understood.

Therefore, the idea is that the outsourcing of sensorimotor processes could be conceived within a broader perspective on 'the narrative of expressive timing', or, alternatively called, 'the expressive narrative'. This narrative, for example, can be conceived as a storyline expressed in music and through dance, as in Tchaikovsky's *Swan Lake*, or it can be an abstract story line, such as the dance sequence in Baroque group dances, which is meant to change partnership among a group of male and female dancers. The narrative element can also be implied by a ritual activity aimed at reaching the divine, such as in the Zekir ritual of the Soefi (Rouget, 1985); or it can be an inherited story line in oral tradition about cattle, providing an ingredient for forward and backward moving in African circular dances (Phyfferoen et al., 2017). The narrative can be anything, as long as it involves sequences of expressive timing. Often, these sequences aim at generating tension arcs in pursuit of an artistic effect. Tension arcs indeed capture the attention of audiences.

In the examples mentioned, we assume that the overall narrative component acts as a guiding principle for intentionality, or goal-directed music–dance action, that creates tension, surprise, and emotional effects through contrasts, both in global timing (the storyline as intentional guide) and local timing (the outsourcing of time through movement). Huron's theory of expectation (2006) is based on the contrast between fast reactive responses and slow appraisal responses. Here we assume that expectations (of timing) are embodied, through the outsourcing of timing in gestures, and that musicians/dancers engage in recruiting these gestures to enact the narrative. As such, the outsourced embodied timing supports the expressive narrative. However, one could also argue that the expressive narrative guides the outsourced embodied timing.

Tensions between biological bias in timing (such as entrainment to beats) and cultural habits in timing (such as the codifications of how beats are accommodated through dance) can be a rich source for artistic expression. This view perhaps challenges a too narrow view on predictive coding as local prediction error minimalization engine. Being guided and misled by musicians or dancers, so that audiences become surprised and novel musical patterns emerge, is likely to be an essential part of expressive and creative dance–music interactions.

Given the current state of the art, we propose two pathways towards a better understanding of expressive timing in short time frames (the sensorimotor perspective) and timing in large time frames (the narrative perspective). The first pathway consists of a gradual expansion of the timescale at which action-perception coupling is studied. The second pathway consists in the development of a theoretical perspective that incorporates sensorimotor prediction mechanisms with the expressive narrative in a perspective that is driven by a dynamic theory.

20.3.1 Embodied Hierarchies

The concept of embodied hierarchies encompasses the idea that dance and music draw upon gestures as a mid-level concept between low-level sensorimotor action and high-level narrative (Godøy & Leman, 2010). Previous work on gesture suggested that gestures can be conceived as a concatenation of basic gestures that compose a gesture narrative, or as a gesture narrative that can be decomposed in units subsuming basic gestures (Leman & Camurri, 2006; Leman & Naveda, 2010; Naveda & Leman, 2010, see also Jensenius et al., 2010). Hilt and colleagues (2019) propose a multilayer approach to group coordination, suggesting that the co-regulation of group behaviour is based on the exchange of information across several layers, each of them tuned to carry specific coordinative signals. Multilayer sensorimotor communication in which several timescales are embedded through several sensory channels (auditory, visual, spatial) may be the key concept for understanding how musicians and, more generally humans, communicate with each other (see also Eerola et al., 2018).

20.3.2 Dynamic Theory

A dynamic theory might help us to understand how expressive timing at the sensorimotor level gets embedded in expressive narratives. Interactions between the two levels are assumed to draw upon balancing mechanisms, creating states of equilibrium (or homeostasis) among involved processes. For example, the tempo of a joint performance can be seen as a state of equilibrium reached through co-regulated expressive timing. This interaction state emerges from a dynamic interaction among performers. Small differences in the timing of one musician or dancer may affect overall tempo-balance at the group level. Several small differences from different musicians or dancers thereby appear as small fluctuations that are compensated for (negative feedback) in view of keeping the balance (i.e. the timing constancy). However, during a performance, one tempo may suddenly have to change to another. That sudden change in tempo would imply another type of regulation (called positive feedback) in the sense that all processes adapt to the newly intended equilibrium state for co-regulated timing. The music and dance ensemble's timing is an example of a system capable of building and maintaining a series of homeostatic co-regulated states that are intrinsically sense-giving, both during the act of creating music and dance and during the act of perceiving both. The latter can be understood as the motivational drive for acting and engaging in music and dance interactions. The narrative can be conceived as an overall structuring element for expressive timing. It can globally define the tempo (e.g. fast or slow), the articulation (e.g. soft or firm), and it can guide the tension of an intended story line (e.g. from fast to slow; from soft to firm). The narrative thus appears as an intentional co-regulating factor, a hyper-parameter that co-steer the parameters that define the semi-automated and automated low-level mechanisms at longer terms. This intentional co-regulation can be understood from the viewpoint of predictive coding as it can probably set expectations for expectations, itself being steered by the possibilities and limitations of the human body.

20.4 Conclusion

Some problems in current dance and music research are concerned with intrinsically different types of knowledge about expressive timing. We reflected on the idea that our scientific knowledge in terms of (subliminal) sensorimotor control and our artistic knowledge in terms of (intended) narrative, can, to some extent, be filled. Thanks to novel technologies and methodologies, artistic intuitions about timing tend to push scientific research further in directions that go beyond classical research topics in sensorimotor timing, such as finger tapping and time-keeping. By looking at expressive timing in music and dance at large time frames, we tend to walk the thin line between order and variation, between prediction and surprise, between tension and release, and between sensorimotor and narrative perspectives. Research that originated in (systematic, cognitive, empirical) musicology has, indeed, contributed many exciting new insights and much understanding of our intuitions about music and dance interactions. Expressive timing has been fully incorporated in modern cognitive (neuro)science. Yet, many challenges remain to be addressed in future research. In this chapter, we suggested that the concept of embodied hierarchies could be helpful as a starting point for understanding multiple time frames of expressive timing. In parallel with this concept, we suggested that expressive timing can be understood from the viewpoint of homeostatic (co-)regulation, which is a dynamic principle.

Clearly, more insights about the relationship and interdependencies of timing on these different temporal scales is needed. Therefore, the further exploration and application of (non-)linear time-series analysis tools that may unveil interdependencies across different temporal scales is important. Consequently, we would gain deeper insights into the biological and cultural principles regulating (interpersonal) timing behaviour, and contribute to the refinement of existing theoretical frameworks. Theory formation will need to integrate the various levels and mechanisms of timing control and co-regulation, ranging from low-level spontaneous coordination based on dynamical principles (Kelso, 1995, 2021; Leman, 2021), to higher-level learning, to predictive processing, and active inference (Gallagher & Allen, 2018; Koban et al., 2019; Sebanz & Knoblich, 2009). In addition, further research is required on the role of variability, deviation, and surprise in human engagement with music and dance. More than other daily activities, for which optimal functioning in terms of behaviour and decision-taking is often crucial, music and art in general offer room for exploring the dynamics of prediction and surprise, of recurrence and variability (Schiavio et al., 2021). Far from being undesirable, surprise and deviation may reveal a diversity of emerging novel patterns in both sound and bodily behaviour, leading to highly rewarding and novel subjective experiences.

New technologies for recording and analysing sound, bodily behaviour, and (neuro)physiological responses have dramatically improved this research on timing in music and dance in the past decades. Recently, new technologies in the domain of extended reality (virtual, augmented, and mixed reality) are being incorporated into the empirical study of embodied music interaction (Turchet et al., 2021; Van Kerrebroeck et al., 2021). They offer radically new possibilities for multisensory, immersive stimulus creation in experimental research on narratives of expressive timing. Advances in (neuro)cognitive research into the fundamental principles underlying the embodied nature of expressive timing, along with emergent new technologies, provide a vibrant context in which research on timing may flourish in the coming years.

References

Amelynck, D., Maes, P.-J., Martens, J. P., & Leman, M. (2014). Expressive body movement responses to music are coherent, consistent, and low dimensional. *IEEE Transactions on Cybernetics, 44*(12), 2288–2301.

Buhusi, C. V., & Meck, W. H. (2005). What makes us tick? Functional and neural mechanisms of interval timing. *Nature Reviews Neuroscience, 6*(10), 755–765.

Cadoz, C., & Wanderley, M. M. (2000). Gesture—music. In M. M. Wanderley & M. Battier (Eds.), *Trends in gestural control of music* (pp. 71–93). Ircam-Centre Pompidou.

Coorevits, E., Maes, P.-J., Six, J., & Leman, M. (2020). The influence of performing gesture type on interpersonal musical timing, and the role of visual contact and tempo. *Acta Psychologica, 210*, 103166.

Davidson, J. W. (1993). Visual perception of performance manner in the movements of solo musicians. *Psychology of Music, 21*(3), 103–113.

Delignières, D., Lemoine, L., & Torre, K. (2004). Time intervals production in tapping and oscillatory motion. *Human Movement Science, 23*(2), 87–103.

Eerola, T., Jakubowski, K., Moran, N., Keller, P. E., & Clayton, M. (2018). Shared periodic performer movements coordinate interactions in duo improvisations. *Royal Society Open Science, 5*(2), 171520.

Elst, O. F., Vuust, P., Kringelbach, M. L., & Foster, N. H. (2021). *The neuroscience of dance: A systematic review of the present state of research and suggestions for future work.* PsyArXiv. https://doi.org/10.31234/osf.io/kfpcx

Gallagher, S., & Allen, M. (2018). Active inference, enactivism and the hermeneutics of social cognition. *Synthese, 196*(6), 2627–2648.

Godøy, R. I., & Leman, M. (2010). *Musical gestures: Sound, movement, and meaning.* Routledge.

Grahn, J. (2012). Neural mechanisms of rhythm perception: Current findings and future perspectives. *Topics in Cognitive Science, 4*(4), 585–606.

Grondin, S. (2010). Timing and time perception: A review of recent behavioral and neuroscience findings and theoretical directions. *Attention, Perception & Psychophysics, 72*(3), 561–582.

Hartmann, M., Mavrolampados, A., Allingham, E., Carlson, E., Burger, B., & Toiviainen, P. (2019). Kinematics of perceived dyadic coordination in dance. *Scientific Reports, 9*(1), 1–14.

Hilt, P. M., Badino, L., D'Ausilio, A., Volpe, G., Tokay, S., Fadiga, L., & Camurri, A. (2019). Multi-layer adaptation of group coordination in musical ensembles. *Scientific Reports, 9*(5854), 1–10.

Huron, D. (2006). *Sweet anticipation: Music and the psychology of expectation.* MIT Press.

Jensenius, A. R., Wanderley, M. M., Godøy, R. I., & Leman, M. (2010). Musical gestures: Concepts and methods in research. In R. I. Godøy & M. Leman (Eds.), *Musical gestures: Sound, movement, and meaning* (pp. 12–35). Routledge.

Keller, P. E. (2014). Ensemble performance: Interpersonal alignment of musical expression. In R. Timmers & E. Schubert (Eds.), *Expressiveness in music performance: Empirical approaches across styles and cultures* (pp. 260–282). Oxford University Press.

Kelso, J. A. S. (1995). *Dynamic patterns: The self-organization of brain and behavior.* A Bradford Book.

Kelso, J. A. S. (2021). Unifying large-and small-scale theories of coordination. *Entropy, 23*(5), 537.

Koban, L., Ramamoorthy, A., & Konvalinka, I. (2019). Why do we fall into sync with others? Interpersonal synchronization and the brain's optimization principle. *Social Neuroscience, 14*(1), 1–9.

Koch, G. K., Oliveri, M., & Caltagirone, C. (2009). Neural networks engaged in milliseconds and seconds time processing: Evidence from transcranial magnetic stimulation and patients with cortical or subcortical dysfunction. *Philosophical Transactions of the Royal Society. Series B, Biological Sciences, 364*(1525), 1907–1918.

Koelsch, S., Vuust, P., & Friston, K. (2019). Predictive processes and the peculiar case of music. *Trends in Cognitive Sciences, 23*(1), 63–77.

Leman, M. (2007). *Embodied music cognition and mediation technology.* MIT Press.

Leman, M. (2010). Music, gesture and the formation of embodied meaning. In R. Godøy & M. Leman (Eds.), *Musical gestures: Sound, movement, and meaning* (pp. 126–153). Routledge.

Leman, M. (2016). *The expressive moment: How interaction (with music) shapes human empowerment.* MIT Press.

Leman, M. (2021). Co-regulated timing in music ensembles: A Bayesian listener perspective. *Journal of New Music Research, 50*(2), 121–132.

Leman, M., & Camurri, A. (2006). Understanding musical expressiveness using interactive multimedia platforms. *Musicae Scientiae, 10*(1 Suppl), 209–233.

Leman, M., Lesaffre, M., & Maes, P.-J. (2017). What is embodied music interaction? In M. Lesaffre, P.-J. Maes, & M. Leman (Eds.), *Routledge companion to embodied music interaction* (pp. 1–10). Routledge.

Leman, M., & Naveda, L. (2010). Basic gestures as spatiotemporal reference frames for repetitive dance/music patterns in Samba and Charleston. *Music Perception, 28*(1), 71–91.

Maes, P.-J., Giacofci, M., & Leman, M. (2015). Auditory and motor contributions to the timing of melodies under cognitive load. *Journal of Experimental Psychology: Human Perception and Performance, 41*(5), 1336–1352.

Maes, P.-J., Wanderley, M. M., & Palmer, C. (2015). The role of working memory in the temporal control of discrete and continuous movements. *Experimental Brain Research, 233*(1), 263–273.

Naveda, L., & Leman, M. (2010). The spatiotemporal representation of dance and music gestures using topological gesture analysis (TGA). *Music Perception, 28*(1), 93–111.

Paton, J. J., & Buonomano, D. V. (2018). The neural basis of timing: Distributed mechanisms for diverse functions. *Neuron, 98*(4), 687–705.

Petter, E. A., Lusk, N. A., Hesslow, G., & Meck, W. H. (2016). Interactive roles of the cerebellum and striatum in sub-second and supra-second timing: Support for an initiation, continuation, adjustment, and termination (ICAT) model of temporal processing. *Neuroscience & Biobehavioral Reviews, 71,* 739–755.

Phyfferoen, D., Stroeken, K., & Leman, M. (2017). The Hiplife zone: Cultural transformation processes in African music seen from the angle of embodied music interactions. In M. Lesaffre, P.-J. Maes, & M. Leman (Eds.), *The Routledge companion to embodied music interaction* (pp. 232–240). Routledge.

Repp, B. H., & Su, Y. H. (2013). Sensorimotor synchronization: A review of recent research (2006–2012). *Psychonomic Bulletin & Review, 20*(3), 403–452.

Robertson, S. D., Zelaznik, H. N., Lantero, D. A., Bojczyk, K. G., Spencer, R. M., Doffin, J. G., & Schneidt, T. (1999). Correlations for timing consistency among tapping and drawing tasks: Evidence against a single timing process for motor control. *Journal of Experimental Psychology: Human Perception and Performance, 25*(5), 1316–1330.

Rouget, G. (1985). *Music and trance: A theory of the relations between music and possession.* University of Chicago Press.

Schiavio, A., Maes, P.-J., & van der Schyff, D. (2021). The dynamics of musical participation. *Musicae Scientiae, 26*(3), 604–626.

Sebanz, N., & Knoblich, G. (2009). Prediction in joint action: What, when, and where. *Topics in Cognitive Science, 1*(2), 353–367.

Toiviainen, P., Luck, G., & Thompson, M. R. (2010). Embodied meter: Hierarchical eigenmodes in music-induced movement. *Music Perception, 28*(1), 59–70.

Torre, K., & Balasubramaniam, R. (2009). Two different processes for sensorimotor synchronization in continuous and discontinuous rhythmic movements. *Experimental Brain Research, 199*(2), 157–166.

Turchet, L., Hamilton, R., & Çamci, A. (2021). Music in extended realities. *IEEE Access, 9,* 15810–15832.

Van Kerrebroeck, B., Caruso, G., & Maes, P.-J. (2021). A methodological framework for assessing social presence in music interactions in virtual reality. *Frontiers in Psychology, 12,* 663725.

Vuust, P., & Witek, M. A. (2014). Rhythmic complexity and predictive coding: A novel approach to modeling rhythm and meter perception in music. *Frontiers in Psychology, 5,* 1111.

Wanderley, M. M. (2002). Quantitative analysis of non-obvious performer gestures. In I. Wachsmuth & T. Sowa (Eds.), *Gesture and Sign Language in Human-Computer Interaction. GW 2001.* (Lecture Notes in Computer Science) (Vol. 2298, pp. 241–253). Springer.

Zelaznik, H. N. (2005). Timing variability in circle drawing and tapping: Probing the relationship between event and emergent timing. *Journal of Motor Behavior, 37*(5), 395–403.

21

Temporal Aspects of Musical Expectancy and Creativity in Improvisation

A Review of Recent Neuroscientific Studies and an Updated Model

Psyche Loui

21.1 Introduction

> A mind is fundamentally an anticipator, an expectation-generator.
>
> (Dennett, 2008, p. 57)

In his seminal work *Emotion and Meaning in Music*, Leonard Meyer (1956) posited that affect in music 'is aroused when an expectation—a tendency to respond—activated by the musical stimulus situation, is temporarily inhibited or permanently blocked' (p. 31). This view has been influential in the study of music, especially in music cognition, because it lends itself to systematic analyses of how musical structure can communicate emotion and meaning without appealing to referential semantics (Pearce & Wiggins, 2012). Developing Meyer's view of expectation, and linking to gestalt theories of perception, Narmour advanced the *Implication–Realization* model for the analysis of melodic structures (Narmour, 1990), where pairs of melodic intervals were designated as implication or realization intervals. While the Implication–Realization model enabled systematic analysis of certain musical structures, it applied only relatively specifically to melodies codified as short sequences of pitches. Expanding on this model, Margulis advanced a model of melodic expectation, where melodic events were assigned expectedness ratings based on their stability, proximity, and direction, with additional contributions from mobility (Margulis, 2005). In a similar vein but using a different approach, Pearce developed the *Information Dynamics of Music* (IDyoM) model, which explicitly quantifies melodic expectancy as a function of information content as it changes over time (Pearce & Wiggins, 2006). The IDyoM model has been used with neuroscience techniques (Cheung et al., 2019; Di Liberto et al., 2020) to show how neural recordings obtained from specific brain regions, including but not limited to the auditory cortex, might encode or reflect melodic expectations. In sum, there has been

Psyche Loui, *Temporal Aspects of Musical Expectancy and Creativity in Improvisation* In: *Performing Time*. Edited by: Clemens Wöllner and Justin London, Oxford University Press. © Oxford University Press 2023. DOI: 10.1093/oso/9780192896254.003.0022 intense interest in music cognition that centres around expectations and predictions and how they are essential to musical experiences.

By contrast, for a model of musical expectations to encompass musical experiences more broadly and flexibly, it should encompass not only specific musical pieces, but rather the capacity to generate and evaluate musical ideas more broadly. This is because a view of musical expectations as applied to specific musical pieces, as is the case in all of the above-mentioned models of musical expectation, requires that the music can be recorded, transcribed, or otherwise reduced to a series of pitches unfolding over time. This reductionism necessarily detracts from the musical experience somewhat. Furthermore, to apply such a model on musical pieces requires that they have already been created. In other words, modelling musical expectancy using established models of musical expectation presumes that the humans that are being studied harbour the same expectations as those quantified by the model. For a forward-looking view of musical expectations, rather than analysing specific pieces of music, it may be useful instead to consider *musicality*, which is the capacity of humans to produce and perceive music (Honing et al., 2015). A model of musical expectations that focuses on musicality is promising as it focuses on the mind and brain that is capable of creating music, thus allowing the possibility of studying more diverse experiences that can more comprehensively encompass what we think of as music. Here, we conceptualize musical expectations in the context of musical improvisation as a real-time form of musical creativity. The central thesis is that musical improvisation, an aspect of musicality, offers a useful window through which to understand real-time creativity (Loui, 2018).

Improvisation differs from other forms of musical creativity, such as composition or a performer's interpretation of an established piece, in significant ways. While composition and interpretation involve reflective processes that can be developed and reworked without the pressure of instantaneously producing the music piece, improvisation is the real-time creation and performance of music (Biasutti, 2015). This real-time view into music creation and performance has prompted others to ask about mental processes that underlie the performance of jazz musicians, and from there, about what constitutes creativity at all (Johnson-Laird, 2002).

Creativity is traditionally defined as the capacity to produce output that is novel, useful, beneficial, and desired by an audience (Runco & Jaeger, 2012). Theories of creativity have focused on four domains, identified as the four Ps—Person, Process, Product, and Press (Rhodes, 1961). The idea that models of musical expectation should focus on musicality mirrors the shift in creativity research from the focus on the Product to a focus on the Process (Rhodes, 1961). Studies in musical creativity, specifically, conceptualize creativity as involving dual processes of idea generation and idea evaluation (Kleinmintz et al., 2014). Training in musical improvisation, then, may release inhibition on the idea generation of novel musical ideas, resulting in greater creativity (Kleinmintz et al., 2014).

21.2 An Updated Model of Musical Creativity

The mind can be characterized as a complex system that lends itself to multiple levels of description. Borrowing from seminal work on vision (Marr, 1982), cognitive scientists have conceptualized the mind at computational, algorithmic, and implementational levels (Figure 21.1, left). At the highest level, the computational level encompasses the overall goals of the system. The algorithmic level is the intermediate level that describes how the computational problems can be solved, and has been termed 'the bridge between computation and brain' (Love, 2015, p. 230). The lowest level is the implementation level; this often refers to the underlying 'hardware' or the neurobiological substrates at work to subserve the cognitive mechanisms specified in the algorithmic level. Here we borrow from this three-level view of the mind and adapt it towards the capacity of the mind to create music, specifically with the goal of understanding musical improvisation, while updating and elaborating on prior iterations of this model (Loui, 2018; Pressing, 1998). The model is shown in Figure 21.1 and is unpacked below.

21.2.1 Computational Level

What are the overall goals of musical improvisation? For Pressing (1998), improvisation involves taking a *referent* and filtering it through a knowledge base. This referent is 'a set of cognitive, perceptual, or emotional structures (constraints) that guide and

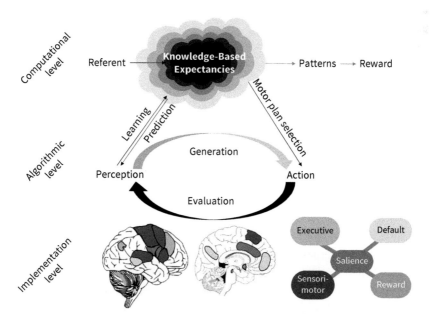

Figure 21.1 A model of expectancy in musical improvisation.

aid in the production of musical materials' (Pressing, 1984, p. 350); this could be a song's form, including its 'licks', and chord progressions, or it could include a theme, an idea, or an emotion. 'The goal of successful improvisations, then, entails filtering the referent through the performer's own knowledge base to generate fluent, cohesive auditory–motor sequences that are intrinsically rewarding' (Loui, 2018, p. 139). One way to think about this knowledge base, as it pertains to musicality, is as a library of expectancies, which are predictions about musical structures (Figure 21.1, top). This comprises the flexible library of information storied in procedural or declarative knowledge, including rhythmic and metric structures, harmonic structures, and melodies, as well as timbre and articulation information that constitute schematic and veridical expectations for music accumulated from one's life experiences (Huron, 2006).

Once the referent is filtered through the knowledge base, the output is musical patterns that are generated by the cognitive system, which are then realized as auditory–motor output. This realization of musical ideas into auditory–motor output validates predictions that the individual finds to be rewarding, while simultaneously adapting to ongoing changes in the musical landscape. This generation of auditory–motor patterns is a creative process, as Limb and Braun (2008) write: 'musical improvisation as a prototypical form of spontaneous creative behaviour, with the assumption that the process is neither mysterious nor obscure, but is instead predicated on novel combinations of ordinary mental processes' (p. 1). As such, the result of musical improvisation that is intrinsically rewarding, fitting Csikszentmihalyi's (1996) description of creative products as 'the result of individual ingenuity that was recognized, rewarded, and transmitted through learning. . . . The results of creativity enrich the culture and so they indirectly improve the quality of all our lives' (p. 10).

21.2.2 Algorithmic Level

The algorithmic level (Figure 21.1, middle) describes the repeated processes that must take place in order to implement the goals of the computational level. In creativity research, dual-process models, such as the *Geneplore* (Generate and Explore) model (Finke et al., 1992), have been used to describe two sets of thinking processes: those involved in the generation of ideas and those involved with their refinement, evaluation, and/or selection (Sowden et al., 2015). Applied to musical improvisation, this involves the linking of perceptual and motor processes in a feedforward and feedback system. This coupling gives rise to idea generation as a feedforward process from perception and action, through the merging of perceptual input with the semantic referent into the knowledge-based library of expectations as described in the computational level section (see Section 21.2.1). Another aspect of the algorithmic level is that idea evaluation is a feedback process that takes the output of motor commands as perceptual input, and continuously evaluates the perceptual input and its associated expectancies relative to expected targets, thus refining the improvised musical patterns by refining predictions and selecting more accurate motor plans over time. This idea-evaluation process closely mirrors the process of 'blind variation and selective retention' hypothesized in creativity research, which again postulates the generation of ideas as combinatorial variation of available ideas, followed by the feedback-dependent pruning of ideas to retain the best ones to be refined at the next iteration (Simonton, 2010). Similar feedforward and feedback processes are hypothesized to be involved in speaking and singing: the *Directions Into Velocities of Articulators* (DIVA) model of speech production posits feedforward and feedback mechanisms, implemented by perceptual mechanisms and motor articulators, that together control speech motor movement production (Guenther, 2017). Analogously, the dual-stream neuroanatomical model of singing posits perceptual–motor coupling to enable feedback and feedforward mechanisms for pitch production (Loui, 2015).

Musical improvisation may appear to unfold with a short time lag (e.g. on the order of seconds) between an idea or a theme being introduced to the cognitive system, and a series of auditory–motor patterns being executed. At the algorithmic and implementational levels, however, such seemingly automatic processes are subserved by efficient coupling between perception and action, which are cognitive (algorithmic) and brain-level (implementation) processes that unfold at an even finer timescale (i.e. on the order of milliseconds). In considering musical improvisation at these different levels, we can scrutinize the finer timescales while simultaneously acknowledging that the phenomenological experience may occur at coarser timescales, such as in seconds or minutes, or over the course of a performance.

21.2.3 Implementational Level

The implementation of such a feedforward and feedback system is at the lowest level of analysis (Figure 21.1, bottom): the implementational level includes brain structures and networks that work together to enable the algorithmic-level functions. Current views of neuroimaging research conceptualize the brain as networks rather than as individual areas that function in isolation, and it is the coactivity and the interactions between these large-scale neuronal networks in the brain that enable cognition (Bressler & Menon, 2010). Specifically, these networks include the sensorimotor network which enables auditory and motor processes, the executive control network which includes lateral frontoparietal areas that are active in most cognitive tasks, and the default mode network which is active typically at rest. Furthermore, the salience network, with the anterior insula and cingulate cortex as crucial hubs, assists multiple brain regions in the generation of appropriate behavioural responses to salient stimuli. These networks are highlighted in Figure 21.1, and will be expanded in the Section 21.3.2 on magnetic resonance imaging (MRI) studies of large-scale brain networks.

More conceptually, neuroscientists have long thought that the nervous system evolved to predict error (Ashby, 1947). A seminal finding that links dopaminergic signalling to prediction error comes from Schultz, Dayan, and Montague (1997), who showed that neurons that carry the neurotransmitter dopamine are not only active when the organism is receiving a reward, but also when it is anticipating a reward. Friston's free-energy principle (Friston et al., 2006) states that the brain minimizes free energy by using hierarchical internal models to generate dynamic and context-sensitive expectations. Following this view, others have written about music as entropy reduction (Hansen & Pearce, 2014), and music as predictive coding (Koelsch et al., 2018). To make musical predictions, then, is to form a mental model that codes for expectations in a specific, refined form. This act of generating predictions is intrinsic to biological systems, and is tied to the same physiological demands that enable survival. With predictive coding, it is gratifying to see that the importance of expectations, first posited by Meyer in 1956, has come full circle to be echoed in neuroscience.

21.3 Musical Time as Psychological Time

Time is an important factor in both predictions and error learning, and the different levels of the model operate on multiple timescales. For example, at the implementational level, the dopaminergic prediction-error mechanism works on the order of milliseconds, observable in human electroencephalography (EEG) studies. Conversely, the default mode network fluctuates in activity at a much slower timescale, on the order of 10 s per cycle (0.1 Hz) (Fox et al., 2005). Similarly, knowledge-based expectancies posited in the computational level may involve moment-to-moment, note-by-note expectations (e.g. as predicted by the IDyoM), as well as long-term knowledge that is refined pedagogically in learning to improvise (Biasutti, 2015). Applied to music, the experience of musical time is determined at least in part by psychological time, which is the subjective experience of time (as opposed to clock time). Psychological time is influenced by attention, memory, and expectation(s). Evidence that psychological time is influenced by prediction and expectation comes from psychophysical studies on subjective duration estimation: unexpected events appear to last longer than expected events. However, the perceived lengthening of the duration of the unexpected event does not transfer to other simultaneous events (Pariyadath & Eagleman, 2007), suggesting that separate neural systems are responsible for duration and timing. The subjective experience of duration has been linked to the amount of neural energy expended to code for a stimulus (i.e. its coding efficiency; see Eagleman & Pariyadath, 2009). As music is an art that unfolds over time, temporally precise neural measures, such as human EEG, are especially useful for relating neural time to psychological time.

I will now review studies on the role of expectancy in musical improvisation at different timescales, ranging from real-time measurements of brain activity with millisecond precision, to coarser-timescale measurements of large-scale neural networks that are affected by long-term effects of improvisation training.

21.3.1 Human EEG Studies

Human EEG yields information with millisecond precision during real-time meaningful experiences, such as live musical performances. Przysinda et al. (2017) directly investigated the role of expectancy as it interacts with the knowledge base (as outlined in the computational level of our model) by comparing electrophysiological and behavioural responses to chord progressions that differed in expectedness given the Western tonal harmonic canon. Comparing electrophysiological responses to these same chord progressions had previously been shown to yield specific neural indices in the event-related potential, including a negative waveform 150–200 ms post stimulus, known as the early right anterior negativity (ERAN), and another positive waveform around 400–800 ms known as the P3 (Koelsch et al., 2000; Koelsch et al., 2002). Here, Przysinda et al. (2017) compared the ERAN and P3 among young adults with jazz improvisational training, with classical (non-improvisational) training, and with no particular musical training. Event-related potentials showed that in response to slightly unexpected musical chord progressions, a larger ERAN was observed in jazz improvising musicians and classical musicians compared to participants with no particular musical training. This begins to suggest that musical training affects expectancy processing, consistent with the hypothesized role of learning on perception as outlined in the model. In response to highly unexpected chord progressions, however, jazz improvising musicians showed a larger ERAN than the other two groups. Furthermore, the P3 showed a further distinction between the earlier, frontocentrally distributed P3a, and a larger, parietally centred P3b component. While this distinction has been highlighted in other work (Polich, 2007), here it emerged as an interaction between expectation and types of musical training. While all three groups showed a P3a in response to highly unexpected chords, only classical musicians showed a robust P3b, whereas jazz improvising musicians showed a *reduced* P3b compared to the other two groups. This persistent expectancy-related activity in the classically trained musicians may be related to perceptual re-evaluation of motor plans that had already been acted upon, that is, the evaluative or feedback part of the perception–action cycle required for musical creativity. When considering preference ratings relative to the expectedness levels of various chord progressions, Przysinda et al. (2017) found that while classically trained and untrained individuals rated highly expected chord progression as preferred and the most unexpected chord progression as disliked, as previously shown (Loui and Wessel, 2007), by contrast, jazz improvising musicians rated the slightly unexpected chord progression as preferred. This interaction between training and expectedness on preference suggests that differently trained individuals find different levels of expectation to be rewarding. Applied to the present model, these results bolster the link between knowledge-based expectancies for auditory–motor patterns and re-ward at the highest computational level. At the algorithmic level, the ERAN can be interpreted as being tied to prediction (Koelsch et al., 2018): the ERAN may be gen-erated as a result of knowledge-based expectancies that inform perception, in the sense of predictive coding as a framework for perception as described by the free-energy model (Friston et al., 2006). The P3a/b is tied to motor plan selection (Polich, 2007; Waller et al., 2021); thus its modulation by knowledge-based expectancies links these expectancies to the action–perception cycle.

Another study in which the same neurophysiological measures were used to examine predictions, but in more flexible contexts, comes from a study on action planning in pianists with different genres of musical training. Bianco et al. (2018) compared electrophysiological indices of action planning between classical and jazz musicians by asking jazz and classical pianists to imitate the hand positions of chord progressions presented without sounds. These chord progressions varied by manner (motor constraints) and by harmonic structure (cognitive constraints). Jazz pianists showed an earlier response to unexpected harmonic structures but were less sensitive to differences in motoric constraints (i.e. which fingers were used to play the chord on the keyboard). These results converge with Przysinda et al. (2017) in highlighting different cognitive constraints for musicians with jazz and classical training.

Goldman et al. (2020) tested the hypothesis that jazz-trained musicians, due to their training in improvisation, would prioritize harmonic function over the identity of specific chords when listening to chord progressions. They found that participants with more improvisation experience responded more quickly and accurately to de-viations in harmonic function, relative to their responses to chord identity per se. Furthermore, they found that the P3b component reliably predicted participants' behavioural performance on discriminating the stimuli. Here again, the P3b com-ponent is linked to action perception, as in the knowledge-based perceptual eval-uation of the consequences of auditory–motor patterns that are presented as chord progressions realized in different manners. While both Goldman et al. (2018) and Przysinda et al. (2017) identified differences in the P3b waveform, Goldman et al. showed larger P3b in experienced improvisers, whereas Przysinda et al. showed larger P3b in non-improvising (classical) musicians. This difference is attributable to the differences in task demands: Goldman et al. employed the task of perceptual dis-crimination between chords, whereas Przysinda et al. used a preference ratings task, thus requiring participants to listen more holistically to the entire chord progres-sion. Thus, both studies point to differences in the organization of knowledge that is intrinsic to musical creativity, but asked for different cognitive modes of engagement between participants and the musical stimuli, thus giving rise to these differences in results. More generally, these differences between studies highlight the exquisitely adaptive way in which our minds can deploy an experience-dependent knowledge base of expectancies within a very short timescale. This flexible deployment of cog-nitive processes, and their underlying neural substrates, enable the combinatorial explosion of ways with which the mind may interact with the environment to give rise to musical creativity.

21.3.2 Large-Scale Brain Networks: MRI Studies

Limb and Braun (2008) examined brain activity during the act of improvising on a keyboard, compared against the control task of playing an overlearned piece or musical scale. They found that improvisation was associated with deactivations as well as activations throughout the mesial and lateral frontal lobe, suggesting the involvement of brain networks that are typically involved in different activities, being active together during musical improvisation. Pinho et al. (2015) asked professional pianists to improvise either with a certain emotion (e.g. 'fearful'), compared to improvising in certain musical pitch sets. During the emotional conditions, they found higher activity in sensorimotor and executive control networks. Belden et al. (2020) compared these intrinsic brain networks between jazz improvising musicians, classically trained (non-improvising) musicians, and minimally musically trained controls in resting-state functional MRI, and their results showed that jazz improvising musicians had highest functional connectivity from sensorimotor regions to both the default mode and the executive control networks. Furthermore, connectivity between the salience network and the superior parietal lobule, which is part of the executive control network, was higher among non-improvising musicians than in the other two groups. The same networks were also higher in functional connectivity among participants who were more creative as defined by (non-musical) laboratory tasks of divergent thinking and idea generation, that is, the *Torrance Tests of Creative Thinking*, a measure taken as an index of more domain-general creativity (Torrance, 1968), which required participants to generate multiple uses of everyday objects. Taken together, these differences in intrinsic connectivity can have consequences for how cognitive processes that enable musical creativity are organized; specifically, the coupling between default mode and executive control networks, mediated by the salience network, is likely linked to the greater ease with which idea generation and evaluation are coupled with each other during musical improvisation.

The findings from Belden et al. (2020) echo the work on more domain-general creativity by Beaty et al. (2018), who took the approach of using individual differences in whole brain functional connectivity to model individual differences in creative thinking, as assessed by a classic divergent thinking task for idea generation. In a large sample of 163 participants, they showed a distinct pattern of functional brain connectivity, including regions distributed across multiple brain networks that related to highly creative behavioural performance. This same pattern of connectivity generalized towards predicting creative behaviour in other functional MRI datasets, including task-free resting-state functional connectivity MRI data, suggesting that creativity involves multiple large-scale brain networks, rather than a single region or network.

Turning from functional to structural neuroimaging studies, Bashwiner et al. (2016) found that musically creative individuals had greater cortical surface area or volume in sensorimotor areas, areas within the default mode network including the medial prefrontal cortex, and areas in the reward network including the amygdala and orbitofrontal cortex. These results dovetail well with those of Belden et al. (2020) and Beaty et al. (2018); however it is notable that the musically creative individuals in that study were identified by self-report, specifically by participants' response to a single multiple-choice question from within a larger survey. In an effort to characterize musical creativity with a more involved behavioural task, Arkin et al. (2019) and Zeng et al. (2018) tested young adults with and without musical training on a simple musical improvisation continuation task, and then associated performance on this task, as rated by experts, with individual differences in brain structure. The improvisation continuation task consisted of 12 musical motifs that were presented to the participants. The participants' task was to first reproduce the presented motifs by playing on indicated keys on a keyboard (continuation), then to improvise on the presented motif (improvisation). The resulting performances garnered a range of creativity ratings from expert improvising musicians. Arkin et al. (2019) found that creativity ratings were negatively associated with grey matter volume in the right inferior temporal gyrus, which is in the default mode network, whereas the duration of improvisation training was negatively associated with grey matter volume in the rolandic operculum, which is in the salience network. Considering white matter associations with performance on the improvisation task, Zeng et al. (2018) found that better performers had higher fractional anisotropy (an indicator of white matter integrity) in the cingulate cortex, a region of the salience network. Since grey matter includes the cell bodies of neurons, whereas white matter includes the axons which are connections between neurons, these results show that both the anatomy and the connectivity of brain regions are related to improvisation. More broadly, these results link improvisatory behaviour to individual differences in brain structure, and show that the relationship between brain and behaviour in musical improvisation is not limited to time-sensitive measures, but also includes more stable brain indices such as volumetric and connectivity differences in specific brain regions.

21.4 Conclusion

This chapter proposes a multilevel model of musical creativity as a complex predictive system that can be described at goal-oriented (computational), cognitive (algorithmic), and neural (implementational) levels, with multiple predictions occurring over a range of timescales. The model seeks to operationalize musical improvisation as part of musicality, rather than to analyse the output of specific musical products. In proposing this model, I have reviewed a growing body of studies in the psychology and neuroscience of musical improvisation. The model also generates certain testable predictions. One testable prediction at the computational level is around the roles of the referent and the knowledge base. Computational modelling studies, for example, may test the extent to which a referent or a sizable knowledge base may be required for generating auditory–motor patterns that are rewarding. At the algorithmic level, future studies may test whether action generation can be decoupled from evaluation and yet still give rise to learning and to the generation of rewarding patterns. At the implementation level, more neuroimaging and brain stimulation studies are needed to test the involvement of each brain network in musical improvisation. Finally, more work should be done to address the links between different levels, such as between activity in the default mode and reward systems and the experience of reward at the highest level. By positing a multilevel organization of musical improvisation, the present model may also inform conceptualizations of musical movement and musical time as discussed in other chapters of the current volume, with the hope of generating and informing ideas for future research.

References

Arkin, C., Przysinda, E., Pfeifer, C. W., Zeng, T., & Loui, P. (2019). Gray matter correlates of creativity in musical improvisation. *Frontiers in human neuroscience*, *13*, 169.

Ashby, W. R. (1947). The nervous system as physical machine: With special reference to the origin of adaptive behavior. *Mind*, *56*(221), 44–59.

Bashwiner, D. M., Bacon, D. K., Wertz, C. J., Flores, R. A., Chohan, M. O., & Jung, R. E. (2020). Resting state functional connectivity underlying musical creativity. *NeuroImage*, *218*, 116940.

Beaty, R. E., Kenett, Y. N., Christensen, A. P., Rosenberg, M. D., Benedek, M., Chen, Q., Fink, A., Qiu, J., Kwapil, T. R., Kane, M. J. & Silvia, P. J. (2018). Robust prediction of individual creative ability from brain functional connectivity. *Proceedings of the National Academy of Sciences of the United States of America*, *115*(5), 1087–1092.

Belden, A., Zeng, T., Przysinda, E., Anteraper, S. A., Whitfield-Gabrieli, S., & Loui, P. (2020). Improvising at rest: Differentiating jazz and classical music training with resting state functional connectivity. *NeuroImage*, *207*, 116384.

Bianco, R., Novembre, G., Keller, P. E., Villringer, A., & Sammler, D. (2018). Musical genre-dependent behavioural and EEG signatures of action planning. A comparison between classical and jazz pianists. *Neuroimage*, *169*, 383–394.

Biasutti, M. (2015). Pedagogical applications of the cognitive research on music improvisation. *Frontiers in Psychology*, *6*, 614.

Bressler, S. L., & Menon, V. (2010). Large-scale brain networks in cognition: Emerging methods and principles. *Trends in Cognitive Sciences*, *14*(6), 277–290.

Cheung, V. K. M., Harrison, P. M. C., Meyer, L., Pearce, M. T., Haynes, J.-D., & Koelsch, S. (2019). Uncertainty and surprise jointly predict musical pleasure and amygdala, hippocampus, and auditory cortex activity. *Current Biology*, *29*(23), 4084–4092.

Csikszentmihalyi, M. (1996). *Creativity: Flow and the psychology of discovery and invention*. Harper Collins Publishers.

Dennett, D. C. (2008). *Kinds of minds: Toward an understanding of consciousness*. Basic Books.

Di Liberto, G. M., Pelofi, C., Bianco, R., Patel, P., Mehta, A. D., Herrero, J. L., de Cheveigné, A., Shamma, S., & Mesgarani, N. (2020). Cortical encoding of melodic expectations in human temporal cortex. *Elife*, *9*, e51784.

Eagleman, D. M., & Pariyadath, V. (2009). Is subjective duration a signature of coding efficiency? *Philosophical Transactions of the Royal Society. Series B, Biological Sciences*, *364*(1525), 1841–1851.

Finke, R. A., Ward, T. B., & Smith, S. M. (1992). *Creative cognition: Theory, research, and applications*. MIT Press.

Fox, M. D., Snyder, A. Z., Vincent, J. L., Corbetta, M., Van Essen, D. C., & Raichle, M. E. (2005). The human brain is intrinsically organized into dynamic, anticorrelated functional networks. *Proceedings of the National Academy of Sciences of the United States of America, 102*(27), 9673–9678.

Friston, K., Kilner, J., & Harrison, L. (2006). A free energy principle for the brain. *Journal of Physiology Paris, 100*(1–3), 70–87.

Goldman, A., Jackson, T., & Sajda, P. (2020). Improvisation experience predicts how musicians categorize musical structures. *Psychology of Music, 48*(1), 18–34.

Guenther, F. H. (2017). *Neural control of speech*. MIT Press.

Hansen, N. C., & Pearce, M. T. (2014). Predictive uncertainty in auditory sequence processing. *Frontiers in Psychology, 5*, 1052.

Honing, H. (2018). *The origins of musicality*. MIT Press.

Honing, H., ten Cate, C., Peretz, I., & Trehub, S. E. (2015). Without it no music: Cognition, biology and evolution of musicality. *Philosophical Transactions of the Royal Society. Series B, Biological Sciences, 370*(1664), 20140088.

Huron, D. (2006). *Sweet anticipation: Music and the psychology of expectation*. MIT Press.

Johnson-Laird, P. N. (2002). How jazz musicians improvise. *Music Perception, 19*(3), 415–442.

Kleinmintz, O. M., Goldstein, P., Mayseless, N., Abecasis, D., & Shamay-Tsoory, S. G. (2014). Expertise in musical improvisation and creativity: The mediation of idea evaluation. *PLoS One, 9*(7), e101568.

Koelsch, S., Gunter, T. C., Friederici, A. D., & Schröger, E. (2000). Brain indices of music processing: Nonmusicians are musical. *Journal of Cognitive Neuroscience, 12*(3), 520–541.

Koelsch, S., Schroger, E., & Gunter, T. C. (2002). Music matters: Preattentive musicality of the human brain. *Psychophysiology, 39*(1), 38–48.

Koelsch, S., Vuust, P., & Friston, K. (2018). Predictive processes and the peculiar case of music. *Trends in Cognitive Sciences, 23*(1), 63–77.

Limb, C. J., & Braun, A. R. (2008). Neural substrates of spontaneous musical performance: An FMRI study of jazz improvisation. *PLoS One, 3*(2), e1679.

Loui, P. (2015). A dual-stream neuroanatomy of singing. *Music Perception, 32*(3), 232–241.

Loui, P. (2018). Rapid and flexible creativity in musical improvisation: Review and a model. *Annuals of the New York Academy of Sciences, 1423*(1), 138–145.

Loui, P., & Wessel, D. (2007). Harmonic expectation and affect in Western music: Effects of attention and training. *Perception & psychophysics, 69*(7), 1084–1092.

Love, B. C. (2015). The algorithmic level is the bridge between computation and brain. *Topics in Cognitive Science, 7*(2), 230–242.

Margulis, E. H. (2005). A model of melodic expectation. *Music Perception, 22*(4), 663–714.

Marr, D. (1982). *Vision: A computational investigation into the human representation and processing of visual information*. W. H. Freeman and Company.

Meyer, L. B. (1956). *Emotion and meaning in music*. University of Chicago Press.

Narmour, E. (1990). *The analysis and cognition of basic melodic structures: The implication-realization model*. University of Chicago Press.

Pariyadath, V., & Eagleman, D. (2007). The effect of predictability on subjective duration. *PLoS One, 2*(11), e1264.

Pearce, M. T., & Wiggins, G. A. (2006). Expectation in melody: The influence of context and learning. *Music Perception, 23*(5), 377–405.

Pearce, M. T., & Wiggins, G. A. (2012). Auditory expectation: The information dynamics of music perception and cognition. *Topics in Cognitive Science, 4*(4), 625–652.

Pinho, A. L., Ullén, F., Castelo-Branco, M., Fransson, P., & de Manzano, Ö. (2015). Addressing a paradox: dual strategies for creative performance in introspective and extrospective networks. *Cerebral Cortex, 26*(7), 3052–3063.

Polich, J. (2007). Updating P300: An integrative theory of P3a and P3b. *Clinical Neurophysiology, 118*(10), 2128–2148.

Pressing, J. (1984). Cognitive processes in improvisation. *Advances in Psychology, 19*, 345–363.

Pressing, J. (1998). Psychological constraints on improvisational expertise and communication. In B. Nettl & M. Russell (Eds.), *In the course of performance* (pp. 47–67). University of Chicago Press.

Przysinda, E., Zeng, T., Maves, K., Arkin, C., & Loui, P. (2017). Jazz musicians reveal role of expectancy in human creativity. *Brain and Cognition, 119*, 45–53.

Rhodes, M. (1961). An analysis of creativity. *The Phi Delta Kappan, 42*(7), 305–310.

Runco, M. A., & Jaeger, G. J. (2012). The standard definition of creativity. *Creativity Research Journal, 24*(1), 92–96.

Simonton, D. K. (2010). Creative thought as blind-variation and selective-retention: Combinatorial models of exceptional creativity. *Physics of Life Reviews, 7*(2), 156–179.

Schultz, W., Dayan, P., & Montague, P. R. (1997). A neural substrate of prediction and reward. *Science, 275*(5306), 1593–1599.

Sowden, P. T., Pringle, A., & Gabora, L. (2015). The shifting sands of creative thinking: Connections to dual-process theory. *Thinking & Reasoning, 21*(1), 40–60.

Torrance, E. P. (1968). Examples and rationales of test tasks for assessing creative abilities. *Journal of Creative Behavior, 2*(3), 165–178.

Waller, D. A., Hazeltine, E., & Wessel, J. R. (2021). Common neural processes during action-stopping and infrequent stimulus detection: The frontocentral P3 as an index of generic motor inhibition. *International Journal of Psychophysiology, 163*, 11–21.

Zeng, T., Przysinda, E., Pfeifer, C., Arkin, C., & Loui, P. (2018). White matter connectivity reflects success in musical improvisation. *BioRxiv*, 218024.

Focus Chapters

22
Experiences of Time in Boring Dance

Anna Pakes

22.1 Introduction: What Is a Boring Dance?

In the midst of the COVID-19 lockdown, it was easy to think back nostalgically to experiences of live theatre dance—the excitement of watching moving dancers run, sweep, and lurch, the visceral thrill of present bodies, brilliant light, and pulsing music. Mostly, I would recall instances of investment and engagement with what was happening on stage—those times when I was kinaesthetically and intellectually caught up in the action, even as a spectator. Such performances seemed either to speed by or take just the time they needed to develop to a satisfying conclusion. But, of course, not all my experiences of theatre dance have been like this. Quite often, despite eager anticipation and my best efforts to approach it with an open mind, I have struggled to enter the world of a dance work. And as the performance unfolds, I have remained detached and distracted, even though numerous possible points of focus may be offered by the dancers' action. In these experiences, time drags—I can't seem to pick up the thread of the performance and I flounder, whatever choreographic intelligence and performative artistry is on display. I get impatient and want it to be over. I find the dance boring.

Why does this happen? Sometimes, dances are experienced as boring because they are repetitive. For example, the same movement phrases recur again and again, with little variation and (crucially) in an apparently contingent way: the repetition does not make an interesting artistic statement, draw aesthetic focus to a related feature or theme (rhythm, duration, or the significance of replication itself), or create a trance-like atmosphere that transcends the mundanity of the movement as such (all ways in which repetition might have artistic purpose and value). Repetition of movement dynamics, images, or structures can also be experienced as boring, if these seem flat, crass, or formulaic (again, in dialectical relation to the artistic point(s) of the work). Meanwhile, sometimes dances are experienced as boring because the performed action develops unreasonably slowly or uneventfully—if, for example, I can't see why things are taking so long or sustain my curiosity about how they will unfold, even when the choreography's duration is obviously purposely extended.

Clearly, such failures or refusals to meet conventional Western aesthetic expectations of originality and variety don't *necessarily* produce experiences of boredom. Alongside the specific artistic context, my psychological framework has a bearing.

Anna Pakes, *Experiences of Time in Boring Dance* In: *Performing Time*. Edited by: Clemens Wöllner and Justin London, Oxford University Press. © Oxford University Press 2023. DOI: 10.1093/oso/9780192896254.003.0023

Indeed, it is unclear whether, in finding a dance boring, I am identifying a property—an objective feature—of the dance itself or commenting on my own attitudes towards it. Lars Svendsen (1999/2005) notes that it is difficult to 'clearly distinguish between whether something *is* boring, or if it only *feels* boring' (p. 108). Wendell O'Brien (2014) characterizes boredom as an unpleasant mental state of uninterested weariness and restlessness, and the property of *being boring* as a tendency to bore, that is, to induce this mental state (pp. 237–238). The property thus appears inextricable from subjective response—a secondary or even tertiary quality rather than a primary one.[1] And yet the object–subject distinction may still be important in parsing different sorts of experience. For example, I can be bored when watching a boring dance ('boring' in the sense that this is the kind of reaction the dance itself seems to invite, whether or not that's a deliberate choreographic choice). But it also seems possible—at least in principle—to be bored when watching an interesting dance, if my head just isn't 'in the game' or if I don't have the wherewithal to appreciate this kind of work. Equally, it seems that I could (perhaps paradoxically) be interested, even stimulated, by watching a boring dance: for example, if I nonetheless find it affecting, or because it says something interesting about choreography, human existence, or some other pressing theme. In such cases, the work has a tendency to bore but somehow I (partly) avoid actually experiencing a mental state of weariness, restlessness, and lack of interest.

22.2 Experiencing Boredom and the Passage of Time

Art deliberately designed to test the patience and endurance of its audiences plays on the latter possibility. Some minimalism exploits repetitive structures and emptiness as a means of challenging or negating expectations of aesthetic plenitude (McDonough, 2017, p. 16). In postmodern dance, for example, Yvonne Rainer's 'No' Manifesto maintains the need to strip extraneous theatricality, expressiveness, and musicality from the dancing body's presentation (Rainer, 1965); dances like *Trio A* flatten dynamic variation in an effort to make them difficult to see, forcing viewers to look and think differently about choreographic rhythm and development.[2] Elsewhere, purposely slow and apparently uneventful performances intentionally amplify and heighten the experience of duration. In Jérôme Bel's *Jérôme Bel* (1995), the naked performers gradually appear, walking slowly onto the stage, and take their time to perform tasks like writing on the back wall in chalk or pulling and stretching at their own skin to create weird images. The pace of the performance is intrinsic to its artistic agenda of reducing dance to *degree zero*, challenging—like many of Bel's works—the apparatus of the theatre and the conventional contract whereby artists are expected to meet the audience's demand to be entertained (Bauer, 2008; Siegmund, 2017, pp. 6–13). When watching such works, I am thrown back on my own reactions, forced to attend to the very process of viewing and to confront the question of how to respond. I am also forced to confront the fact of time passing and my relationship to that fact and to the experience of passage. In watching dance, as in other domains, boredom may result 'whenever, from the relative emptiness of content of a tract of time, we grow attentive to the passage of time itself' (James, 1890, p. 626).

Theatre dance is (typically) presented in a way that clearly delineates a tract of time, which it promises to fill with choreographic content. In attending a performance event, the viewer agrees to spend the designated time focused on the content presented, living through an externally defined duration (usually of 1 or 2 hr for the entire show, although the length of individual works may vary considerably). The producer, choreographer, or convention decides the extent of the duration, rather than me. Dance is, in this sense, like other performing arts but unlike visual arts that manifest in static objects, and where the viewer can usually determine for herself how long to spend with the work. Equally, as the viewer of a sculpture or painting, I can walk away from (and return to) a work as and when I like (within the constraints of the exhibition format), just as I can put down (and pick up) a novel at will. Even if I'm not literally tied down to my seat in the theatre, it is more difficult to walk away from a boring dance: I may be reluctant to forgo the possibility that it may become more interesting and maybe also the opportunity to see the dance at all, especially given that I've (usually) paid to be present. Also, my action risks being read by performers and audience as a statement of rejection, and I may not want to spotlight my response in this way, especially if I worry that finding the dance boring is a somewhat shameful reaction, interpretable as a sign of cultural incompetence. The feeling of confinement is often identified as a key element of boredom (see, e.g., Toohey, 2011), particularly situational or situative boredom, one category into which bored responses to dance most readily fall.[3] O'Brien's analysis emphasizes lack of interest 'in something to which one is *subjected*' (2014, p. 237, my emphasis). The framework of theatre dance accentuates this aspect of boredom because the viewer feels trapped in the time and space of the event.

Perhaps the experience of boring dance can be interpreted more positively, however. Perhaps, by enabling me to pay renewed attention to the passage of time and my own relation to it, boredom opens a fruitful space of reflection. Superficially (and as in other experiences of boredom beyond the dance context), my attention becomes focused on the limited time I have, and on the importance of spending it wisely: whether that be by looking more deeply or broadly to the affordances offered by the (apparently) boring dance in front of me, or by avoiding spending future time on performances that will likely go the way of this one (although it remains unclear how I could identify such, given the complexities of boringness as a secondary or tertiary quality). More radically, adapting a Heideggerian perspective, perhaps experiencing boredom in the theatre (as elsewhere) enables the fundamental temporality of human being to be revealed and grasped philosophically, in turn enabling a more authentic existence. On this view, boredom 'removes a veil of meaning from things and allows them to appear as empty and ephemeral [...] Even fully immersed in nothingness, *Dasein* is still there, and Being can then reveal itself to *Dasein*' (Svendsen, 1999/2005, p. 130).

22.3 Heideggerian Boredom

Martin Heidegger's (1983/1995) analysis posits three different levels of boredom, which become progressively more profound. The first level is the experience of being bored *by* something (a kind of situative boredom), in which time drags and we are held in limbo: Heidegger's example is the experience of passing unexpected hours at a railway station waiting for a delayed train, but we might substitute that of being stuck in the theatre watching a dance and waiting for it to capture one's interest. Although there are many things 'at hand' in this situation—which should present plenty of possibilities for perceptual and intellectual action to pass the time—somehow they offer nothing, rather leaving us empty. Indeed, '[u]ltimately the dragging, oppressive time that holds us in limbo is what permits the station [or the dance] not to offer what it ought to' (Heidegger, 1983/1995, p. 104). And we are held in limbo because these things 'stand at the disposal of time [. . .] are bound to time'. Heidegger's second level of boredom is the experience of being bored *with* something: he gives the example of spending a pleasant evening among friends, and only subsequently realizing that one was in fact bored by the experience. Likewise, one might seem pleasantly occupied on a night in the theatre, but later feel an unsatisfactory emptiness, concomitant with a thinning of the meaningfulness and value of the experience. In such cases, says Heidegger, we have given ourselves time by deciding to attend, but the time passes inconspicuously: 'in such casualness there arises a slipping away, away from ourselves toward whatever is happening', and so the emptiness is equivalent to 'a being left behind of our proper self' (1983/1995, p. 120).

Heidegger's third level of boredom—it being 'boring for one' (where I am bored by boredom itself)—is the deepest. 'In profound boredom, one is left empty by everything—even by oneself' and so, one is 'forced to take one's own freedom into account instead of attempting to forget it while engaging in various pastimes' (Svendsen, 1999/2005, p. 122). As Svendsen notes, no example is forthcoming in Heidegger's text because this most profound level of boredom is all-encompassing rather than related to specific situations. It therefore becomes problematic to try to apply the idea to particular dance experiences, or to imagine that a boring dance could provoke emptiness of this degree and scope, where 'everything collapses into one indifferent whole' (Svendsen, 1999/2005, p. 123). Indeed, it is hard to see how specific activities like dance—which is, after all, one way of passing the time—could continue to be differentiated as the ontic contents of human experience are emptied out. This at least limits the usefulness of the analysis to the attempt to understand boring dance. It might also contribute to the sensation that Heidegger 'commit[s] a highly questionable sublimation of boredom' (Svendsen, 1999/2005, p. 131), insisting on the metaphysical grandeur of what is in fact a common phenomenon without necessarily any great significance for the temporality of being.

22.4 Concluding Thoughts

Even if art does seek (in Heideggerian vein) to push me to understand the true nature of my being, there is something peculiarly frustrating and patronizing about insisting on boring me in order to do it. No doubt the capacity of dance performance to test and stretch duration and endurance presents a valuable counterpoint to everyday temporality and the dominance of clock time. In this, dance participates in contemporary art's soliciting of 'an *interested* time—one that is amplified, heightened, divergent and confronting', thereby contrasting with 'the time of numbers and measures' (Bretkelly-Chalmers, 2019, p. 4). But Bretkelly-Chalmers' vision of this alternative time as one of 'dynamism and becoming' (p. 4; and perhaps also the notion of 'interested' time) appears to nonetheless assume a sustained engagement on the part of the viewer, precisely the kind of engagement that is disrupted when I become bored. Several commentators describe how a reflex action of a bored person is to look at her watch—an act that is not in itself a way of passing time, but 'indicates, by its helpless gesture, our failure to pass the time' (Heidegger, 1983/1995, p. 97; see also Svendsen, 1999/2005, p. 117–118). And the state of being bored comes about 'not because the progress of time is slow, but because it is *too* slow', prompting us to 'fight against this peculiar vacillating and dragging of time' (Heidegger, 1983/1995, p. 97). So, either I have to somehow pull myself out of my bored state of mind, or the dance needs to give me enough meaningful content off which to hang the experience, for its potential to reflect on duration itself to be fulfilled. Even then, consciousness of— and anxiety about—my own finitude may nag at the periphery of the renewed attention to time that the dance demands.

Notes

1. See also Heidegger (1983/1995, pp. 83–86.) The distinction between primary and secondary qualities derives from John Locke (1690/1997) and has been criticized by (among others) George Berkeley, David Hume, and Immanuel Kant, although there is insufficient space to explore the debate here. Primary–secondary and secondary–tertiary distinctions arguably also inform the more contemporary contrast between non-aesthetic and aesthetic qualities (Sibley, 2001), equally relevant to understanding how the (aesthetic) quality of being boring may be related to (non-aesthetic) perceptual features like repetitiveness.
2. This dance is described in detail and analysed in Banes (1987), pp. 44–55, and in articles by a range of authors in *Dance Research Journal*, 2009, *41*(2).
3. Martin Doehlemann (1991) offers a typology of four types of boredom: (a) situative boredom (boredom generated by a particular situation or object); (b) boredom of satiety (where there is too much of the same thing); (c) existential boredom (where the individual feels empty and that the

world lacks meaning); and (d) creative boredom (where the experience generates new action). See also Svendsen (1999/2005), pp. 41–42.

References

Banes, S. (1987). *Terpsichore in sneakers: Post-modern dance* (Rev. ed.). Wesleyan University Press.

Bauer, U. (2008). The movement of embodied thought. The representational game of the stage zero of signification in *Jérôme Bel. Performance Research*, *13*(1), 35–41. https://doi.org/10.1080/1352816080 2465508

Bel, J. (Choreographer) (1995). *Jérôme Bel* [Dance]. First performed at the Brigittines international festival, Brussels, 1 September. Video of performance in Ghent (December 1998). www.jeromebel.fr

Bretkelly-Chalmers, K. (2019). *Time, duration and change in contemporary art*. Intellect.

Doehlemann, M. (1991). *Langeweile? Deutung eines verbreiteten Phänomens*. Suhrkamp.

Heidegger, M. (1995). *Fundamental concepts of metaphysics* (W. McNeill & N. Walker, Trans.). Indiana University Press. (Original work published 1983)

James, W. (1890). The perception of time. In *Principles of psychology* (Vol. 1, pp. 605–642). Henry Holt & Co.

Locke, J. (1997). *An essay concerning human understanding*. Penguin Books. (Original work published 1690)

McDonough, T. (Ed.). (2017). *Boredom: Documents of contemporary art*. Whitechapel Gallery.

O'Brien, W. (2014). Boredom. *Analysis*, *74*(2), 236–244. https://doi.org/10.1093/analys/anu041

Rainer, Y. (1965). Some retrospective notes on a dance for 10 people and 12 mattresses called 'Parts of Some Sextets'. *Tulane Drama Review*, *10*(2), 168–178. https://doi.org/10.2307/1125242

Rainer, Y. (Choreographer). (1966). *Trio A*. [Dance] First performed as The Mind is a Muscle, Part 1, at Judson Church, New York, 10 January. Video documentation/reconstruction (1978). http://vdb.org/titles/trio

Sibley, F. (2001). *Approach to aesthetics: Collected papers on philosophical aesthetics*. Oxford University Press.

Siegmund, G. (2017). *Jérôme Bel: Dance, theatre and the subject*. Palgrave Macmillan.

Svendsen, L. (2005). *A philosophy of boredom* (J. Irons, Trans.). Reaktion Books. (Original work published 1999)

Toohey, P. (2011). *Boredom: A lively history*. Yale University Press.

23

Evaluating the Psychological Reality of Alternate Temporalities in Contemporary Music

Empirical Case Studies of Gérard Grisey's *Vortex Temporum*

Jason Noble, Tanor Bonin, Roger Dean, and Stephen McAdams

23.1 Introduction

> To the complex time of a piece of music . . . we must finally relate another as-
> pect of time, infinitely more complex: that of the person who perceives.
>
> (Grisey, 1987, p. 273)

Musical expressions of different temporalities have preoccupied many 20th- and 21st-century composers, one of the most prominent being Gérard Grisey (1946–1998). He poetically invoked 'the time of humans (the time of language and breathing), the time of whales (the spectral time of sleep rhythms), and the time of birds or insects (extremely contracted time where contours fade)' (Hervé, 2001, p. 19), and used these as structuring principles in his compositions (Baillet, 2000). The temporalities developed and conveyed in Grisey's music have captured the imaginations of many. The present work investigates how perceptually salient these phenomenologies are to listeners of his music.

Vortex Temporum (1994–1996) manifests Grisey's times of humans, birds, and whales explicitly, with distinct musical profiles for each conveyed by attributes such as the durations of musical gestures and sustained tones (longest in 'whale time', shortest in 'bird time'), frequency ranges (lowest in 'whale time', highest in 'bird time'), and the presence or absence of pulse, metre, and motivic patterns (present in 'human time', absent elsewhere). Listeners are likely aware of these material differences, but it remains to be seen whether or not they associate them with different temporalities.

In this chapter, we report selected findings from a larger study on temporal experiences of recent music. Our theoretical framework draws on Noble (2018), which related experiences of musical timelessness to the temporal structure of auditory

Jason Noble, Tanor Bonin, Roger Dean, and Stephen McAdams, *Evaluating the Psychological Reality of Alternate Temporalities in Contemporary Music* In: *Performing Time*. Edited by: Clemens Wöllner and Justin London, Oxford University Press.
© Oxford University Press 2023. DOI: 10.1093/oso/9780192896254.003.0024

perception. Our analytical framework draws on several studies by Dean and colleagues, which applied time series analysis to perceptions of change and segmentation in recent music (Dean & Bailes, 2016; Dean et al., 2014, 2019; Olsen et al., 2016). Our experimental method adapts procedures used by Carol Krumhansl (1998) in a study on the psychological reality of musical topics, in which participants' ratings of memorability, emotion, and openness in pieces by Mozart and Beethoven were used to corroborate topical analyses (Agawu, 2014). We wondered if continuous self-reports of temporal phenomenology may map onto Grisey's temporalities in the same way as Krumhansl's participants' self-reports of emotion, closure, and memorability mapped onto Agawu's topics.

We analysed participants' continuous real-time responses to excerpts of recent music, including two from *Vortex Temporum*, using a joystick paradigm adapted from Knowles (2016; see also Knowles & Ashley, this volume). We reasoned that if Grisey's temporalities have perceptual reality, then changes in musical attributes corresponding to the implied temporalities should be reflected in participants' real-time indications of their temporal experiences. We further wondered if participants' responses may reveal differences in temporality not coterminous with Grisey's formal structure, such as smaller-scale shifts in temporal phenomenology within formal sections. Finally, we wondered if examining continuous joystick data may reveal different rating strategies indicated by coherent clusters of response profiles. If so, we could analyse the recordings for different attributes that map onto these clusters, potentially offering an account of plural but non-arbitrary temporal associations with the same musical excerpts.

23.2 Experimental Findings

The full study employed 20 excerpts drawn from commercial recordings. In this chapter, we discuss only the two excerpts from Grisey's *Vortex Temporum*: 0:00–1:00 of movement I, and 10:30–11:40 of movement III from Ensemble Recherche's recording (Grisey, 1996/2001). For more information, including technical details and results for several other excerpts, see Noble and colleagues (2020). Participants were presented with the following description:

- Musical experience is often related to the subjective experience of the flow of time. Some classes of profound musical experience have even been described in terms of 'timelessness', in which the subjective experience of time is suspended or annihilated.
- The goal of the experiment is to investigate which properties of contemporary music may underlie musical time or timelessness.

They were instructed to use the joystick to report their experiences of the pace of time while listening to musical excerpts, leaving it in a central position to indicate 'normal' time, and moving it forward to indicate time speeding up or backward to indicate time slowing down (proportionate to the extent of alteration), providing continuous data on a scale of 0–1 with 0.5 as the central position. For each example, they were prompted to rate how strong their respective senses of time and timelessness were on 5-point Likert scales (ranging from 'a weak sense of time' to 'a strong sense of time' and from 'a weak sense of timelessness' to 'a strong sense of timelessness'). Ratings for time and timelessness were reported separately to allow for varied experiences over the course of the excerpts, and to avoid forcing participants to treat them as mutually exclusive opposites (in case, as in complex emotions, apparently contradictory experiences are simultaneously present for some people).

Our participants' responses[1] ($N = 78$) revealed significantly different experiences of time and timelessness between the two excerpts. In the excerpt from *Vortex I* (all in 'human time'), the mean rating for sense of time (3.53, SD = 1.53) was significantly higher ($p < .001$) than the mean rating for sense of timelessness (2.26, SD = 1.42). In the excerpt from *Vortex III* (including sections of 'whale', 'human', and 'bird' times; a more detailed account of the musical excerpts and corresponding real-time responses is given below), the mean rating for sense of time (2.81, SD = 1.44) was lower than the mean rating of the sense of timelessness (3.13, SD = 1.61) but the statistical significance was marginal ($p = .078$). Comparing ratings for the two excerpts, *Vortex III* yielded a significantly weaker sense of time and a significantly stronger sense of timelessness than *Vortex I* ($p < .001$).

Continuous joystick data also revealed different profiles, which we interpret in relation to the musical properties of each excerpt. The excerpt from *Vortex I* consists of nine musical phrases that all begin strongly accented and then progressively diminuendo, as readily visible in its waveform (Figure 23.1a). Overall, coordination between the waveform profile and participants' continuous joystick responses was quite strong, as confirmed by a tangle graph (Figure 23.1b; showing all individual responses, normalized to each individual's response range). Time series models were made for each individual and excerpt using autoregressive moving averages, along with several acoustical and musical parameters as potential predictors. The models showed that measured acoustic intensity was only a strong predictor of responses in two participants for *Vortex I* and six participants for *Vortex III* respectively; rather, a range of spectral properties (that generally changed also in coordination with the waveform) was more widely influential. The predictor coefficients from these individual time series models were used as the basis for hierarchical clustering analysis, which revealed coherent clusters of responses between participants following several different patterns (Figure 23.1c). The largest cluster ($N = 21$, turquoise line) closely followed the waveform (see Knowles & Ashley, this volume, for a related finding). Another cluster ($N = 12$, green line) followed rhythmic groupings: after a baseline pattern of eight-note repeating figures has been established in the first four phrases, ratings for this cluster go up in response to shorter (six-note) or more complex (14-note, 10-note) rhythmic patterns, and back down when the baseline pattern returns. Two other clusters, each with 18 participants, showed opposite tendencies over the

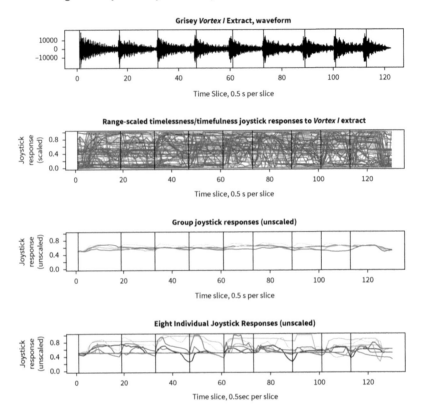

Figure 23.1 (a) Waveform of the excerpt from *Vortex I*. (b) Tangle graph showing responses for all participants (normalized to the range of each individual's responses). (c) Mean ratings for response clusters (unscaled). (d) Eight individual responses (unscaled).

first eight phrases, with one showing a gradual overall decrease (purple line) and the other an increase (red line). For comparison, eight randomly selected individual responses are shown in Figure 23.1d.

Formal divisions in *Vortex III* are fewer but more dramatic, with shifts between Grisey's three temporalities. Although the boundaries are clearly demarcated in a formal analysis based on the composer's sketches (Baillet, 2000), the transitions between them vary in the musical realization, with some gradual transitions and some abrupt shifts. The excerpt begins in 'whale time' with long sustained tones grounded in a medium-low register. From 0:20–0:25 (corresponding to 40–50 in the graph) the music shifts to 'human time' with the emergence of a repeating motive with a clear pulse in a middle register, which dominates until 0:32 (64). From 0:32–0:38 (64–76), the pulse gradually dissolves and the music moves into a higher register, until 'human time' is ruptured and 'bird time' appears suddenly with very high, loud, rapid gestures interspersed with very soft sustained tones. These temporalities appear strongly in participants' joystick data (Figure 23.2). The same analytical procedures described above revealed four response clusters containing eight, 29, four, and 36 participants, respectively. Although the nuanced contours differ, the overall

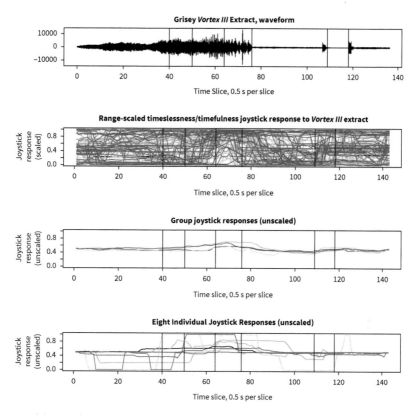

Figure 23.2 (a) Waveform of the excerpt from *Vortex III*. (b) Tangle graph showing responses for all participants (normalized to the range of each individual's responses). (c) Mean ratings for response clusters (unscaled). (d) Eight individual responses (unscaled).

trajectories between clusters are much more similar than those for *Vortex I*. All of them begin with relatively low ratings for 'whale time', sharply increase through 'human time' and/or the transition to it, and return to low ratings in 'bird time'. An additional section from 0:55–0:59 (corresponding to 110–118 in the graph) is noteworthy: it is almost completely silent, and many participants returned the joystick to the middle position here (as they were instructed to do at the end of excerpts). Since it seems likely that some participants mistakenly thought the excerpt was over, we exclude this section from our discussion.

Following the experiment, participants were asked to describe their rating strategies. A full textual analysis of these data is beyond the scope of this chapter, but we anecdotally present a few representative responses. As these comments demonstrate, while no single musical parameter emerges as the determinant of temporal phenomenologies among all subjects, participants did individually report clear relations between properties of the music and their experiences of different temporalities:

- 'A pulse helps to keep track of time, but dynamics also influence the flow of time.'

- 'The flow of time: find the downbeat.'
- 'Timelessness: continuous sound, no beat presented.'
- 'When the music gets tension like cresc or accel [sic] and the musical line is descending or ascending, I can feel the flow of time. If the music (or the motif) is repeating again [and] again, or there is just one instrument playing a very long note, the timelessness can be felt.'

23.3 Discussion and Conclusion

These results suggest that when prompted, listeners can provide responses reflecting the different temporalities Grisey attempts to portray in this music. Participants' Likert ratings indicate a much stronger overall sense of timelessness in *Vortex III*, which includes 'whale time', 'human time', and 'bird time', than in *Vortex I*, which presents only 'human time'. The *Vortex III* joystick data clearly reflect the temporalities in the compositional design, with both 'whale' and 'bird' times deviating from 'human' time in participants' joystick data. The effect appears to be slightly stronger on average in bird time, but as this may be influenced by the order of presentation and compositional form as well as the properties of each section, it is not clear whether or not this reflects a general tendency. Participants' verbal responses anecdotally suggest that people can and do interpret musical attributes as signifiers of temporal phenomenologies, at least when prompted to do so in this experimental context.

An interesting plurality of response types was revealed in coherent clusters of participant responses. In *Vortex I*, some participants linked the pace of time closely with dynamic intensity, while others linked it more with rhythmic groupings. Another group reported a progressively increasing pace of time, perhaps conveying that the continuous transformation of motivic patterns and phrase structure builds excitement over time, while still another group reported a progressively decreasing pace of time, perhaps focusing on the high degree of repetition, which, according to Elizabeth Margulis (2013), can cause 'a satisfying pull toward the present moment' (p. 18). The inverse relationship between the contours for these two clusters intriguingly highlights the tension between difference and repetition in Grisey's music, which is compellingly analysed by Joshua Mailman (2020).

Interpretations of subjective self-report responses are of course speculative to some degree, and we imply neither that the responses of any cluster are entirely explicable by the descriptive terms offered here, nor that the clusters are mutually exclusive in the attributes that influenced their ratings. The important point to note is that responses are neither random nor unanimous: different clusters that appear to map plausibly onto different musical attributes suggest plural but non-arbitrary mappings between musical stimuli and temporal phenomenology.

A limitation of this study is that in order to cover a wide range of excerpts during data collection we used minute-long clips instead of full movements or pieces. We thereby undermined the larger-scale formal context in which the music is intended to be experienced, which may have significantly constrained our participants' temporal experiences in this study. We deemed this necessary in order to survey a larger sample of the many interesting approaches to temporality found in contemporary music. Building upon the encouraging results reported here, it would be valuable to repeat the experiment with fewer but longer stimuli such as entire pieces or movements. Conversely, it would be interesting to use shorter excerpts (e.g. 5–10 s) to examine the range of temporal experiences they can engender (see Wöllner, this volume). It would also be valuable to test excerpts from music presumed to express more normative experiences of time, such as many examples of classical and popular music, to see how perceptions of those excerpts of music may compare with contemporary music that intentionally presents alternate temporalities.

Finally, we acknowledge that much more remains to be said about this complex subject. While Grisey's 'whale time' and 'bird time' appear to be perceptually different from 'human time', it remains to be demonstrated how different they are from one another. It also remains to be demonstrated whether repeated occurrences of the same temporality within a piece have the same psychological value, how they may evolve over greatly extended durations (as in *Vortex II*—not studied in this experiment—which prolongs 'whale time' for over 8 min), how subjective listening behaviours may affect experiences of these temporalities, and so forth. We hope that many future studies will explore the array of germane perspectives on temporality in contemporary music, which, as Grisey (1987) famously stated, 'is only a place of exchange and coincidence between an infinite number of different times' (p. 274).

Note

1. Participants varied in their musicianship as well as their scores on the Absorption in Music Scale (Sandstrom & Russo, 2013); additionally, there were two different groups whose instructions were worded slightly differently to reflect the perception–induction distinction (Juslin & Laukka, 2004). Discussing the differences between all of these groups is beyond the scope of this short chapter and will be the subject of a future paper; here we treat all participants as a single group.

References

Agawu, V. K. (2014). *Playing with signs: A semiotic interpretation of classic music* (Princeton Legacy Library). Princeton University Press.

Baillet J. (2000). *Gérard Grisey: Fondements d'une écriture* (Collection musique et musicologie). L'Itinéraire.

Dean, R. T., & Bailes, F. (2016). Relationships between generated musical structure, performers' physiological arousal and listener perceptions in solo piano improvisation. *Journal of New Music Research, 45*(4), 361–374. https://doi.org/10.1080/09298215.2016.1207668

Dean, R. T., Bailes, F., & Drummond, J. (2014). Generative structures in improvisation: Computational segmentation of keyboard performances. *Journal of New Music Research, 43*(2), 224–236. https://doi.org/10.1080/09298215.2013.859710

Dean, R. T., Milne, A. J., & Bailes, F. (2019). Spectral pitch similarity is a predictor of perceived change in sound- as well as note-based music. *Music & Science, 2*, 1–14. https://doi.org/10.1177/2059204319847351

Grisey, G. (1987). Tempus ex machina: A composer's reflections on musical time. *Contemporary Music Review, 2*(1), 239–275. https://doi.org/10.1080/07494468708567060

Grisey, G. (2001). Vortex Temporum [Song]. Performed by Ensemble Recherche, conducted by K. Ryan. On *Vortex Temporum; Taléa.* Accord. (Original work published 1996)

Hervé J.-L. (2001). *Dans le vertige de la durée: Vortex Temporum de Gérard Grisey* (Collection musique et musicologie). L'Itinéraire.

Juslin, P., & Laukka, P. (2004). Expression, perception, and induction of musical emotions: A review and a questionnaire study of everyday listening. *Journal of New Music Research, 33*(3), 217–238. https://doi.org/10.1080/0929821042000317813

Knowles, K. (2016). *The boundaries of meter and the subjective experience of time in post-tonal, unmetered music.* [PhD dissertation, Northwestern University].

Krumhansl, C. L. (1998). Topic in music: An empirical study of memorability, openness, and emotion in Mozart's string quintet in C major and Beethoven's string quartet in a minor. *Music Perception, 16*(1), 119–134. https://doi.org/10.2307/40285781

Mailman, J. (2020). *Process philosophy overcoming itself: Modeling Grisey's Vortex Temporum.* [Video] https://youtu.be/qLICBP9FczQ

Margulis, E. H. (2013). *On repeat: How music plays the mind.* Oxford University Press.

Noble, J. (2018). What can the temporal structure of auditory perception tell us about musical 'timelessness'? *Music Theory Online, 24*(3). https://doi.org/10.30535/mto.24.3.5

Noble, J., Bonin, T., & McAdams, S. (2020). Experiences of time and timelessness in electroacoustic music. *Organised Sound, 25*(2), 232–247. https://doi.org/10.1017/S135577182000014X

Olsen, K. N., Dean, R. T., & Leung, Y. (2016). What constitutes a phrase in sound-based music? A mixed-methods investigation of perception and acoustics. *Plos One, 11*(12), 0167643. https://doi.org/10.1371/journal.pone.0167643

Sandstrom, G. M., & Russo, F. A. (2013). Absorption in music: Development of a scale to identify individuals with strong emotional responses to music. *Psychology of Music 41*(2), 216–228. https://doi.org/10.1177/0305735611422508

24

Measuring Experienced Time While Listening to Music

Kristina L. Knowles and Richard Ashley

24.1 Time and Musical Structure: Prior Knowledge and Methodological Problems

Studies on the subjective experience of time have had to address two interrelated problems: (a) the extent to which the structure of events in time, both internal and external, influence temporal experience; and (b) how best to capture or represent an individual's perception or experience of time. Previous research demonstrates that an individual's allocation of attentional resources (Brown & Boltz, 2002; Zakay, 1989), attending mode (Boltz, 1991; Jones & Boltz, 1989), encoding of information into memory (Block, 1989; Ornstein, 1969), and emotional responses to a stimulus or event (Droit-Volet et al., 2013) can differentially impact perceived time and can interact dynamically with structural aspects of a stimulus or event, such as the degree of temporal coherency (Boltz, 1998; Jones & Boltz, 1989) or complexity (Block, 1992; Block et al., 2010). Additionally, differences in methods used to collect responses, including duration estimation versus reproduction tasks and prospective versus retrospective paradigms, can lead to widely differing results (Block & Zakay, 1997; Brown, 1985). These two interrelated issues are compounded when considering the impacts of music on experienced time. As an art form that 'structures time' (Epstein, 1981; see Wöllner, this volume), music is a highly coherent temporal stimulus (Jones, 2018) where successive events are often related at both local and global levels.

A growing body of research on music and the subjective experience of time has demonstrated that the temporal regularity afforded by metre and tonal harmony, along with their interaction, has a significant influence on our perception of time. Studies have suggested that coupling and decoupling temporal cues provided by metre and tonal harmony can influence duration judgements for melodies of the same length (Jones & Boltz, 1989), as can disrupting the regularity of rhythmic and harmonic phrasing to create 'incoherent' melodies (Boltz, 1992, 1998). In contrast, studies on the impact of other musical parameters on perceived time including mode (Bueno & Ramos, 2007; Kellaris & Kent, 1992), tonal versus atonal pitch structures (Ziv & Omer, 2011), complexity (Bueno et al., 2002), and loudness (Kellaris &

Kristina L. Knowles and Richard Ashley, *Measuring Experienced Time While Listening to Music* In: *Performing Time*. Edited by: Clemens Wöllner and Justin London, Oxford University Press. © Oxford University Press 2023. DOI: 10.1093/oso/9780192896254.003.0025

Altsech, 1992) are problematic. Results of these studies are often inconclusive or contradictory due to differences in methodology, stimuli, and operationalization of the target musical structure as well as complex covariances among musical parameters (Eitan & Granot, 2006). Consequently, beyond the ability of metric and harmonic structures to provide temporal information and cue listeners 'when' and 'what' is most likely to happen next in a musical passage, we know relatively little about the impact of other musical parameters on experienced time.

These issues are compounded by a shared methodological problem in both prospective and retrospective paradigms––namely that both methods ask participants to provide responses after the presentation of the duration or stimulus. As a result, most studies regarding music's impact on the subjective experience of time are only able to capture a single data point for a musical passage, representing a static, post hoc response to a temporally dynamic stimulus (see Loui, this volume). Such an approach is limiting given that the various interacting parameters that generate musical structure are dynamic, generating both small and large structural changes at the local and global levels. In this chapter, we propose the use of a continuous response methodology to collect subjective responses to perceived time while participants listen to music, allowing us to explore the perceived pacing of musical events within their larger musical contexts and their impact on the experience of time while listening.

24.2 A New Methodology to Study the Relationship Between Music and Experienced Time

A continuous response methodology offers several advantages over traditional subjective time estimation tasks for studying experienced time in music. First, it enables the collection of 'real-time' responses to musical structures as they unfold, affording a direct comparison between changes in musical structures and potential shifts in response patterns. Second, it affords multiple data points for each musical passage rather than the single data point collected from more traditional estimation, reproduction, or bisection tasks. And third, while it has been used previously to explore listener responses to silence in musical passages (Margulis, 2007a), it mirrors similar continuous response methods used in studying changes in expressivity (Sloboda & Lehman, 2001), valence and arousal (Bachorik et al., 2009), and tension (Farbood, 2012; Fredrickson, 2000; Lehne et al., 2013; Lerdahl & Krumhansl, 2007) in response to music, making it possible to draw comparisons across these subjective dimensions to gain a more holistic picture of an individual's listening experience and study potential interactions between them.

In this exploratory study, we chose musical excerpts that contained contrasts in paired musical parameters, including alternations between sound and silence, loud and soft dynamics, and metric and ametric passages, following research emphasizing the role of contrast or perceptible change on the subjective experience of time (Block & Reed, 1978; James, 1890). Post-tonal excerpts (excerpts from George Crumb's *Vox Balaenae* and 'Dream Images', and Igor Stravinsky's *Symphonies of Wind Instruments*) were chosen to minimize the potential impact of tonal harmony on perceived time (Boltz, 1998; Schmuckler & Boltz, 1994) and range from ametric to fully metric. Participants were musicians, with an average of 13.2 years of formal training. A joystick was used to collect continuous responses along the participant's sagittal axis (Boroditsky, 2001), with participants instructed to attend to their perception of time while listening and push the joystick forwards when they perceived time moving faster and pull it backwards when they perceived time moving slower. Participants were free to use as much or as little of the joystick range as they liked; the joystick returned to a central 'zero' position when no force was applied. After a practice trial to familiarize themselves with the methodology, participants heard the excerpts presented in a randomized order. After finishing the experiment, participants completed a questionnaire on their musical background and listening habits.

24.3 Results: Connections Between Musical Structure and Temporal Perception

Responses were averaged across participants (*Vox Balaenae* and *Symphonies*, n = 32; 'Dream Images', *n* = 10). The position of the joystick was sampled at a rate of 10 Hz (100 ms) and coded on a scale from 0 to 480 with 240 as the midpoint, or resting position, of the joystick. Lower numbers correspond to the joystick being pulled backwards (temporal deceleration), higher numbers to the joystick being pushed forward (temporal acceleration). As silences are arguably the simplest musical structure to examine, we chose to focus first on the musical excerpt featuring alternations between motives and silences.

Existing theories pertaining to attention (Zakay, 1989) and event density (Block & Zakay, 1997) suggest silences may result in a perception of time moving slower when compared to motives, as silences have a lower event density and contain less nontemporal information. However, studies on the filled duration illusion have found that in some contexts filled durations are perceived as longer than empty durations (e.g. Repp & Bruttomesso, 2009), which would suggest a perception of time moving slower for motives when compared to silences. The excerpt chosen comes from the end of Crumb's *Vox Balaenae* (1971), has a total duration of 40 s, and contains four repetitions of the same motive alternating with pauses that get progressively longer over the course of the passage (3.2–12.5 s). In performance, these pauses allow motives to gradually decay into silences, and therefore are not 'dead air', but contain soft reverberations. However, given contextual cues such as the length of the pauses and their role in creating group boundaries between motivic utterances (Knowles, 2016), they are likely to elicit a categorical perception of silence despite the presence of acoustic artefacts. In other words, while these are not *acoustic* silences they are likely to be heard and interpreted as *perceived* silences (Margulis, 2007b). Results of a paired t-test revealed that Motives (M = 192.5, SD = 109.0) were rated as significantly faster than Silences (M 170.0, SD = 124.2), paired t (31) = 2.40, p < .04, Cohen's d = 0.26, a small effect according to Cohen's (1988) norms. This finding suggests that silences generally evoke a perception of time moving slower in comparison to motives, a different finding from the filled duration illusion, but related to the prediction generated from studies on attention and event density. It is plausible that the decay of motives into silences mitigated responses to silences, resulting in a smaller effect size. A graph of the response profile (Figure 24.1a) shows that responses to silences and motives varied both across the duration of the relevant structure and with regard to the structure's location in relation to the larger excerpt. A linear regression confirms a trend towards deceleration over the course of the excerpt, $F(1, 447)$ = 489.3, p < .001, r^2 =0.52, y = 214.8–0.151×(time), suggesting a compounding effect of the repeating and lengthening silences.

The second excerpt—Stravinsky's *Symphonies of Wind Instruments* (1920), Rehearsal 42–47—features two distinct blocks (Horlacher, 2011) differing in both dynamics and articulation (Block 1 = piano/legato, Block 2 = forte/staccato). Blocks alternate twice across the excerpt, for a total of four distinct sections (total duration = 25.7 s). As we are using a pre-existing piece and recording, decibel differences within each block vary. Mean decibel difference between blocks is 7.4 dB, with the greatest contrast in decibels occurring at the point of transition between Block 1 (soft), and Block 2 (loud), with a mean difference of 16 dB. Following prior research showing that louder music increases both perceived duration and the perceived pace of a stimulus (Kellaris & Altsech, 1992), we hypothesize that joystick responses to Block 2 will be higher on average than responses to Block 1. Results of a paired t-test confirmed our hypothesis, with participants rating Block 2 (M = 302.8, SD = 135.9) as faster than Block 1 (M = 234.7, SD = 106.4), paired t (31) = 5.90, p < .001, Cohen's d = 0.97, a large effect according to Cohen's norm. A graph of the response profile (Figure 24.1b) shows a striking difference in responses to Block 1 (soft) and Block 2 (loud). The change in slope (positive to negative) midway through the first appearance of Block 2 corresponds to a *subito piano* in the recording, suggesting participant responses to this excerpt may be largely driven by changes in dynamics.

The third and final excerpt examined comes from the beginning of Crumb's 'Dream Images', *Makrokosmos Volume 1* (1972) and features a contrast between a repeating ametric and post-tonal passage which surround a quotation from Chopin's *Fantasie-Impromptu* (tonal, metric). Given previous findings concerning effects of familiarity for tonal versus atonal music (Ziv & Omer, 2011) and the differences in attending modes afforded by the contrast of ametric/post-tonal and metric/tonal structures (Boltz, 1991; Jones & Boltz, 1989), we hypothesize that the metric and tonal passage will result in a perception of time moving faster than the ametric and post-tonal passages (Knowles, 2016, 2020). Results of a paired t-test did not reveal a significant difference between ametric (M = 166.35, SD = 136.51) and metric (M = 224.63, SD = 136.51) passages, paired t (9) = 1.84, p = .099, Cohen's d = 0.50, a medium effect size according to Cohen's (1988) norms, likely due to the

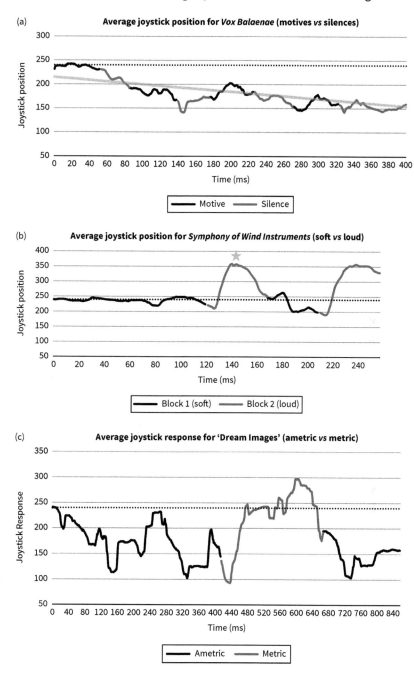

Figure 24.1 (a) Average joystick response profile to *Vox Balaenae* excerpt, along with a linear regression showing a trend towards deceleration (y = 214.8−0.151x). (b) Average joystick response profile for *Symphonies of Wind Instruments* excerpt. A star indicates the location of a *subito piano* partway through the first appearance of Block 2 and a corresponding change in the overall slope (positive to negative). (c) Average joystick response profile for 'Dream Images'. For all graphs, time is given on the x-axis, where 1 = 100 ms, and position of the joystick is given on the y-axis, with the midpoint of the joystick (y = 240) indicated with a dotted line.

smaller sample size. While this test did not achieve statistical significance, results are trending in the direction following our hypothesis. A graph of the response profile can be seen in Figure 24.1c. Similar to the response profile for *Vox Balaenae*, responses varied across the relevant structure, and appear to show a repeating pattern in response to repetition of motives within the ametric passage, although further analysis and a larger sample size would be necessary in order to identify what may be driving these response patterns.[1]

24.4 Conclusion: Towards a Multivariable Model

Results of this preliminary study support the feasibility of a continuous response method for studying the subjective experience of time in music, with differences in the perceived pace of contrasting structures following trends reported in previous studies on comparable structures using more traditional subjective time estimation methods where applicable. However, use of the continuous response method affords a greater level of detail regarding participant in-time temporal responses to musical structures. This enables an examination of responses to both local and global structures, providing more information regarding the impact of music on perceived time than traditional subjective time estimation methods. The use of ecologically valid stimuli in this case study does present several confounds. As noted previously, many of the contrasts examined result from a combination of musical parameters, making it difficult to isolate how much of the response is driven by any one musical parameter. While this complicates the interpretation of the presented results, our findings can be used to inform future studies using composed or manipulated stimuli to isolate the impact of the various musical structures discussed. Results of such future studies could be used to inform the development of a multivariable model for experienced time in music, factoring in the differential impact of co-varying and contrasting musical parameters and contributing to our understanding of musical experience.

Acknowledgements

This research was supported by research grants from Arizona State University and Northwestern University. We would like to thank K. J. Patten for his help and advice on the statistical analysis.

Note

1. Space precludes discussion of participant and piece effects.

References

Bachorik, J. P., Bangert, M., Loui, P., Larke, K., & Berger, J. (2009). Emotion in motion: Investigating the time-course of emotional judgements of musical stimuli. *Music Perception*, 26(4), 355–364. https://doi.org/10.1525/mp.2009.26.4.355

Block, R. A. (1989). Experiencing and remembering time: Affordance, context and cognition. In I. Levin & D. Zakay (Eds.), *Time and human cognition* (pp. 333–363). Elsevier Science. https://doi.org/10.1016/S0166-4115(08)61046-8

Block, R. A. (1992). Prospective and retrospective duration judgment: The role of information processing and memory. In F. Macar (Ed.), *Time, action and cognition* (pp. 141–152). Kluwer Academic Publishers. https://doi.org/10.1007/978-94-017-3536-0_16

Block, R. A., Hancock, P. A., & Zakay, D. (2010). How cognitive load affects duration judgments: A meta-analytic review. *Acta Psychologica*, 134(3), 330–343. https://doi.org/10.1016/j.actpsy.2010.03.006

Block, R. A., & Reed, M. A. (1978). Remembered duration: Evidence for a contextual-change hypothesis. *Journal of Experimental Psychology: Human Learning and Memory*, 4(6), 656–665. https://doi.org/10.1037/0278-7393.4.6.656

Block, R. A., & Zakay, D. (1997). Prospective and retrospective duration judgments: A meta-analytic review. *Psychonomic Bulletin & Review*, 4(2), 184–197. https://doi.org/10.3758/BF03209393

Boltz, M. (1991). Time estimation and attentional perspective. *Perception & Psychophysics*, 49(5), 422–433. http://dx.doi.org.ezproxy1.lib.asu.edu/10.3758/BF03212176

Boltz, M. G. (1992). The remembering of auditory event durations. *Journal of Experimental Psychology: Learning, Memory, and Cognition*, 18(5), 938–956. https://doi.org/10.1037/0278-7393.18.5.938

Boltz, M. G. (1998). The processing of temporal and nontemporal information in the remembering of event durations and musical structure. *Journal of Experimental Psychology: Human Perception and Performance*, 24(4), 1087–1104. https://doi.org/10.1037/0096-1523.24.4.1087

Boroditsky, L. (2001). Does language shape thought? Mandarin and English speakers' conceptions of time. *Cognitive Psychology*, 43(1), 1–22. https://doi.org/10.1006/cogp.2001.0748

Brown, S. W. (1985). Time perception and attention: The effects of prospective versus retrospective paradigms and task demands on perceived duration. *Perception & Psychophysics*, 38(2), 115–124. https://doi.org/10.3758/BF03198848

Brown, S. W., & Boltz, M. G. (2002). Attentional processes in time perception: Effects of mental workload and event structure. *Journal of Experimental Psychology: Human Perception and Performance*, 28(3), 600–615. http://dx.doi.org.ezproxy1.lib.asu.edu/10.1037/0096-1523.28.3.600

Bueno, J. L. O., Firmino, É. A., & Engelman, A. (2002). Influence of generalized complexity of a musical event on subjective time estimation. *Perceptual and Motor Skills*, 94(2), 541–547. https://doi.org/10.2466/PMS.94.2.541-547

Bueno, J. L. O., & Ramos, D. (2007). Musical mode and estimation of time. *Perceptual and Motor Skills*, 105(3, Pt 2), 1087–1092. https://doi.org/10.2466/pms.105.4.1087-1092

Cohen, J. (1988). *Statistical power analysis for the behavioral sciences* (2nd ed.). Erlbaum.

Droit-Volet, S., Ramos, D., Bueno, L. J., & Bigand, E. (2013). Music, emotion, and time perception: The influence of subjective emotional valence and arousal? *Frontiers in Psychology*, 4, 417. https://doi.org/10.3389/fpsyg.2013.00417

Eitan, Z., & Granot, R. Y. (2006). How music moves: Musical parameters and listeners images of motion. *Music Perception: An Interdisciplinary Journal*, 23(3), 221–248. https://doi.org/10.1525/mp.2006.23.3.221

Epstein, D. (1981). On musical continuity. In J. T. Fraser, N. Lawrence, & D. Park (Eds.), *The study of time IV: Papers from the Fourth conference of the International Society for the Study of Time* (pp. 180–197). Springer-Verlag.

Farbood, M. M. (2012). A parametric, temporal model of musical tension. *Music Perception*, 29(4), 387–428. https://doi.org/10.1525/mp.2012.29.4.387

Fredrickson, W. E. (2000). Perception of tension in music: Musicians versus nonmusicians. *Journal of Music Therapy*, 37(1), 40–50. http://dx.doi.org.ezproxy1.lib.asu.edu/10.1093/jmt/37.1.40

Horlacher, G. (2011). *Building blocks: Repetition and continuity in the music of Stravinsky*. Oxford University Press.

James, W. (1890). *The principles of psychology* (Vol. 1). Dover Publications Inc.

Jones, M. R., & Boltz, M. (1989). Dynamic attending and responses to time. *Psychological Review, 96*(3), 459–491. https://doi.org/10.1037/0033-295X.96.3.459

Jones, M.-R. (2018). *Time will tell: A theory of dynamic attending*. Oxford University Press.

Kellaris, J. J., & Altsech, M. B. (1992). The experience of time as a function of musical loudness and gender of listener. *Advances in Consumer Research, 19*, 725–729.

Kellaris, J. J., & Kent, R. J. (1992). The influence of music on consumers' temporal perceptions: Does time fly when you're having fun? *Journal of Consumer Psychology, 1*(4), 365–376. https://doi.org/10.1016/S1057-7408(08)80060-5

Knowles, K. (2020). 'No doubt they are dream-images': Meter and memory in George Crumb's 'Dream-Images'. In M. Aydintan, F. Edler, R. Graybill, & L. Kramer (Eds.), *Gegliederte Zeit: 15. Jahreskongress der Gesellschaft für Musiktheorie Berlin 2015* (pp. 238–248). Verlag Olms.

Knowles, K. (2016). *The boundaries of meter and the subjective experience of time in post-tonal, unmetered music* [PhD dissertation, Northwestern University].

Lerdahl, F., & Krumhansl, C. L. (2007). Modeling tonal tension. *Music perception, 24*(4), 329–366. https://doi.org/10.1525/mp.2007.24.4.329

Lehne, M., Rohrmeier, M., Gollmann, D., & Koelsch, S. (2013). The influence of different structural features on felt musical tension in two piano pieces by Mozart and Mendelssohn. *Music Perception, 31*(2), 171–185. http://dx.doi.org.ezproxy1.lib.asu.edu/10.1525/mp.2013.31.2.171

Margulis, E. H. (2007a). Silences in music are musical not silent: An exploratory study of context effects on the experience of musical pauses. *Music Perception, 24*(5), 485–506. https://doi.org/10.1525/mp.2007.24.5.485

Margulis, E. H. (2007b). Moved by nothing: Listening to musical silence. *Journal of Music Theory, 51*(2), 245–276. https://doi.org/10.1215/00222909-2009-003

Ornstein, R. (1969). *On the experience of time*. Penguin Books.

Repp, B., & Bruttomesso, M. (2009). A filled duration illusion in music: Effects of metrical subdivision on the perception and production of beat tempo. *Advances in Cognitive Psychology, 5*, 114–134. https://doi.org/10.2478/v10053-008-0071-7

Schmuckler, M., & Boltz, M. (1994). Harmonic and rhythmic influences on musical expectancy. *Perception & Psychophysics, 56*(3), 313–325. https://doi.org/10.3758/BF03209765

Sloboda, J. A., & Lehman, A. C. (2001). Tracking performance correlates of changes in perceived intensity of emotion during different interpretations of a Chopin piano prelude. *Music Perception, 19*(1), 87–120. https://doi.org/10.1525/mp.2001.19.1.87

Zakay, D. (1989). Subjective time and attentional resource allocation: An integrated model of time estimation. In I. Levin & D. Zakay (Eds.), *Time and human cognition: A life-span perspective* (pp. 365–397). North-Holland. https://doi.org/10.1016/S0166-4115(08)61047-X

Ziv, N., & Omer, E. (2011). Music and time: The effect of experimental paradigm, musical structure and subjective evaluations on time estimation. *Psychology of Music, 39*(2), 182–195. https://doi.org/10.1177/0305735610372612

25

The Experience of Musical Groove

Body Movement, Pleasure, and Social Bonding

Jan Stupacher, Michael J. Hove, and Peter Vuust

25.1 Introduction

> With the groove our only guide, we shall all be moved.
>
> > (Funkadelic, 1978: 'One Nation Under a Groove')

Some musical rhythms immediately grab our attention. Once we figure out how these rhythms organize time, they draw us in and compel us to participate in the form of foot tapping, head bobbing, or even unbridled dance. This pleasurable drive to move in time with a rhythm has been defined as the psychological construct of groove (Janata et al., 2012; Madison, 2006; Senn et al., 2020). Experiencing groove in music is essentially predicting and enjoying how time is structured by sound. In this chapter, we argue that the experience of groove—alone and in groups—depends on a fine balance between predictability and surprise.

25.2 Sensorimotor Integration in Groove Experiences

Converging evidence indicates that the human motor system is involved in rhythm processing. Listening to music without overt movement engages motor-related brain regions, such as the basal ganglia, supplementary motor area, premotor cortex, and cerebellum (Chen et al., 2008; Grahn & Brett, 2007). Additionally, moving in time with a rhythm improves beat perception (Su & Pöppel, 2012) and increases beat-related steady-state evoked potentials in the electroencephalogram signal (Stupacher, Witte et al., 2016). Importantly, behavioural and neurophysiological studies suggest higher motor-system activation when processing musical rhythms with a strong groove. The accuracy of sensorimotor synchronization and the amount of spontaneous movement increase when moving with high-groove compared to low-groove music (Janata et al., 2012). Similarly, musicians' motor corticospinal excitability is increased when sitting still and listening to music that was rated as high

Jan Stupacher, Michael J. Hove, and Peter Vuust, *The Experience of Musical Groove* In: *Performing Time*. Edited by: Clemens Wöllner and Justin London, Oxford University Press. © Oxford University Press 2023. DOI: 10.1093/oso/9780192896254.003.0026 groove compared to low groove (Stupacher et al., 2013). Non-musicians, conversely, show less motor excitability when listening to high-groove music, potentially reflecting motor inhibition arising from a lower ability to decouple imagined and executed rhythmic movements (Stupacher et al., 2013).

The sonic properties of high-groove music can be investigated in music-information retrieval studies, which demonstrate that the urge to move to a musical rhythm is positively associated with audio features such as salient beats, repetitive patterns, high event density, percussiveness of sounds, and variability of the energy in the bass frequency spectrum (Stupacher, Hove, & Janata, 2016). Additionally, expressive timing deviations from strict positions on the metric grid, called *microtiming*, are often discussed as an important feature of groove, as they can contribute to a sense of collective participation (Keil, 1995). However, empirical evidence on the influence of microtiming on groove ratings is inconclusive, with various studies finding negative, positive, or null effects (for an overview, see e.g. Senn et al., 2016). Musicians and producers often employ the above-mentioned features—for example, by creating dense percussive patterns with syncopation (Madison & Sioros, 2014), or a pumping bass that lays down the beat (Hove et al., 2020)—potentially because musical pieces that make us move and dance are more likely to end up at a high chart position (Askin & Mauskapf, 2017).

In sum, the literature on sensorimotor integration suggests that motor activation and accuracy in rhythm processing relate to the temporal and sonic features of music. Music with a clear beat, pumping bass, moderate amount of syncopation, and high percussiveness can enhance motor activation and promote the experience of groove.

25.3 Predictability and Surprise: Pleasure in Groove Experiences

The same musical features that enhance our groove experience also make it easier to predict how a rhythm unfolds and develops over time. Predicting future events in music is rewarding and essential for experiencing pleasure (Salimpoor et al., 2015). Consequently, the experience of groove depends on predictive models of musical rhythm.

How accurately an individual's internal model predicts future events in a rhythm depends on the rhythm's complexity, on the one hand, and the individual's cultural and personal experiences with music and dance, on the other. This distinction between stimulus-driven bottom-up perception and model-based top-down interpretation is a central assumption of the predictive coding framework, which assumes that the brain uses Bayesian inference to minimize prediction errors when comparing a real-time generative model with the sensory input (Friston, 2005). Applied to rhythm perception and action, this means that the predictive model of a rhythm (e.g. beat and metre) is constantly checked and updated by comparing it to the actual musical input (Vuust & Witek, 2014).

The predictive coding approach can be used to explain the experience of groove. Empirical findings show that moderately complex rhythms elicit a stronger desire to move than very simple or very complex rhythms, resulting in an inverted U-shaped relationship between rhythmic complexity and groove experience (Matthews et al., 2019; Stupacher et al., 2022; Witek et al., 2014; Figure 25.1a). Given a rhythm with moderate rhythmic complexity, an individual can create an internal prediction model that is close to, but not identical with, the actual musical input. Depending on the individual's background in music and dance, this model may result in prediction errors caused by unpredicted rhythmic events that are then used to update the model in real time. In the predictive coding framework, updating the internal model can be seen as sharpening predictions, increasing engagement, and facilitating the affective and embodied experiences that define groove, pleasure, and reward (Vuust & Witek, 2014). However, if a rhythm is very simple, the prediction model and the input often match almost perfectly. Thus, fewer prediction errors occur, and the predictive

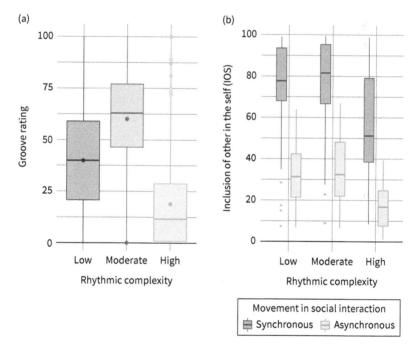

Figure 25.1 The inverted U-shape of rhythmic complexity in relation to groove ratings and social connectedness (Inclusion of Other in the Self (IOS)) in interpersonal interactions with music. (a) Replicating findings by Matthews and colleagues (2019), groove ratings are highest for rhythms with moderate rhythmic complexity, followed by low and high rhythmic complexity (Stupacher et al., 2022). Dots in the boxplots represent mean values; horizontal lines represent median values. (b) Social connectedness to another person, as measured by ratings of IOS, showed an inverted U-function over rhythmic complexity, similar to the pattern in groove ratings (Stupacher et al., 2020). Ratings of IOS were highest for music with moderate followed by low and high complexity and higher when moving in synchrony compared to asynchrony with a virtual other person.

model is not updated regularly, which can lead to habituation and boredom. In contrast, if a rhythm is very complex, prediction errors are unlikely to occur because the individual is either unable to create an appropriate predictive model or the model breaks down too quickly.

The physical properties of music most closely associated with the experience of groove fit into the predictive coding framework. Salient beats and repeating patterns facilitate the creation of a predictive model for perception and action, while dense percussive elements allow for variation and syncopation. This variation produces prediction errors that challenge and update the listener's model, keeping the listening experience rewarding, engaging, and active (Koelsch et al., 2019). High-groove music might therefore create just the right amount of tension between predictability through repetition and surprise through deviation.

Moderate tension between predictability and surprise in rhythm perception and action may hit the sweet spot, not only for the experience of groove, but also for that of *flow*. Flow is a pleasurable experience driven by an optimal balance between challenge and skill, which, like the experience of groove, largely depends on sensorimotor integration. Comparable to the inverted U-shape of groove experience and rhythmic complexity, recent findings demonstrated that the flow dimension *fluency of performance* is positively associated with sensorimotor synchronization accuracy for moderately and highly syncopated rhythms, but not for very simple rhythms without any syncopation (Stupacher, 2019). This finding suggests that a sensorimotor integration task has to be complex enough to challenge an individual's skill set to induce flow-related attributes, such as positive affect, motivation, creativity, concentration, and satisfaction (Csikszentmihalyi & LeFevre, 1989). The pleasure that comes with groove experiences might therefore be partly related to the positive affect associated with flow.

In conclusion, empirical evidence and the predictive coding theoretical approach both suggest that experience of groove and the related experience of flow in music perception and action are most intense when the rhythmic complexity is low enough to enable the creation of predictive models but high enough to challenge these predictions. This optimal balance between predictability and surprise becomes evident in the inverted U-shaped relationship between groove and rhythmic complexity and may enhance an individual's engagement, entrainment, and pleasure. Of course, what defines a moderately complex rhythm depends on personal taste, musical expertise, cultural background, and the social situation.

25.4 Groove as a Shared Experience in Social Interactions

> Probably because a collective emotion cannot be expressed collectively
> without some order that permits harmony and unison of movement . . .

gestures and cries tend to fall into rhythm and regularity, and from there into songs and dances.

(Durkheim, 1912/1995, as cited in Clayton, 2012)

The two main aspects of an individual's experience of groove—pleasure and the drive to move—may be amplified when experiencing groove with other people. Elements of this idea can be found in Durkheim's description of 'collective emotion' and 'unison of movement' in song and dance, as well as in Phillips-Silver and Keller's (2012) definition of *affective* and *temporal* entrainment in joint musical action. When listening to music in a social environment, the rhythm's interplay between repetition and novelty, between predictability and surprise, not only influences how we feel and move, but also how we perceive others. When moving together with a rhythm, as in dance, another person's behaviour becomes less predictable if it does not follow one's own internal model of beat and metre, potentially diminishing—or even hindering—feelings of affiliation and trust. As shown in Figure 25.1b, social connectedness increases when individuals virtually walk in time with music and a synchronized other person, compared to a partner who is asynchronized (Stupacher et al., 2020). This effect of movement synchrony on social closeness also occurs with visual stimuli (Hove & Risen, 2009), and might be stronger for music compared to a metronome (Stupacher, Maes, et al., 2017; Stupacher, Wood, & Witte, 2017). Importantly, social connectedness follows a similar inverted U-shape function when plotted against three levels of rhythmic complexity as groove ratings (Figure 25.1). How, exactly, the affective and sensorimotor aspects in individual groove experiences relate to the feeling of interpersonal connectedness in social situations is a question for future research. Another open question is whether *individual* groove experiences differ from *shared* groove experiences in a quantitative or qualitative way.

One feature of musicality may be that the metre allows a group of dancing individuals to contribute to a shared activity in a similar way, while still leaving room for creative behaviour (Savage et al., 2021). From a predictive coding perspective, moving to the metre promotes a shared predictive model that increases unity, while subtle rhythmic variations in dance allow for expressions of individuality that add an 'individual flourish' to the monotony of the basic rhythm (Merker et al., 2009). Ambiguous rhythms, polyrhythms, and syncopated rhythms use this feature and offer various metric models that can playfully disrupt unity. Following the inverted U-shaped relationship between groove and rhythmic complexity, high-groove music can provide an ideal stimulus for creating unity by repeating rhythmic patterns but also allowing individuality and creative expressions in social interactions through syncopation and playful violations of temporal predictions. Thus, moderately complex rhythms might result in individuals feeling most strongly socially connected when moving together with another person (Figure 25.1b; Stupacher et al., 2020).

25.5 Future Directions

In the song 'One Nation Under a Groove', the band Funkadelic (1978) promotes social and racial progress through musical rhythm. This becomes especially clear in the line 'With the groove our only guide, we shall all be moved'. A question for future research is whether it is possible to encourage synchrony with high-groove music to enable shared time, shared ideas, and social cohesion in large groups. Another future direction of groove studies is the use of physiological and implicit measures. A promising implicit measure of affiliation and sympathy in social entrainment featuring music is helpful behaviour towards others (Kokal et al., 2011; Stupacher, Wood, & Witte, 2017). Physiologically, stronger flow experiences are associated with increased heart rate variability, respiratory depth, and activity of the zygomaticus major muscle, which is involved in smiling (de Manzano et al., 2010). These and other physiological measures, such as pupil dilation (Bowling et al., 2019), might also be related to the experience of groove. Applied to group-data collection, physiological and implicit measures could provide important insights into groove as an individual and a shared experience. The discussion about the effects of microtiming on the experience of groove may especially profit from physiological and implicit measurements, which can capture subtle and unconscious changes in body and mind related to slight variations in musical rhythm.

25.6 Conclusion

An essential part of listening and dancing to music is predicting future events with minimal error. To do so, we build internal models of a rhythm's metric structure that we update when we are surprised by an unforeseen deviation. Music that makes us experience groove, that is, music that engages our motor system, hits the captivating sweet spot between predictability (through repetitive rhythmic patterns) and surprise (through deviations from strict isochrony). This fine-tuned tension keeps us engaged, and is one of the reasons that groove experiences are so rewarding and pleasurable. The balance between predictability and surprise is also essential for social interactions with music. The repetitive patterns of high-groove music allow for shared and predictable movements that can enhance trust and affiliation, while rhythmic deviations allow for unpredictable expressions of individuality.

References

Askin, N., & Mauskapf, M. (2017). What makes popular culture popular? Product features and optimal differentiation in music. *American Sociological Review, 82*(5), 910–944. https://doi.org/10.1177/0003122417728662

Bowling, D. L., Graf Ancochea, P., Hove, M. J., & Fitch, W. T. (2019). Pupillometry of groove: Evidence for noradrenergic arousal in the link between music and movement. *Frontiers in Neuroscience, 12,* 1039. https://doi.org/10.3389/fnins.2018.01039

Chen, J. L., Penhune, V. B., & Zatorre, R. J. (2008). Listening to musical rhythms recruits motor regions of the brain. *Cerebral Cortex, 18*(12), 2844–2854. https://doi.org/10.1093/cercor/bhn042

Clayton, M. (2012). What is entrainment? Definition and applications in musical research. *Empirical Musicology Review, 7*(1–2), 49–56. https://doi.org/10.18061/1811/52979

Csikszentmihalyi, M., & LeFevre, J. (1989). Optimal experience in work and leisure. *Journal of Personality and Social Psychology, 56*(5), 815–822. https://doi.org/10.1037//0022-3514.56.5.815

de Manzano, Ö., Theorell, T., Harmat, L., & Ullén, F. (2010). The psychophysiology of flow during piano playing. *Emotion, 10*(3), 301–311. https://doi.org/10.1037/a0018432

Durkheim, E. (1995). *The elementary forms of religious life* (K. E. Fields, Trans.). The Free Press. (Original work published 1912).

Friston, K. (2005). A theory of cortical responses. *Philosophical Transactions of the Royal Society of London. Series B, Biological Sciences, 360*(1456), 815–836. https://doi.org/10.1098/rstb.2005.1622

Funkadelic. (1978). One nation under a groove [Song]. On *One nation under a groove.* Warner Bros. Records.

Grahn, J. A., & Brett, M. (2007). Rhythm and beat perception in motor areas of the brain. *Journal of Cognitive Neuroscience, 19*(5), 893–906. https://doi.org/10.1162/jocn.2007.19.5.893

Hove, M. J., Martinez, S. A., & Stupacher, J. (2020). Feel the bass: Music presented to tactile and auditory modalities increases aesthetic appreciation and body movement. *Journal of Experimental Psychology: General, 149*(6), 1137–1147. https://doi.org/10.1037/xge0000708

Hove, M. J., & Risen, J. L. (2009). It's all in the timing: Interpersonal synchrony increases affiliation. *Social Cognition, 27*(6), 949–960. https://doi.org/10.1521/soco.2009.27.6.949

Janata, P., Tomic, S. T., & Haberman, J. M. (2012). Sensorimotor coupling in music and the psychology of the groove. *Journal of Experimental Psychology: General, 141*(1), 54–75. https://doi.org/10.1037/a0024208

Keil, C. (1995). The theory of participatory discrepancies: A progress report. *Ethnomusicology, 39*(1), 1–19. https://doi.org/10.2307/852198

Koelsch, S., Vuust, P., & Friston, K. (2019). Predictive processes and the peculiar case of music. *Trends in Cognitive Sciences, 23*(1), 63–77. https://doi.org/10.1016/j.tics.2018.10.006

Kokal, I., Engel, A., Kirschner, S., & Keysers, C. (2011). Synchronized drumming enhances activity in the caudate and facilitates prosocial commitment—If the rhythm comes easily. *PLoS One, 6*(11), e27272. https://doi.org/10.1371/journal.pone.0027272

Madison, G. (2006). Experiencing groove induced by music: Consistency and phenomenology. *Music Perception, 24*(2), 201–208. https://doi.org/10.1525/mp.2006.24.2.201

Madison, G., & Sioros, G. (2014). What musicians do to induce the sensation of groove in simple and complex melodies, and how listeners perceive it. *Frontiers in Psychology, 5,* 894. https://doi.org/10.3389/fpsyg.2014.00894

Matthews, T. E., Witek, M. A. G., Heggli, O. A., Penhune, V. B., & Vuust, P. (2019). The sensation of groove is affected by the interaction of rhythmic and harmonic complexity. *PloS One, 14*(1), e0204539. https://doi.org/10.1371/journal.pone.0204539

Merker, B. H., Madison, G. S., & Eckerdal, P. (2009). On the role and origin of isochrony in human rhythmic entrainment. *Cortex, 45*(1), 4–17. https://doi.org/10.1016/j.cortex.2008.06.011

Phillips-Silver, J., & Keller, P. E. (2012). Searching for roots of entrainment and joint action in early musical interactions. *Frontiers in Human Neuroscience, 6,* 26. https://doi.org/10.3389/fnhum.2012.00026

Salimpoor, V. N., Zald, D. H., Zatorre, R. J., Dagher, A., & McIntosh, A. R. (2015). Predictions and the brain: How musical sounds become rewarding. *Trends in Cognitive Sciences, 19*(2), 86–91. https://doi.org/10.1016/j.tics.2014.12.001

Savage, P. E., Loui, P., Tarr, B., Schachner, A., Glowacki, L., Mithen, S., & Fitch, W. T. (2021). Music as a coevolved system for social bonding. *Behavioral and Brain Sciences, 44,* e59. https://doi.org/10.1017/S0140525X20000333

Senn, O., Bechtold, T., Rose, D., Câmara, G. S., Düvel, N., Jerjen, R., Kilchenmann, L., Hoesl, F., Baldassarre, A., & Alessandri, E. (2020). Experience of groove questionnaire. *Music Perception*, *38*(1), 46–65. https://doi.org/10.1525/mp.2020.38.1.46

Senn, O., Kilchenmann, L., von Georgi, R., & Bullerjahn, C. (2016). The effect of expert performance microtiming on listeners' experience of groove in swing or funk music. *Frontiers in Psychology*, *7*, 1487. https://doi.org/10.3389/fpsyg.2016.01487

Stupacher, J. (2019). The experience of flow during sensorimotor synchronization to musical rhythms. *Musicae Scientiae*, *23*(3), 348–361. https://doi.org/10.1177/1029864919836720

Stupacher, J., Hove, M. J., & Janata, P. (2016). Audio features underlying perceived groove and sensorimotor synchronization in music. *Music Perception*, *33*(5), 571–589. https://doi.org/10.1525/mp.2016.33.5.571

Stupacher, J., Hove, M. J., Novembre, G., Schütz-Bosbach, S., & Keller, P. E. (2013). Musical groove modulates motor cortex excitability: A TMS investigation. *Brain and Cognition*, *82*(2), 127–136. https://doi.org/10.1016/j.bandc.2013.03.003

Stupacher, J., Maes, P.-J., Witte, M., & Wood, G. (2017). Music strengthens prosocial effects of interpersonal synchronization—If you move in time with the beat. *Journal of Experimental Social Psychology*, *72*, 39–44. https://doi.org/10.1016/j.jesp.2017.04.007

Stupacher, J., Witek, M. A. G., Vuoskoski, J. K., & Vuust, P. (2020). Cultural familiarity and individual musical taste differently affect social bonding when moving to music. *Scientific Reports*, *10*, 10015. https://doi.org/10.1038/s41598-020-66529-1

Stupacher, J., Witte, M., Hove, M. J., & Wood, G. (2016). Neural entrainment in drum rhythms with silent breaks: Evidence from steady-state evoked and event-related potentials. *Journal of Cognitive Neuroscience*, *28*(12), 1865–1877. https://doi.org/10.1162/jocn_a_01013

Stupacher, J., Wood, G., & Witte, M. (2017). Synchrony and sympathy: Social entrainment with music compared to a metronome. *Psychomusicology: Music, Mind, and Brain*, *27*(3), 158–166. https://doi.org/10.1037/pmu0000181

Stupacher, J., Wrede, M., & Vuust, P. (2022). A brief and efficient stimulus set to create the inverted U-shaped relationship between rhythmic complexity and the sensation of groove. *PLoS One*, *17*(5), e0266902.

Su, Y.-H., & Pöppel, E. (2012). Body movement enhances the extraction of temporal structures in auditory sequences. *Psychological Research*, *76*(3), 373–382. https://doi.org/10.1007/s00426-011-0346-3

Van Dyck, E., Moelants, D., Demey, M., Deweppe, A., Coussement, P., & Leman, M. (2013). The impact of the bass drum on human dance movement. *Music Perception*, *30*(4), 349–359. https://doi.org/10.1525/mp.2013.30.4.349

Vuust, P., & Witek, M. A. G. (2014). Rhythmic complexity and predictive coding: A novel approach to modeling rhythm and meter perception in music. *Frontiers in Psychology*, *5*, 1111. https://doi.org/10.3389/fpsyg.2014.01111

Witek, M. A. G., Clarke, E. F., Wallentin, M., Kringelbach, M. L., & Vuust, P. (2014). Syncopation, body-movement and pleasure in groove music. *Plos One*, *9*(4), e94446. https://doi.org/10.1371/journal.pone.0094446

SECTION 5
CONCLUSIONS

Capturing Time in Performance and Science

Anchor Chapters

26

Embodied Time

What the Psychology and Neuroscience of Time Can Learn From the Performing Arts

Marc Wittmann

26.1 Introduction

The famous dispute between Albert Einstein and Henri Bergson on the nature of time in 1922 has often been interpreted as Einstein's rigorous scientific victory over an irrational thinker. Einstein's catchy phrase that there were only a physics of time and a psychology of time and thereafter 'the time of the philosophers did not exist' (Canales, 2015, p. 5; '*Il n'y a donc pas un temps des philosophes*') summarizes this interpretation. For a philosopher like Bergson, there is no independent approach to understand time. Time can only be studied through physics (objective time) and psychology (subjective time).

In a recent analysis of the debate, we tried to vindicate Bergson (Wittmann & Montemayor, 2021). We argued that Bergson employed a phenomenological approach when he elaborated on experienced duration (*la durée*) as experiential time, which he considered primarily non-quantifiable (compare this with Kozak's view, this volume). Dainton (2017) similarly treats Bergson as a phenomenologist when he juxtaposes Bergson's analysis in the *Essaie sur les données immédiates de la conscience* (*Time and Free Will: An Essay on the Immediate Data of Consciousness*)— 'inner duration, perceived by consciousness, is nothing else but the melting of states of consciousness into one another' (Bergson, 1913, p. 107)—with a description of the stream-like structure of consciousness: 'A is experienced as flowing into B, B is experienced as flowing into C, and C into D' (Dainton, 2017, p. 101).

Even when considering monist approaches to the brain–consciousness problem, the time of the psychologist is primarily informed by phenomenal experience ('this musical performance lasted painfully long') (Velmans, 2009). The phenomenology of time thereafter strongly overlaps with physical and psychological time, that is, judgements of subjective duration in relation to clock time. Though hardly studied at the time of the debate, Bergson's idea of an emotional and visceral vitality underlying all cognition and, specifically, the feeling of time passing, is now in the focus of contemporary cognitive neuroscience, and related to the notion of embodiment (e.g. Craig, 2015; Damasio, 1999; Tsakiris & de Preester, 2018).

Marc Wittmann, *Embodied Time* In: *Performing Time*. Edited by: Clemens Wöllner and Justin London, Oxford University Press.
© Oxford University Press 2023. DOI: 10.1093/oso/9780192896254.003.0027

Bergson considered time to be a vital force in our lives that cannot be reduced to metric relations, such as simultaneity, temporal order, or clock-based duration. Although empirical researchers do study the underlying processes and structures, one must begin in any type of analytic method with the irreducible experience of time as flow and passage, which manifests itself at its clearest in the visceral and empathic reactions we associate with conscious awareness (Montemayor & Haladjian, 2015). Psychologists and cognitive neuroscientists are interested in the mechanisms underlying the phenomenal dynamics, which provide a basis for understanding phenomenal consciousness.

Such a dual mode of analysis of phenomena, on the one hand, and mechanisms, on the other, is naturally pursued in music. Experienced music can be regarded as a stream of emotional movements, as 'the melting of states of consciousness into one another' (Bergson, 1913, p. 107). Music is also analysed according to the intrinsic temporalities of rhythm and metre. This dual nature of music is what Clemens Wöllner refers to when he states that 'music is an ephemeral form of art that works simultaneously on different structural levels' (see Wöllner, this volume). Music is immediately experienced as an emotional stream by the listener. Psychologists interested in music perception investigate the underlying temporal mechanisms on different levels. If researchers have inquisitive minds, they do not adhere to the strict demarcation imposed by the dual mode of phenomena and mechanisms; they do not restrict themselves to the quantitative side of music, but also attempt to capture the qualitative aspects of experience.

26.2 Embodied Experience of Temporal Perception and Music and Dance

As we argued (Wittmann & Montemayor, 2021), Henri Bergson's dynamic notion of consciousness as constituting subjective time corresponds well with the embodied approach to the sense of time. Subjective feelings depend on bodily signals, the ongoing visceral and somatosensory stimulation from the peripheral nervous system. The phenomenologist Maurice Merleau-Ponty (1945), who referred to the prevailing neuropsychological research, explicitly stated that subjective time emerges through the sense of an enduring self across time as an embodied entity. A number of studies indicate the relationship between affective physical states and subjective time (Droit-Volet et al., 2013; Mella et al., 2011; Wittmann, 2009). For example, relatively higher physical arousal levels, as psycho-physiologically measured with heart rate variability indices, lead to an overestimation of temporal duration (Ogden, Henderson, McGlone, & Richter, 2019), while relatively more relaxation leads to an underestimation of time (Ogden, Henderson, Slade, et al., 2019). Many direct associations between changes in specific physical parameters and time estimates have been demonstrated. In two separate studies, the heart steadily slowed down and skin conductance levels progressively decreased during the temporal reproduction of auditory (Meissner & Wittmann, 2011) and visual (Otten et al., 2015) intervals in the range of several seconds. In another, the heart rate evoked potential in the electro-encephalogram was recorded during a time perception task, and an early negative component of the heart rate evoked potential amplitude appeared to be related to the accuracy in estimating the time interval (Richter & Ibáñez, 2021). When presenting video clips in slow motion, as contrasted with video clips presented in real time, a relatively lower respiration rate was induced and a smaller pupillary diameter recorded, both of which were associated with a relative underestimation of duration (Wöllner et al., 2018).

Regarding the neural basis of subjective time, that is, the question of *how* and *where* time is processed in the brain, no unequivocal conceptualization exists, which corresponds to models of the neural basis of space representation regarding grid and border cells in hippocampal and parahippocampal structures (Moser et al., 2017). Meta-analyses of neuroimaging studies reveal that many different areas in the brain are involved in time perception. Depending on the involvement of motor action in timing tasks, sensorimotor loops in the brain which are modulated by the dopamine system are activated (Buhusi & Meck, 2005). The duration of the interval to be timed is also crucial. Relatively more activation in cortical, as opposed to subcortical, regions is typically detected with supra-second stimuli (Nani et al., 2019). In the following, we highlight the contribution of the insular cortex to the perception of time, as it represents one of the areas in the brain repeatedly identified as crucial in neuroimaging studies (Nani et al., 2019; Richter & Ibáñez, 2021; Teghil et al., 2019). The insula is the primary interoceptive cortex, the primary region in the cortex that processes signals from the body organs; as such, it plays the key role in the embodied shaping of perception and cognition (Craig, 2015; Evrard, 2019). The insula demonstrates ramp-like activity during time estimation tasks with multiple-second durations (Wittmann, 2013). Resting-state functional connectivity with the insular cortex during a time perception task was related to increased body awareness, as assessed by a personality trait questionnaire across individuals (Teghil et al., 2020). To summarize the probed and tested ideas presented here, ascending bodily signals from the periphery and the internal organs produce a dynamic series of conscious emotional moments. These are integrated in the neural system connected with the insular cortex and are thus related to the conscious sense of time passage.

Music and dance, as experienced and understood by the embodied and active listener, temporally unfold in exactly that way as 'a dynamic series of conscious emotional moments'. This emotional flux creates episodes of lived time full of sensibilities and tensions (see Kozak, this volume; Maes & Leman, this volume). We typically experience this 'dynamic series of conscious emotional moments' continuously through our waking hours from the first-person perspective. We are more or less immersed in what we are doing; there are marked fluctuations in arousal and attention, automaticity of behaviour, and self-awareness (Khoshnoud et al., 2020). One way to objectively control for variations in the flow of events is to assess corresponding subjective feeling states while people play video games (Rutrecht et al.,

2021). Musical excerpts provide the prime medium to induce a dynamic embodied experience and, thereby, control and measure an individual's reaction from a third-person perspective (see Maes & Leman, this volume). Similarly, dance can be used to assess spectators' mental states and bodily reactions as empathic reactions to the dynamic qualities of the choreographed movement (Vatakis et al., 2014). As a kin-aesthetic art, dance induces automatic reactions in the entire body of the spectator (Hagendoorn, 2004). On seeing dance movements, an observer internally re-enacts the action in the same brain regions which are active when someone moves their own body (Bläsing et al., 2012; Calvo-Merino et al., 2005). Such a re-enactment can even be provoked with static images which influence subjective time for participants in laboratory studies. For example, in the context of dance performance photos, the viewing of static postures requiring more movement on the part of the dancer was estimated to last longer than photos of postures requiring less movement (Nather & Bueno, 2012; Nather et al., 2011; for a comprehensive review of laboratory dance studies, see Bläsing, this volume).

Neurophenomenological methods can be applied to align subjective awareness with neuroscientific and behavioural methods (Thompson, 2010). Although an increasing number of researchers emphasize the need for first-person data, only a few studies have been conducted that systematically combine the first- and third-person perspectives. One such study concerned the neural correlates of viewing and reporting the emergence of a three-dimensional illusory geometric shape out of random-dot patterns (Lutz et al., 2002), while another combined neural signal and subjective report analysis of a highly experienced meditator conducting the famous Libet task examining free will, in which a subject produces self-timed button presses (Jo et al., 2014).

A methodological attempt to assess and juxtapose music experience with at least one objective behavioural dimension is presented in a study by Knowles and Ashley (see Knowles & Ashley, this volume). In typical time perception studies, participants are only asked after the stimulus has been presented. This is a natural approach because subjects can only judge the duration of the event after it has ter-minated. Here, the participants, who were experienced musicians, used a joystick to give continuous responses while they were listening to music excerpts. When they felt that the musical piece accelerated, they pushed the joystick forward; when they felt it decelerated, they pulled it backward. This provided a plotted, subjective profile of temporal experience which covered the duration of different musical ex-cerpts lasting several minutes (see Knowles & Ashley, this volume, Figure 24.1). This continuous-response method is one attempt to capture the subjective ex-perience of local and global structures in music. Researchers in psychology and the cognitive neurosciences could learn from this approach, as it can be used in a variety of contexts where ongoing subjective experience must be recorded and correlated with behavioural and neural responses over the course of several sec-onds and minutes. Several different dimensions could be tested and compared; for example, the speed of time passage could be related to a sensed faster time passage corresponding to increased arousal (see Wöllner, this volume). One question could be whether subjects who indicate their arousal levels produce a similar signature of joystick movements over time compared to subjects asked to indicate subjective time passage. In the work by Noble and colleagues, a similar method was used to assess the pace of time in a specific musical piece; leaving it in the central position indicated 'normal time', moving it forward meant a speeding up of time, backward, a slowing down (see Noble et al., this volume). The different methods reveal the need to investigate and develop valid measures to assess dynamic temporal experience.

The continuous-response method could complement the prevalent method of asking participants after an interval has ended (i.e. a retrospective evaluation). Passage of time judgements and duration estimates in combination with questions about affective states assessed after exposure to a condition can be related to the dynamics of the continuous response plot. Such an approach has actually been undertaken when measuring pain perception; the retrospective evaluation of total pain experienced during a colonoscopy was related to the temporal profile of patients' verbal intensity ratings assessed every 60 s (Redelmeier & Kahneman, 1996). Patients' memories (the retrospective evaluation) regarding the painful procedure reflected the peak intensity of pain during the procedure and the final part of the colonoscopy experience. Retrospective affective music experience could similarly reflect certain aspects of the dynamics of the continuous evaluation of the listening experience. Many studies exist concerning time perception in subjects listening to music who report their impressions after the excerpt ended (e.g. Bailey & Areni, 2006; Firmino et al., 2020), or individuals were requested to reproduce the duration of presented music recordings differing in tempo, where slower tempi resulted in fewer perceived events and shorter reproduced durations (Hammerschmidt et al., 2021). With a similar reproduction method, subjective durations of presented music have been studied under the influence of ayahuasca, a hallucinogen consumed during a shamanistic ritual (Campagnoli et al., 2020). In future studies, the momentary impression of time passage while listening to music could be further assessed and correlated with typical retrospective judgements.

Retrospective duration evaluations in psychological research have been obtained from participants after waiting situations (Witowska et al., 2020), after exposure to different environments over an extended period (Ehret et al., 2020; Pfeifer et al., 2019; 2020), and after playing a video game, both on screen and in virtual reality (Rutrecht et al., 2021). One research group is combining first-person reports in collective dance improvisations with the analysis of recorded third-person kinematics in dancers, both individuals and groups (Himberg et al., 2018). The underlying assumption is that the dancers are creating an entanglement of individual intrinsic temporalities and thus 'making time together' (see Laroche et al., this volume). Subjective reports vary dynamically when the dancer is embedded in the social dynamics of lived time—temporal social interactions which are constitutional for us humans.

In a recent study of ours (Deinzer et al., 2017) we were inspired by an experimental setup of the dance researchers Bachrach and colleagues (2015), which contained a slow-movement piece based on Myriam Gourfink's work. These dance movements are in extremely slow motion, and without changes in speed. We contrasted this movement type with a fast-movement piece consisting of smooth body motions capturing a steady flow. Both dances were based on the same script with a fixed movement sequence but presented at different speeds. In our experimental design we presented the two conditions (very slow, fast) in two 5-min live dances, which were choreographed and eventually performed by a professional dancer in front of a theatre audience with a total of 52 spectators on two separate evenings. We counterbalanced the order of dances on the two evenings. The dances were presented silently, as music would have introduced a strong confounding factor.

The spectators preferred the fast dance to the slow one. During the former, the participants showed higher levels of absorption; they also focused more on the dancer's breathing and less on their own body. A typical sign of flow is the relative loss of the sense of self and of time passage while one is mentally absorbed in an activity (Rutrecht et al., 2021). Accordingly, spectators reported that time seemed to pass more quickly during the fast dance. Interestingly, participants estimated the faster dance to have lasted longer, which we interpreted as retrospective memory effect on time judgement (for details of the discussion, see Deinzer et al., 2017). Longer duration judgements in the fast condition were related to more memorable (i.e. pleasant) experiences while observing the dance. In the retrospective model of time perception, the more stored experiences are retrieved, the longer subjective duration becomes (Zakay & Block, 2004). We conducted statistical path analyses and discovered that when spectators paid more attention to their bodily signals this mediated the feeling of time passage in the slow dance. That is, due to increased attention to the body, time passed more slowly, which fits the embodied model of time perception (Wittmann, 2009, 2013). The slow dance seemed to have evoked states of boredom; the audience tended to experience more unpleasant feelings and were more aware of time passage. They were thrown back on their own affective and bodily reactions, which, as Pakes argues, can lead us to one of the three types of boredom which Heidegger discussed in his *Fundamental Concepts of Metaphysics* (see Pakes, this volume). Since our study only employed a retrospective evaluation after each dance, future studies could employ the above-mentioned methods and plot subjective profiles of temporal experience produced with a joystick in real time (see Knowles & Ashley, this volume)—potentially in co-registration of physiological signals of heart and breathing rates.

26.3 Temporal Processing Levels in Perception and Music

The assessments of arousal, valence, and felt passage of time inform us about the overall lived experience of listening to music. More detailed analyses of temporal structures in music reveal smaller building blocks of what constitutes and enables this lived experience (see Kozak, this volume). The human temporal information processing inherent in music perception can be described in the following ways: (a) through a micro-processing level related to nuances in expressive musical effects in the range of tens to hundreds of milliseconds, and (b) an intermediate processing level related to melodic, harmonic, and rhythmic patterns with intervals up to 3–5 s (see Kozak, this volume; Wöllner, this volume). There are even longer musical structures which represent larger units of a performance. These units enable a listener to elaborate a mental schema of the music, which can be symbolized by a mental line consisting of segments (Deliège, 1995).

The micro and intermediate temporal processing levels identified in music perception correspond to two general temporal integration mechanisms in sensorimotor processing. One is identified in the range of milliseconds as *functional moments* which define whether two events are perceived as simultaneous or as successive (Elliott & Giersch, 2016). The other is in a range of around 2–3 s, an *experienced moment* related to temporal integration when events are experienced as presently happening (Lubashevsky & Plavinska, 2021; Pöppel, 1997, 2009; Singhal & Srinivasan, 2021; Wittmann, 2011). Wöllner argues that 'there are certain temporal boundaries for "optimal" musical experiences of performers, listeners, and dancers' (see Wöllner, this volume). These boundaries need to be delimited by the temporal processing mechanisms of the body and brain. Music with inter-beat intervals that are too short (the music is too fast) or with intervals exceeding a few seconds (the music is too slow) are typically experienced as unpleasant (Wittmann & Pöppel, 1999). A similar reasoning for the existence of temporal integration levels is applied to sensorimotor processing, in general. Discretely operating processing mechanisms must come into play when considering the spectrum of cognitive processes in human perception and interpersonal behaviour, that is, when communicating with others (Trevarthen, 1999; Tschacher et al., 2013). Successful interactions with other humans are limited by certain temporal constraints: operating not too fast (to accurately perceive) and not too slow (for being in time). The function of an extended and shared moment is related to inter-subjective synchronization and communication by means of a common temporal platform (Kimura et al., 2020). Consider a musical performance where a quartet or, indeed, a whole orchestra must synchronize for the music to be perceived as pleasant, or of the exact timing of movements necessary for a couple to dance in synchrony. The temporal structure of auditory (music), visual, and body movement synchronization creates togetherness among performers such as musicians and dancers, as well as the feeling of a common fate with the audience (see Bläsing, this volume; Doelling et al., this volume; Goebl & Bishop, this volume).

26.3.1 Present-Moment Experience

Regarding the intermediate level of temporal processing, analyses of representative occidental music have revealed that a rhythmic *gestalt* of up to 2–4 s is typical, such as in the famous themes of Beethoven's Fifth Symphony or the Dutchman's theme in Wagner's *Flying Dutchman* (Epstein, 1995; Pöppel, 1989). The composition genre of *minimal music* uses timing gestalts of pattern repetition by explicitly producing and stressing the sense of circular motion in such an approximate time range. Tonal surfaces that violate this implicit rule of composition nevertheless exist, such as in musical creations by Luigi Nono and Klaus Lang, where tonal events persist longer than 2–4 s. But, in those cases, a different aesthetic impression is generated precisely through this violation (Wittmann & Pöppel, 1999).

The largest overlap between research in experimental psychology and music psychology on the intermediate level of temporal processing probably lies in research on metronome speed and related experience. The sequence of 'ticks' a metronome produces at a moderate speed are automatically integrated and accentuated to 'tick-tacks' every n-th beat (1–2, 1–2, 1–2, or 1–2–3, 1–2–3, etc.). The beats form rhythmic units which are perceptual constructs, since they do not physically exist (Pöppel, 1997, 2009; Szelag, 1997). A certain speed range defines whether individual 'ticks' are perceived as part of a temporal gestalt. Inter-beat intervals shorter than 200–300 ms define a lower limit (fastest speed) and an interval of around 2 s an upper limit, the slowest possible speed (London, 2002; Povel, 1984). If the metronome is too fast, a train of 'ticks' is perceived, and no temporal integration occurs. If the metronome speed is too slow, only individually separated events are heard (1–1–1; Linares Gutiérrez et al., 2019; Szelag et al., 1996). The perceived units of integration of such accent patterns depend on the tempo of the sequence, but the maximum temporal gestalt lies at approximately 2–3 s (Bååth, 2015; Szelag, 1997). Several other experimental paradigms have been developed to assess behavioural and neural indices relating to subjective impressions of discontinuities (Benussi, 1913; Nakajima et al., 1980; Wang et al., 2015). Although the outcomes of this research vary to some extent in the duration of the detected units, they nevertheless converge on a range of a few seconds (Lubashevsky & Plavinska, 2021; Singhal & Srinivasan, 2021; White, 2017).

When the motor component comes into play on this intermediate temporal processing level—that is, when subjects are instructed to follow the metronome beats by tapping their fingers on a button each time a beat occurs—this sensorimotor task can be accomplished effortlessly and accurately within a similar time range of inter-beat intervals (Fraisse, 1984; Mates et al., 1994; Peters, 1989). A tempo with inter-beat intervals shorter than around 250 ms is too fast for subjects to be able to accurately synchronize the taps to the beats. A self-paced tapping tempo typically has inter-tap intervals longer than 250 ms, the personal tapping speed inter-individually ranging with a mode in the distribution of 2 Hz (Fraisse, 1984; Hammerschmidt et al., 2021; Wittmann et al., 2004). The spread of intervals produced in the personal tapping task thus lie within an approximate range of metronome speeds that are judged to be neither too fast nor too slow: the majority of inter-tap intervals fall in a broad range between 400 and 1200 ms (Hammerschmidt et al., 2021, Figure 1), and the majority of metronome intervals that are perceived as pleasant tempos fall between 500 and 900 ms (Frischeisen-Köhler, 1933; Parncutt, 1994).

If metronome intervals between ticks exceed the duration of 2–3 s, behavioural variance increases, and the button is often pressed either far too early or too late (the latter being reaction times). Only when using a counting strategy—like a musician who keeps track of the rhythmic framework in music—can one accurately synchronize one's own taps with the 'ticks'. Counting and rhythmic body movements subdivide longer intervals into smaller units, reducing the variability of synchronization with a very slow metronome (Repp, 2010). Body movements synchronized to sound function as an external timekeeper (see Maes & Leman, this volume). Importantly, the indicated time range is not to be seen as a fixed interval, but rather stems from underlying biological mechanisms that exhibit high variability.

The metronome and metronome-tapping tasks naturally come closest to actual music performance, which requires accurate and precise timing, whether playing solo or with others. Therefore, the metronome paradigm could ideally be probed and tested with musicians. It might be even more appropriate to use the task with trained musicians, as investigations with non-musically trained subjects have produced diverse outcomes, since some individuals have difficulty understanding the task (Linares Gutiérrez, 2021). Similarly, professional dancers, as compared to non-dancers, are more proficient in judging duration. In one study they could more accurately and precisely judge the passage of time of movement sequences presented in a series of static images (Sgouramani & Vatakis, 2014).

Concerning embodiment of the present moment, correlations between autonomic nervous activity indices and performance in the metronome task have been demonstrated in individuals with meditation experience. Stronger vagal (parasympathetic) activity in participants who had just meditated was related to a larger integration interval with metronome intervals of 300-ms duration, the fastest of presented frequencies. Longer respiratory periods after meditation also led to longer integration intervals for 1-s inter-stimulus intervals (Linares Gutiérrez et al., 2019). Experienced meditators are more present-oriented and body-centred, especially directly after meditation (Matko & Sedlmeier, 2021). These correlations indicate a meditation-induced embodiment effect on the experienced present moment. Musicians, by definition, are skilled motor timers and natural candidates for metronome studies, that is, to study the known facilitatory role of body movement in the entrainment to auditory rhythms (Su & Pöppel, 2012). For example, amateur musicians who performed timing tasks were better able than non-musicians to modulate performance precisely, that is, to synchronize with complex multimodal rhythms, mentally bisect metronome intervals, and tap only at the bisection points (anti-phase tapping) (Repp, 2010; Su, 2014).

26.3.2 Perception of Sequence and Temporal Order

For temporal processing at the micro level, the most basic experiences are those of simultaneity and successiveness and of temporal order (Pöppel, 1997). The lowest detection threshold observed in psychophysical tasks is found in the auditory system, where two short acoustic stimuli only 2–3 ms apart are detected as appearing non-simultaneously (Lotze et al., 1999). The visual and the tactile systems have higher succession thresholds (lower temporal resolution) in the range of some tens of milliseconds, inter-modal (auditory–visual) stimulation leading to the highest thresholds (Fraisse, 1984). Temporal order thresholds for two light flashes, two tactile stimuli, or two sounds lie at similar time ranges between 20 and 60 ms; inter-modal temporal order thresholds are slightly higher (Exner, 1875; Fostick et al., 2019). When the temporal order of more than two complex stimuli have to be identified, the inter-onset intervals between individual stimuli must be at least 200–300 ms for one to be able to tell the correct sequence (Ulbrich et al., 2009; Warren and Obusek, 1972). Natural variations in detected thresholds can be explained by the physical properties of the two stimuli to be judged, such as their complexity, intensity, and frequency, which have an influence (see Wöllner, this volume). Similarly, in several musical styles (e.g. hip-hop) the contextual nature of what is heard influences the micro-level of groove; for example, 'muddy' sounds obscure the exact temporal location of the beat (see Danielsen, this volume).

The detection of temporal order can be interpreted as a primary experiential datum, as it connects the subjective experience of succession with physical order (Wackermann, 2007). The notions of time and duration are based on the elementary temporal relationship between two events, A and B. The two events are perceived in their temporal order as 'A occurs before B' or 'B occurs before A'. The experience of duration is only possible when one can demarcate the onset A and offset B of the temporal interval. The detection of the correct temporal order of auditory signals is essential in music and spoken language. For example, patients with damage to the left hemisphere have problems detecting the temporal order of clicks and tones (Wittmann et al., 2004). They also have difficulties distinguishing certain stop consonants which are identifiable through the detection of the correct sequence of spectral events in the speech signal (Fink et al., 2006). In one study with musically untrained subjects, temporal order detection was significantly better for speech than for musical stimuli. The authors concluded that non-selected individuals are more sensitive to temporal order in speech than in musical stimuli (Vatakis & Spence, 2006).

Despite the identification of these discrete levels of temporal integration on a micro (milliseconds) and an intermediate (seconds) level, experience is a continuous and unified whole. This is best exemplified when listening to music. The temporal order of musical events (milliseconds) and the integration of these events into meaningful units of musical themes (seconds) constitute the basis for lived affective experience across time. Experienced continuity may well be established through short-term/working-memory processes which create a platform of *mental presence* in the range of multiple seconds (Wittmann, 2011, 2016). Mental presence is characterized by the ongoing dynamic transition from momentary experiences to the fading out of this mental content within the boundaries of working memory. As summarized by an expert neuroscientist in the field, the integrative property of working memory 'provides a temporal bridge between events—both those that are internally generated and environmentally presented—thereby conferring a sense of unity and continuity to conscious experience' (Goldman-Rakic, 1997, p. 559). Short-term retention of what one has just experienced is subjected to a gradual loss as time passes; in experimental studies, the correct recall of items decreases with increasing delay (Rubin & Wenzel, 1996). Mental presence is a sliding window, with experiences constantly appearing as novel events and, in turn, fading out as memory contents (James, 1890, Chapter XIV). With respect to music perception, within mental presence an 'expressive narrative' can be maintained that acts as a guiding principle for intentionality and creates an overarching emotional effect—music as lived experience (see Maes & Leman, this volume).

26.4 Conclusion

The predominant methodology in research on time perception and sensorimotor timing does not contain musical and dance elements, which is to say it does not use music as a stimulus or examine performance contexts. Yet, music and dance are ideal ways to evoke a lived experience in an embodied listener and spectator, or to generate a synchronized experience for musicians and dancers, themselves. Since a set of empirical studies in the time perception literature point to the relation between affective bodily states and subjective time, music and dance could be used to assess time experience on a macroscopic level, in the range of many seconds and minutes. A micro and an intermediate level of temporal integration of the present moment, which mechanistically underlie lived experience, could be subjected to experimental tests in a range between milliseconds and seconds. These underlying mechanistic levels of temporal integration could have upstream effects on the macro level of experience. In contrast, contextual effects of macro-level music experience could have downstream effects on the lower levels of processing. Individuals not specifically trained to play an instrument, sing, or dance could be compared to trained performers, in much the same way that studies have assessed embodiment and time perception in people trained in meditation techniques. Henri Bergson rightly described emotional movements through time as 'the melting of states of consciousness into one another' (1913, p. 107), so music is an ecological valid stimulus to probe for time consciousness.

References

Bååth, R. (2015). Subjective rhythmization: A replication and an assessment of two theoretical explanations. *Music Perception, 33*(2), 244–254.

Bachrach, A., Fontbonne, Y., Joufflineau, C., & Ulloa, J. L. (2015). Audience entrainment during live contemporary dance performance: Physiological and cognitive measures. *Frontiers in Human Neuroscience, 9*, 179.

Bailey, N., & Areni, C. S. (2006). When a few minutes sound like a lifetime: Does atmospheric music expand or contract perceived time? *Journal of Retailing*, *82*(3), 189–202.

Benussi, V. (1913). *Psychologie der Zeitauffassung*. Carl Winters Universitätsbuchhandlung.

Bergson, H. (1913). *Time & free will*. George Allen.

Bläsing, B., Calvo-Merino, B., Cross, E. S., Jola, C., Honisch, J., & Stevens, C. J. (2012). Neurocognitive control in dance perception and performance. *Acta Psychologica*, *139*(2), 300–308.

Buhusi, C. V., & Meck, W. H. (2005). What makes us tick? Functional and neural mechanisms of interval timing. *Nature Reviews Neuroscience*, *6*(10), 755–765.

Calvo-Merino, B., Glaser, D. E., Grèzes, J., Passingham, R. E., & Haggard, P. (2005). Action observation and acquired motor skills: An fMRI study with expert dancers. *Cerebral Cortex*, *15*(8), 1243–1249.

Campagnoli, A. P. S., Pereira, L. A. S., & Bueno, J. L. O. (2020). Subjective time under altered states of consciousness in ayahuasca users in shamanistic rituals involving music. *Brazilian Journal of Medical and Biological Research*, *53*(8), e9278.

Canales, J. (2015). *The physicist and the philosopher: Einstein, Bergson, and the debate that changed our understanding of time*. Princeton University Press.

Craig, A. D. (2015). *How do you feel? An interoceptive moment with your neurobiological self*. Princeton University Press.

Dainton, B. (2017). Bergson on temporal experience and durée réelle. In: I. Phillips (Ed.), *The Routledge handbook of philosophy of temporal experience* (pp. 93–106). Routledge.

Damasio, A. R. (1999). *The feeling of what happens: Body and emotion in the making of consciousness*. Houghton Mifflin Harcourt.

Deinzer, V., Clancy, L., & Wittmann, M. (2017). The sense of time while watching a dance performance. *SAGE Open*, *7*(4), 2158244017745576.

Deliège, I. (1995). Cue abstraction and schematization of the musical form. *Scientific Contributions to General Psychology*, *14*, 11–28.

Droit-Volet, S., Fayolle, S., Lamotte, M., & Gil, S. (2013). Time, emotion and the embodiment of timing. *Timing & Time Perception*, *1*(1), 99–126.

Ehret, S., Trukenbrod, A. K., Gralla, V., & Thomaschke, R. (2020). A grounded theory on the relation of time awareness and perceived valence. *Timing & Time Perception*, *8*(3–4), 316–340.

Elliott, M. A., & Giersch, A. (2016). What happens in a moment. *Frontiers in Psychology*, *6*, 1905.

Epstein, P. (1995). *Shaping time*. Schirmer.

Evrard, H. C. (2019). The organization of the primate insular cortex. *Frontiers in Neuroanatomy*, *13*, 43.

Exner, S. (1875). Experimentelle Untersuchung der einfachsten psychischen Processe. III. Abhandlung. *Pflügers Archiv für die Gesamte Physiologie*, *11*, 403–432.

Fink, M., Churan, J., & Wittmann, M. (2006). Temporal processing and context dependency of phoneme discrimination in patients with aphasia. *Brain and Language*, *98*(1), 1–11.

Fink, M., Ulbrich, P., Churan, J., & Wittmann, M. (2006). Stimulus-dependent processing of temporal order. *Behavioral Processes*, *71*(2–3), 344–352.

Firmino, É. A., Campagnoli, A. P., & Bueno, J. L. (2020). Temporal order of musical keys and subjective estimates of time. *Acta Psychologica*, *202*, 102959.

Fostick, L., Lifshitz-Ben-Basat, A., & Babkoff, H. (2019). The effect of stimulus frequency, spectrum, duration, and location on temporal order judgment thresholds: Distribution analysis. *Psychological Research*, *83*(5), 968–976.

Fraisse, P. (1982). Rhythm and tempo. In: D. Deutsch (Ed.), *Psychology of music* (pp. 149–180). Academic Press.

Fraisse, P. (1984). Perception and estimation of time. *Annual Review of Psychology*, *35*, 1–37.

Frischeisen-Köhler, I. (1933). Feststellung des weder langsamen noch schnellen (mittelmäßigen) Tempos. *Psychologische Forschung*, *18*(1), 291–298.

Goldman-Rakic, P. (1997). Space and time in the mental universe. *Nature*, *386*(6625), 559–560.

Hagendoorn, I. G. (2004). Some speculative hypotheses about the nature and perception of dance and choreography. *Journal of Consciousness Studies*, *11*(3–4), 79–110.

Hammerschmidt, D., Frieler, K., & Wöllner, C. (2021). Spontaneous motor tempo: Investigating psychological, chronobiological, and demographic factors in a large-scale online tapping experiment. *Frontiers in Psychology*, *12*, 2338.

Hammerschmidt, D., Wöllner, C., London, J., & Burger, B. (2021). Disco time: The relationship between perceived duration and tempo in music. *Music & Science, 4*, 205920432098638. https://doi.org/10.1177/2059204320986384

Himberg, T., Laroche, J., Bigé, R., Buchkowski, M., & Bachrach, A. (2018). Coordinated interpersonal behaviour in collective dance improvisation: The aesthetics of kinaesthetic togetherness. *Behavioral Sciences, 8*(2), 23.

James, W. (1890). *The principles of psychology.* MacMillan.

Jo, H. G., Wittmann, M., Borghardt, T. L., Hinterberger, T., & Schmidt, S. (2014). First-person approaches in neuroscience of consciousness: Brain dynamics correlate with the intention to act. *Consciousness and Cognition, 26*, 105–116.

Khoshnoud, S., Igarzábal, F. A., & Wittmann, M. (2020). Peripheral-physiological and neural correlates of the flow experience while playing video games: A comprehensive review. *PeerJ, 8*, e10520.

Kimura, K., Ogata, T., & Miyake, Y. (2020). Effects of a partner's tap intervals on an individual's timing control increase in slow-tempo dyad synchronisation using finger-tapping. *Scientific Reports, 10*(*1*), 1–8.

Linares Gutiérrez, D. (2021). *Effects of meditation-induced mental states and individual differences on subjective time* [Doctoral dissertation, University of Freiburg]. https://doi.org/10.6094/UNIFR/218296

Linares Gutierrez, D., Kübel, S., Giersch, A., Schmidt, S., Meissner, K., & Wittmann, M. (2019). Meditation-induced states, vagal tone, and breathing activity are related to changes in auditory temporal integration. *Behavioral Sciences, 9*(5), 51.

London, J. (2002). Cognitive constraints on metric systems: Some observations and hypotheses. *Music Perception, 19*(4), 529–550.

Lotze, M., Wittmann, M., von Steinbüchel, N., Pöppel, E., & Roenneberg, T. (1999). Daily rhythm of temporal resolution in the auditory system. *Cortex, 35*(1), 89–100.

Lubashevsky, I., & Plavinska, N. (2021). *Physics of the human temporality.* Springer.

Lutz, A. (2002). Toward a neurophenomenology as an account of generative passages: A first empirical case study. *Phenomenology and the Cognitive Sciences, 1*, 133–167.

Mates, J., Müller, U., Radil, T., & Pöppel, E. (1994). Temporal integration in sensorimotor synchronization. *Journal of Cognitive Neuroscience, 6*(4), 332–340.

Matko, K., Ott, U., & Sedlmeier, P. (2021). What do meditators do when they meditate? Proposing a novel basis for future meditation research. *Mindfulness, 12*, 1791–1811.

Mella, N., Conty, L., & Pouthas, V. (2011). The role of physiological arousal in time perception: Psychophysiological evidence from an emotion regulation paradigm. *Brain and Cognition, 75*(2), 182–187.

Meissner, K., & Wittmann, M. (2011). Body signals, cardiac awareness, and the perception of time. *Biological Psychology, 86*, 289–297.

Merleau-Ponty, M. (1945). *Phénoménologie de la perception.* La Librairie Gallimard.

Montemayor, C., & Haladjian, H. H. (2015). *Consciousness, attention, and conscious attention.* MIT Press.

Moser, E. I., Moser, M. B., & McNaughton, B. L. (2017). Spatial representation in the hippocampal formation: A history. *Nature Neuroscience, 20*(11), 1448–1464.

Nakajima, Y., Shimojo, S., & Sugita, Y. (1980). On the perception of two successive sound bursts. *Psychological Research, 41*(4), 335–344.

Nani, A., Manuello, J., Liloia, D., Duca, S., Costa, T., & Cauda, F. (2019). The neural correlates of time: A meta-analysis of neuroimaging studies. *Journal of Cognitive Neuroscience, 31*(12), 1796–1826.

Nather, F. C., Bueno, J. L., Bigand, E., & Droit-Volet, S. (2011). Time changes with the embodiment of another's body posture. *PLoS One, 6*(5), e19818.

Nather, F. C., & Bueno, J. L. O. (2012). Exploration time of static images implying different body movements causes time distortions. *Perceptual and Motor Skills, 115*(1), 105–110.

Ogden, R. S., Henderson, J., McGlone, F., & Richter, M. (2019a). Time distortion under threat: Sympathetic arousal predicts time distortion only in the context of negative, highly arousing stimuli. *PloS One, 14*(5), e0216704.

Ogden, R. S., Henderson, J., Slade, K., McGlone, F., & Richter, M. (2019). The effect of increased parasympathetic activity on perceived duration. *Consciousness and Cognition*, *76*, 102829.

Otten, S., Schötz, E., Wittmann, M., Kohls, N., Schmidt, S., & Meissner, K. (2015). Psychophysiology of duration estimation in experienced mindfulness meditators and matched controls. *Frontiers in Psychology*, *6*, 1215.

Parncutt, R. (1994). A perceptual model of pulse salience and metrical accent in musical rhythms. *Music Perception*, *11*(4), 409–464.

Peters, M. (1989). The relationship between variability of intertap intervals and interval duration. *Psychological Research*, *51*(1), 38–42.

Pfeifer, E., Fiedler, H., & Wittmann, M. (2020). Increased relaxation and present orientation after a period of silence in a natural surrounding. *Nordic Journal of Music Therapy*, *29*(1), 75–92.

Pfeifer, E., Geyer, N., Storch, F., & Wittmann, M. (2019). 'Just think'—Students feel significantly more relaxed, less aroused, and in a better mood after a period of silence alone in a room. *Psych*, *1*(1), 343–352.

Pöppel, E. (1989). The measurement of music and the cerebral clock: A new theory. *Leonardo*, *22*(1), 83–89.

Pöppel, E. (1997). A hierarchical model of temporal perception. *Trends in Cognitive Sciences*, *1*(2), 56–61.

Pöppel, E. (2009). Pre-semantically defined window for cognitive processing. *Philosophical Transactions of the Royal Society of London. Series B, Biological Sciences*, *364*(1525), 1887–1896.

Povel, D. J. (1984). A theoretical framework for rhythm perception. *Psychological Research*, *45*(4), 315–337.

Redelmeier, D. A., & Kahneman, D. (1996). Patients' memories of painful medical treatments: Real-time and retrospective evaluations of two minimally invasive procedures. *Pain*, *66*(1), 3–8.

Repp, B. H. (2010). Self-generated interval subdivision reduces variability of synchronization with a very slow metronome. *Music Perception*, *27*(5), 389–397.

Richter, F., & Ibáñez, A. (2021). Time is body: Multimodal evidence of crosstalk between interoception and time estimation. *Biological Psychology*, *159*, 108017.

Rubin, D. C., & Wenzel, A. E. (1996). One hundred years of forgetting: A quantitative description of retention. *Psychological Review*, *103*(4), 734–760.

Rutrecht, H., Wittmann, M., Khoshnoud, S., & Igarzábal, F. A. (2021). Time speeds up during flow states: A study in virtual reality with the video game Thumper. *Timing & Time Perception*, *9*(4), 353–376.

Sgouramani, H., & Vatakis, A. (2014). 'Flash' dance: How speed modulates perceived duration in dancers and non-dancers. *Acta Psychologica*, *147*, 17–24.

Singhal, I., & Srinivasan, N. (2021). Time and time again: A multi-scale hierarchical framework for time-consciousness and timing of cognition. *Neuroscience of Consciousness*, *2021*(2), niab020.

Su, Y. H. (2014). Audiovisual beat induction in complex auditory rhythms: Point-light figure movement as an effective visual beat. *Acta Psychologica*, *151*, 40–50.

Su, Y. H., & Pöppel, E. (2012). Body movement enhances the extraction of temporal structures in auditory sequences. *Psychological Research*, *76*(3), 373–382.

Szelag, E. (1997). Temporal integration of the brain as studied with the metronome paradigm. In: H. Atmanspacher & E. Ruhnau (Eds.), *Time, temporality, now: Experiencing time and concepts of time in an interdisciplinary perspective* (pp. 121–131). Springer.

Szelag, E., von Steinbüchel, N., Reiser, M., Gilles de Langen, E., & Pöppel, E. (1996). Temporal constraints in processing of nonverbal rhythmic patterns. *Acta Neurobiologiae Experimentalis*, *56*(1), 215–225.

Teghil, A., Boccia, M., D'Antonio, F., Di Vita, A., de Lena, C., & Guariglia, C. (2019). Neural substrates of internally-based and externally-cued timing: An activation likelihood estimation (ALE) meta-analysis of fMRI studies. *Neuroscience & Biobehavioral Reviews*, *96*, 197–209.

Teghil, A., Di Vita, A., D'Antonio, F., & Boccia, M. (2020). Inter-individual differences in resting-state functional connectivity are linked to interval timing in irregular contexts. *Cortex*, *128*, 254–269.

Thompson, E. (2010). *Time in life: Biology, phenomenology, and the sciences of mind*. Harvard University Press.

Trevarthen, C. (1999). Musicality and the intrinsic motive pulse: Evidence from human psychobiology and infant communication. *Musicae Scientiae, 3* (1 Suppl), 155–215.

Tsakiris, M., & de Preester, H. (Eds.). (2018). *The interoceptive mind: From homeostasis to awareness.* Oxford University Press.

Tschacher, W., Ramseyer, F., & Bergomi, C. (2013). The subjective present and its modulation in clinical contexts. *Timing & Time Perception, 1*(2), 239–259.

Ulbrich, P., Churan, J., Fink, M., & Wittmann, M. (2009). Perception of temporal order: The effects of age, sex, and cognitive factors. *Aging, Neuropsychology and Cognition, 16*(2), 183–202.

Vatakis, A., Sgouramani, H., Gorea, A., Hatzitaki, V., & Pollick, F. E. (2014). Time to act: New perspectives on embodiment and timing. *Procedia—Social and Behavioral Sciences, 126*, 16–20.

Vatakis, A., & Spence, C. (2006). Audiovisual synchrony perception for speech and music assessed using a temporal order judgment task. *Neuroscience Letters, 393*(1), 40–44.

Velmans, M. (2009). *Understanding consciousness.* Routledge.

Wackermann, J. (2007). Inner and outer horizons of time experience. *Spanish Journal of Psychology, 10*(1), 20–32.

Wang, L., Lin, X., Zhou, B., Pöppel, E., & Bao, Y. (2015). Subjective present: A window of temporal integration indexed by mismatch negativity. *Cognitive Processing, 16*(1), 131–135.

Warren, R. M., & Obusek, C. J. (1972). Identification of temporal order within auditory sequences. *Perception & Psychophysics, 12*(1), 86–90.

White, P. A. (2017). The three-second 'subjective present': A critical review and a new proposal. *Psychological Bulletin, 143*(7), 735–756.

Witowska, J., Schmidt, S., & Wittmann, M. (2020). What happens while waiting? How self-regulation affects boredom and subjective time during a real waiting situation. *Acta Psychologica, 205*, 103061.

Wittmann, M. (2009). The inner experience of time. *Philosophical Transactions of the Royal Society of London. Series B, Biological Sciences, 364*(1525), 1955–1967.

Wittmann, M. (2011). Moments in time. *Frontiers in Integrative Neuroscience, 5*, 66.

Wittmann, M. (2013). The inner sense of time: How the brain creates a representation of duration. *Nature Reviews Neuroscience, 14*(3), 217–223.

Wittmann, M. (2016). The duration of presence. In: B. Mölder, V. Arstila, & P. Øhrstrøm (Eds.), *Philosophy and psychology of time* (pp. 101–113). Springer.

Wittmann, M., Burtscher, A., Fries, W., & von Steinbüchel, N. (2004). Effects of brain-lesion size and location on temporal-order judgment. *NeuroReport, 15*(15), 2401–2405.

Wittmann M., & Montemayor C. (2021). Reinterpreting the Einstein-Bergson debate through contemporary neuroscience. In: A. Campo & S. Gozzano (Eds.). *Einstein vs. Bergson: An enduring quarrel of time* (pp. 347–372). De Gruyter.

Wittmann, M., & Pöppel, E. (1999). Temporal mechanisms of the brain as fundamentals of communication—with special reference to music perception and performance. *Musicae Scientiae, 3*(1 Suppl), 13–28.

Zakay, D., & Block, R. A. (2004). Prospective and retrospective duration judgments: An executive-control perspective. *Acta Neurobiologiae Experimentalis, 614*(3), 319–328.

27

Learning to Feel the Time

Reflections of a Percussionist

Russell Hartenberger

27.1 Watching, Listening, Imitating

> Education is an admirable thing. But it is well to remember from time to time that nothing that is worth knowing can be taught.
>
> (Oscar Wilde, 1894, p. 533)

Perhaps Oscar Wilde's aphorism could be amended for our use to say: 'it is well to remember that *time* cannot be taught'. Learning time is an oral tradition. Even with notated Western music, one must see and hear how accomplished players interpret rhythms and how they place their attacks in time. My introduction to learning time began with drum lessons when I was 11 years old. My teacher, Alan Abel, played everything with me, providing the perfect template for learning. I could see and hear his drumming alongside mine as I attempted to imitate his strokes, rhythms, and time feel. He told me the most important thing about developing time feel is: 'You need to discipline your hands so they do what your mind and ear say should be done' (A. Abel, personal communication, 10 November 1998).

Just as I imitated Mr Abel's every movement, all musicians need a template to follow in interpreting time feel and rhythmic placement. Jazz musicians traditionally learn from listening to other jazz musicians—either live or on recordings—to understand the special feel for their genre. This is also the case in many non-Western traditions. I asked Bob Becker, my colleague in Nexus, about learning time. He said if he taught young students, he 'would play with them . . . even if it is just exercises' (B. Becker, personal communication, 6 February 1998). Becker then explained that he wasn't taught that way when he was young, but added:

> I started doing that after Sharda Sahai [the esteemed *guru* of the Benares *tabla gharana*] did it with me. It is standard in North Indian teaching for the teacher or advanced students to sit and play with the younger students and not say a word about what they are supposed to learn through instruction. They just play and you do your best to keep up with them . . . It forces you into a state of incredible anxiety, but awareness, too. You're really

Russell Hartenberger, *Learning to Feel the Time* In: *Performing Time*. Edited by: Clemens Wöllner and Justin London, Oxford University Press. © Oxford University Press 2023. DOI: 10.1093/oso/9780192896254.003.0028 listening hard, and it makes you try to memorize as quickly as you can, otherwise you don't get the material.

Becker continued:

> But it's also entrainment . . . It's like a vibration gets transmitted even if it's only by small amounts that . . . somehow get into synchronization. When you're playing along with someone who is better than you, they somehow have a pull on you. It forces you, without you knowing or trying, as long as you are listening, to match their spacing and clarity and rhythmic accuracy. (Personal communication, 6 February 1998)

Trichy Sankaran, the virtuoso *mrdangam* player and scholar from South India, said:

> I come from a tradition where the music is memorized and learned at the feet of the teacher in the old *gurukala* system. This system is really to prepare you for *self-discovery*; it is great training for the brain. I cannot over-emphasize the importance of this oral tradition method by which we retain many of the intricate patterns all in our memory. (Personal communication, 20 August 2014)

My experience learning West African drumming was also one of watching, listening, and imitating. My teacher, Abraham Adzenyah, patiently played patterns over and over until I was able to imitate his attack placement. I then repeated my rhythm until my muscle memory took over. The Akan drums we played had a design carved into the side that Adzenyah called the eye of the drum. He told me to point the eye towards him while I drummed to emphasize the importance of watching and listening.

27.2 Metronome, Technical Control

Accomplished musicians have a variety of ways they incorporate a metronome into their teaching and learning processes, none of which is intended to develop an accurate sense of time. Western musicians who are learning a new piece of music use a metronome to gauge their progress in attaining a desired speed. Western and non-Western musicians often use a metronome to determine tempo. Alan Abel said a metronome 'is not so much to develop steadiness as it is to get the tempo of a piece . . . It is something to use until you can do it on your own' (personal communication, 10 November 1998). Bob Becker expressed a similar sentiment when he said: 'I really started working with a metronome when I started playing *tabla*, and it was as much for tempo as anything at that point' (personal communication, 6 February 1998). Sharda Sahai stated he uses a metronome with young students 'if their time is not getting perfect. In India everyone can't have a metronome because it is too expensive' (personal communication, 23 October 1997). He added that a metronome is useful 'for a little while, but not forever. Indian music is not very much like a metronome. Sometime if you are perfect in time, the other people are not perfect in time' (personal communication, 23 October 1997).

I use a metronome in the above ways, but I find it more valuable in simulating what it is like to play with another person or to enable my mind to hear music in a different way. For example, I set a metronome at various speeds and play halfway between the clicks. Musicians call this playing on the up-beat, after-beat, or off-beat. Once you become comfortable playing on the off-beat, you realize it is a more solid time feel than trying to play exactly with the on-beat clicks. This is the reason it feels more musical to clap to a piece of music on two and four rather than on one and three. It has also been shown to give greater precision in time estimation (Repp, 2005). A good mental exercise is to try to feel the metronome clicks as off-beats. Africanist scholar David Locke calls this a *gestalt* flip, something that occurs regularly while playing West African music (Locke, 1998, p. 7). It describes the sensation of hearing a rhythmic pattern one way in relation to a pulse and then changing perception of the same pattern to hear it a new way in relation to a different pulse (Hartenberger, 2020, p. 84). It is also how *amadinda* xylophone players from Uganda manage to play on-beat, off-beat patterns at such a fast speed (Kubik, 1994, pp. 65–66), or similar to the way Balinese *gamelan* players play the rapid interlocking patterns called *kotekan* (Tenzer, 2000, pp. 212–231).

In Steve Reich's *Music for 18 Musicians*, two piano players and two marimba players alternate a down-beat, up-beat pulse for much of the hour-long composition. Most players of the up-beat pulse continue to feel their parts off the beat throughout the piece. Pianist Philip Bush, whose assignment in the Reich ensemble is to play the up-beat piano part, told me he did not feel confident maintaining a consistent evenness while thinking of his chords as off-beats, so he decided to convince himself that he was playing *on* the beat (personal communication, 29 July 2015). Of course, this meant he heard an entirely different piece than the rest of the ensemble or, for that matter, even the audience.

Jim Blackley, drum set teacher and author of two fundamental publications for drum set (Blackley, 1961, 2001), famously insisted his students play the jazz ride cymbal pattern at quarter note = MM 40 for their first few weeks of study before he allowed them to play with recordings or other people (R. Moore, personal communication, 7 January 2022). Blackley's exercise is not intended to teach time; however, it does achieve two important elements of time feel. First, it helps students develop control of their hands. Alan Abel emphasized the importance of this control when he said: 'There could be people who just have a much better sense of time than others, but it is all affected by one's hand control' (A. Abel, personal communication, 10 November 1998).

The second result of Blackley's metronome exercise is that at this agonizingly slow pace, the player must develop the ability to subdivide empty space into discernible chunks, essentially creating a mental grid in which to place attacks. This is not unlike the sense of *tala* that seems to be eternally in the minds of Indian musicians as they organize rhythm in a certain way, even when performing in a Western musical context (T. Sankaran, personal communication, 20 August 2014).

27.3 Tempo

In my early snare drum studies, I approached the development of technique by gradually increasing the speed of a particular exercise. In the world of snare drum, there is a lexicon of rudiments that all aspiring drummers learn. We practise these rudiments, such as the paradiddle, ratamacue, and double-stroke roll, in what is called rudimental form: beginning very slowly and accelerating to the fastest speed we can play each pattern, then returning gradually to the initial speed. As it turns out, this format may result in some technical development on the instrument, but it may not be a very good way to develop a sense of time or a thorough understanding of how multiples of two factor into music. By practising technical exercises with an *accelerando*, the player does not establish a solid time base and in fact grows accustomed to speeding up while playing; no metric relationship is created at different speeds. By playing an exercise at a very slow tempo, then doubling the speed and quadrupling the speed, the player can feel a connection between a rhythmic pattern and a sense of time (Allingham & Wöllner, 2022; see London, this volume). This was made clear to me in my Karnatak music studies.

In my first lessons with my South Indian *mrdangam* teacher, Ramnad Raghavan, I was shown the four basic strokes on the instrument—*ta, di, thom, num*—played alternately, left hand, right hand, left hand, right hand. I played these strokes extremely slowly and loudly to set the mechanics of the stroke manipulation in my hands and against the *Adi tala* cycle of eight beats. Once I could play the strokes correctly, Raghavan told me to double the speed. A few lessons later, when I was able to accomplish this doubling, he told me to double the speed again so I would be playing four times the speed of my original pattern, always within the *Adi tala* cycle. This basic exercise set the stage for my awareness of time in Karnatak music. There are three speeds, slow, medium, and fast, and all rhythms are played in relation to a *tala* cycle. Sankaran explained the doubling principle this way:

> This general concept of doubling can be more precisely related to what I refer to as *The Three-Speed Formula*. There are many different terms which can be used to express the simple mathematical relationship of these three different speeds, but the concept remains the same regardless of terminology—slow speed, medium speed, and fast speed; one to two to four; 1:2:4. It's important to bear in mind that the relationship between these different speeds is not arbitrary or a simple question of one speed being somewhat faster than another. There is a precise geometrical relationship between the three speeds. (T. Sankaran, personal communication, 20 August 2014)

27.4 Groove, Energy, Empty Spaces

I have often been asked to bring a shaker or other small percussion instrument to a commercial recording session and overdub on top of a track of electronically produced music to 'humanize' the groove. The producers of these recordings understand that the quantized groove of electronic music has an artificial time feel. The percussionist Thomas Brett wrote: 'a good drummer generates a sense of kinetic, forward-moving musical motion—colloquially called a good 'groove'—by *not* being perfectly steady, but by being subtly elastic' (Brett 2011; see Danielsen, this volume; Stupacher et al., this volume). Charles Keil calls these pushes and pulls on the time 'participatory discrepancies' (Keil & Feld, 1994, p. 96).

An excellent example in Western music of a good groove is the opening drum solo in Paul Simon's '50 Ways to Leave Your Lover'. Musicians familiar with jazz and popular music recognize immediately that the drummer is the great Steve Gadd. Gadd plays with a strong sense of time, clarity, technical proficiency, and a centred sound that projects through the music and gives energy to the ensemble. Part of the reason for this energy is the precision of his execution; it allows the listener to hear the spaces between the attacks. In a conversation with Haruki Murakami, conductor Seiji Ozawa said:

> In Japan we talk about *ma* in Asian music—the importance of those pauses or empty spaces—but it's there in Western music, too. You get a musician like Glenn Gould, and he's doing exactly the same thing. Not everybody can do it—certainly no ordinary musician. But somebody like him does it all the time. (Murakami, 2016, p. 22)

Murakami asked, 'Ordinary musicians don't do it?' Ozawa replied:

> No, never. Or if they do, the spaces don't fit in as naturally as this. It doesn't grab you—you don't get drawn in as you do here. That's what putting in these spaces, or *ma*, is all about isn't it? You grab your audience and pull them in. East or West, it's all the same when a virtuoso does it. (Murakami, 2016, p. 22)

27.5 Negotiation in Ensemble Performance

A musician playing pulse-based music with another person must constantly be aware of the other musician's sense of time while still expressing a forceful feel. When Nexus performs with Abraham Adzenyah, we find that we have to negotiate the time feel among ourselves rather than having every member of the group make an individual connection with Adzenyah's time. Nexus member Bill Cahn described it this way: 'Time is a negotiated thing . . . it is a social phenomenon, too . . . In other words, [learning time] is learning to relate to other people, and that's a negotiated thing' (personal communication, 14 December 1997).

Martin Clayton explained: 'For me, music cannot simply reflect time in general: rather, musical time is the result of negotiation between physical and psychological constraints on the one hand, and human individuals' attempts to describe their experience on the other' (Clayton, 2000, p. 7).

Asserting one's individuality while participating in a collective creation is indeed a paradox as well as a lesson in personal negotiation (Makota, 1987). An example of this negotiating paradox is the time issue raised in Steve Reich's *Drumming*. For a performance of *Drumming* to be successful there should be a unified time feel among the musicians. As Steven Schick expressed:

> Beyond pointing to a model of cultural coexistence, *Drumming* also demonstrates a new way of interaction within a chamber ensemble. This is simple to describe: no one leads *Drumming*. In fact, nowhere in the entire chamber music repertoire for percussion is there an example of such a mutually dependent and communally reinforced musical structure. Stewardship of the piece is a group concern, progressing as one player after another completes his or her specific task(s) from building up to phasing to playing resultant patterns . . . The great parable of this music—that the health and vitality of the whole is tied to the health and vitality of the smallest of its parts—requires the presence of human beings who need each other and who make space for each other. (Schick, 2006, p. 241)

27.6 Magic Time

In the early 1970s, I began rehearsals with the Steve Reich ensemble as Reich was composing his iconic minimalist composition, *Drumming*. Reich taught *Drumming* by rote: through the process of imitation and repetition I played the patterns that he demonstrated, memorized them, and attached them to the material I learned at the previous rehearsal. I had never learned a composition this way, and I was fascinated by the fact that Reich employed the same learning process used by my teachers of non-Western music. Around the same time, my percussion group Nexus was formed and began playing concerts that included musicians from a variety of musical cultures. This concurrence of musical experiences piqued my interest in time and rhythm. I began to research these concepts in the hope that my own performance and understanding of time would improve, and that I would discover how musicians think about and learn time. *Drumming* provided an ideal template for this examination of rhythm and time. Time feel is the key to a successful performance of *Drumming*, and it is no accident that it is a crucial element in Reich's music. He said:

> I used to go to Birdland . . . and I remember seeing my idol, Kenny Clarke [the innovative bebop drummer]. The reason he was my idol was that he had this almost magical sense of time, though he just played ride cymbal and a few kick drum accents. What was magical about him was not his technique but the actual feeling of his playing the time—floating Miles Davis and the whole band on his ride cymbal . . . He had this feeling of *magic time*. It was the simplicity and the quality of him playing the ride cymbal. Nobody could play it the way he did. (S. Reich, personal communication, 18 December 2003)

When Reich taught *Drumming* to the percussionists in his ensemble, he demonstrated each pattern and gave it a certain lilt trying to achieve this sense of magic time. The percussionists imitated his approach, adding their concepts of sound, and this became the basis for the performance style of all Reich's early compositions.

27.7 Time Perception, Phasing

In *Drumming*, phasing occurs when two or more players play the identical rhythmic pattern and one of those players moves gradually ahead of the other(s) until arriving at the next interlocking position. Reich described the process of phasing as 'essentially a form of canon using irrational numbers' (2002, p. 5). The term irrational can also be applied to the way I feel when I am in the midst of a phase. I lose all sense of time and feel my hands moving fast while my mind is moving slowly. I feel like I am entering a space–time continuum and losing all contact with the other player, the music, time, and my hands. My concept of steady time and of time in general is suspended during the phasing process (see Doelling et al., this volume; Loui, this volume).

In 2013, I attended a lecture by Justin London who described a research project with Rainer Polak in which they recorded and analysed a piece by Mande drummers from Mali (Polak & London, 2014). At one point in the music, the drummers made an *accelerando* and London and Polak devised a way to chart it. Their analysis inspired me to attempt to determine what actually happens in a phase as opposed to what I think happens. In June 2014, I arranged to record the bongo phases in *Drumming* with Bob Becker at the LIVE Lab at McMaster University. Ray Dillard, recording engineer for Nexus records, supervised the audio recording and created a system for attaching piezo electric transducers to each bongo in order to capture individual attacks. Michael Schutz then transferred the data into plots that would display the phases in a clear format (Schutz, 2016, 2019). (For detailed information on the phasing analysis please visit www.maplelab.net/reich.)

In our performance of the first bongo phase, there were 67 repetitions of the *Drumming* pattern, and each repetition took 1267 ms or about 1.2 s. At this rate, the phase took approximately 75.6 s to complete. Over the 67 repetitions of the rhythmic pattern, the moving part averaged 0.25% faster in tempo (approximately 0.5 ms/beat). In contrast to my expectations, the separation and re-alignment of the two parts was neither smooth nor consistent. At least one-fifth of the cycle repetitions in the moving voice *actually moved backward* while Becker's steady part also had fluctuations of movement. The analysis confirmed my feeling and Becker's contention that he pushes slightly when I phase in order to create time resistance, and that I push and pull during phasing (Figure 27.1).

This empirical study of phasing confirmed some of my feelings while raising other points that I had not considered. It is clear that a phase between two players, at least by Becker and me, is not a process generated entirely by the person playing the moving

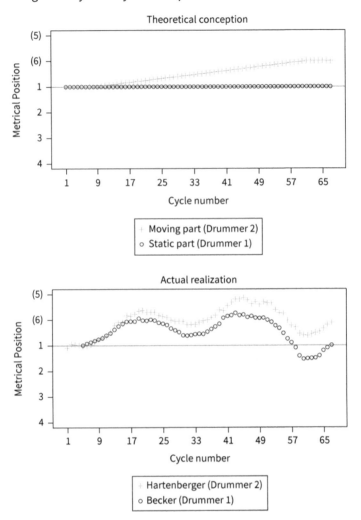

Figure 27.1 Plots depicting theoretical conception and actual realization of *Drumming* phase (m. 19). Used by kind permission of Michael Schutz.

part but is a give-and-take manoeuvre between both players. The moving part proceeds in an irregular stop-and-start fashion while stretching and compressing the rhythmic pattern throughout the phase. The steady part is only nominally steady and generally pushes the overall tempo during a phase.

The intense scrutiny of the phasing process in this experiment caused both Becker and me to be aware of the change of tension in our hands and arms as we shifted mentally from interlocking mode to phasing mode. This focus in physical tension precipitated by a change in mental attitude was an unanticipated result that was brought to conscious awareness by the project. I now have more knowledge of the phasing process, but I also am more sensitive to the changes that occur in my mind and body as I prepare to begin a phase; I am reminded of the yogic principle of the elimination of outside distractions in focusing on simple physical actions. For a percussionist, the attention to a single stroke is sound creation at its most fundamental level and the beginning of the understanding of time (Hartenberger, 2016, pp. 90–107).

27.8 Conclusion

It is clear from this phasing experiment and from comments made by accomplished musicians that time in pulse-based music is learned and felt by playing with other people; and even then, mysteries abound. The joy in learning time is discovering its feel; but can all musicians experience this discovery? When I asked Sharda Sahai if time feel is natural or learned, he replied, 'If they don't have this natural time sense, they can't have freedom. If you have to teach it to them, they can't have freedom. When we have a natural time sense, then we have freedom'. As to why some people have it and some people don't, Sahai said, 'It is God gifted' (personal communication, 23 October 1997). When asked to describe time, my Nexus colleague John Wyre answered spontaneously, 'Dance partner!' (personal communication, 15 December 1997). What better way to go through life than dancing with time!

References

Allingham, E., & Wöllner, C. (2022). Slow practice and tempo-management strategies in instrumental music learning: Investigating prevalence and cognitive functions. *Psychology of Music, 50*(6), 1925–1941.https:// doi/10.1177/03057356211073481

Blackley, J. (1961). *Syncopated rolls for the modern drummer* (Rev. ed.). Blackley Publications.

Blackley, J. (2001). *The essence of jazz drumming.* Southern Percussion.

Brett, T. (2011, 26 April). *On musical time and drummers' brains.* Brettworks. https://brettworks.com/2011/04/26/on-musical-time-and-drummers-brains/

Chernoff, J. M. (1979). *African rhythm and African sensibility.* University of Chicago Press.

Clayton, M. (2000). *Time in Indian Music.* Oxford University Press.

Hartenberger, R. (2016). *Performance practice in the music of Steve Reich.* Cambridge University Press.

Hartenberger, R. (2020). A different kind of virtuosity. In R. Hartenberger & R. McClelland (Eds.), *The Cambridge companion to rhythm* (pp. 75–89). Cambridge University Press.

Keil, C., & Feld, S. (1994). *Music grooves: Essays and dialogues.* University of Chicago Press.

Kubik, G. (1994). *Theory of African music, Vol. 1.* University of Chicago Press.

Locke, D. (1990). *Drum Damba: Talking drum lesson.* White Cliffs Media.

Locke, D. (1998). *Drum Gahu.* White Cliffs Media.

Locke, D. (2020). The musical rhythm of Agbadza songs. In R. Hartenberger & R. McClelland (Eds.), *The Cambridge companion to rhythm* (pp. 217–240). Cambridge University Press.

Makota, Ō. (1987). *Renga—Linked poems.* In Ō. Makota & T. Fitzsimmons (Eds.), *A play of mirrors* (pp. 201–206). Katydid Books.

Murakami, H. (2016). *Absolutely on music: Conversations with Seiji Ozawa* (J. Rubin, Trans.). Alfred A. Knopf.

Polak, R., & London, J. (2014). Timing and meter in Mande drumming from Mali. *Music Theory Online, 20*(1). https://mtosmt.org/issues/mto.14.20.1/mto.14.20.1.polak-london.php

Reich, S. (2002). *Writings on music, 1965–2000* (P. Hillier, Ed.). Oxford University Press.

Reich, S. (2016). Thoughts on percussion and rhythm. In R. Hartenberger (Ed.), *The Cambridge companion to percussion* (pp. 173–184). Cambridge University Press.

Repp, B. H. (2005). Sensorimotor synchronization: A review of the tapping literature. *Psychonomic Bulletin and Review, 12*(6), 969–992.

Schick, S. (2006). *The percussionist's art: Same bed, different dreams.* University of Rochester Press.

Schutz, M. (2016). Lessons from the laboratory. In R. Hartenberger (Ed.), *The Cambridge companion to percussion* (pp. 267–280). Cambridge University Press.

Schutz, M. (2019). What really happens in Steve Reich's *Drumming? Percussive Notes, 57*(4), 86–89.

Tenzer, M. (2000). *Gamelan gong kebyar.* University of Chicago Press.

Wilde, O. (1894). Nineteen maxims [Published anonymously]. *Saturday Review: Of Politics, Literature, Science, and Art, 78,* 17 November.

Focus Chapters

28
Performing and Feeling Time in Contemporary Dance

Henry Daniel in conversation with Justin London

28.1 Creating and Experiencing Temporal Complexity

JUSTIN LONDON (JL): To start with an impossibly broad question, can you reflect on how you think about time in creating your dance works?

HENRY DANIEL (HD): Working within the mediums of dance and choreography, I treat time conceptually as something that has a start followed by a period of development before gesturing towards some kind of ending. If it is a thought, it can begin in a millisecond, generate other thoughts or ideas that have their own unique time scales, and eventually last an entire lifetime. In this way, one can think of rhythms as patterns created by how that thought (or those thoughts) unfolds, rebounds, resonates, obstructs, or is obstructed by other entities in its journey through space and time. The dancer, choreographer, participant, or audience member can sense these rhythms as synchronous and harmonious, or asynchronous and dissonant.

The Montreal-based Franco-Congolese Canadian dancer, writer, choreographer, scholar, and teacher of Contemporary West African Dance Zab Maboungou once confessed that all her efforts in dance consisted in 'trying to create time', and that her manner of dealing with rhythm—or rather rhythms—was as if they were 'embodied entities' that had the possibility of connecting various elements in time (Maboungou, 2005). Here I believe Mme Maboungou was elaborating on a technique of putting two or three conflicting rhythms together in African polyrhythmic drumming. She explains that these rhythms often confused dancers from the West, who would apprehend them as 'dissonant'. Maboungou also claims that these rhythms had the capacity to free the body from being bound by the constraints of a limited earthly existence, and by understanding—in an embodied manner—that we are complex creatures with the capacity to move in a rhythmically complex manner, and that the dancer and the musician can engage in rhythmic interplay that allows them to experience heightened states of awareness.

Rhythmic complexity can therefore be seen as the simultaneous unfolding of different processes at different rates on both micro and macro scales, processes

Henry Daniel in conversation with Justin London, *Performing and Feeling Time in Contemporary Dance*
In: *Performing Time*. Edited by: Clemens Wöllner and Justin London, Oxford University Press. © Oxford University Press 2023.
DOI: 10.1093/oso/9780192896254.003.0029

that have implications for and resonances in the human body. As such, experiencing temporal 'dissonance' could mean that our system may not be attuned to this larger framework of time. In other words, our bodies and listening apparatuses are not able in that moment to accommodate overlapping rhythms with different beginnings, middles, and endings. As a dancer, one needs a rigorous practice to facilitate such an attunement. Recent research by Laroche and colleagues (2021) extends the tradition of dance improvisation—within a more scientific frame—that was so important for the choreographers who formed the Judson Dance Theatre collective in the downtown New York dance scene between the early to mid-1960s (Banes, 1993; Burt, 2006). Giving oneself up to these environmental rhythms, as these choreographers did, meant opening the body to events and experiences outside the frame of more formal or institutionalized dance structures. For example, complex polyrhythmic sounds linked to cycles of the breath become vehicles or embodied entities that can take one into new and different temporal frameworks.

Having grown up dancing to these types of complex rhythms in a Caribbean context, I had somehow transformed them into a mode of being. In other words, I had developed a way to hold different thoughts, ideas, and emotional states rhythmically and simultaneously in my body. I could thus understand that these so-called dissonant rhythms of that mode of 'being' or 'becoming' were not dissonant at all if one understood the larger framework within which they were created and how they subsequently developed and unfolded. Thus I had to find—and at other times create—new points of alignment in my experience of different dance forms, choreographic styles, foreign languages, cultures, disciplinary frameworks, and even ways of speaking so that others could understand the complex ideas I was developing about bodies and their movements through space/time. In short, my 'performances' expanded beyond the theatre stage into the larger everyday world, a concept that has been integral to the discipline of performance studies (Carlson, 2018; Goffman, 1959; Harding & Rosenthal, 2011; Schechner, 2020). The cognitive structures associated with my ability to perceive and conceptualize time—my choreographic impetus—had moved beyond the reflexive to something that was much more complex (Furey & Fortunato, 2017). The point here is that bodies create time in their complex movements through space; they have their own unique signatures that say a lot about how their identities are formed and the circumstances or structural frameworks that influence that development.

28.2 Time in Rehearsal Versus Time in Performance

JL: It seems to me that not all musical/dance experiences of time, from the performer's point of view, are the same. That is, certain kinds of temporal experiences happen *in performance*, but not in rehearsal or when we are practising. In the practice room we're very close to ordinary time; we're worried about getting our work done—'Do I have the twenty minutes I need to learn this passage?'—and then we have to go on to something else.

HD: You are right. One has different experiences of time in the rehearsal studio and on the performance stage. In the studio we are trying to establish a framework that we can then perform onstage in front of a live audience. The energy is quite different and so is our conception of time.

JL: Yes. So, the performance context itself gives a very different time frame, such that moments of selflessness or flow tend to happen more in performance than in rehearsal. So, when we're in that moment, in performance, does it make any sense to say is it 'longer' than regular time or 'shorter'?

HD: We measure our time because of physical manifestations, like the movements of the planetary bodies and their effects on light and temperature during different seasons. We also measure our time according to how much we've divided those measured sequences into—hours, minutes, and seconds—or how long we have to do a particular task, and so induce ourselves into a specific kind of time frame. But if you were to ask me, during one of those special performance moments, 'How long were you in that zone, or having that sense of flow?', I couldn't really tell you. That kind of time depends on what is happening in the environment at that moment: the audience you have, the state of mind you are in, the place you are performing in, for example.

JL: So do you think, then, along the lines of this kind of altered temporal experience that a performer can have, can the audience have anything like it, or is the temporal experience of an audience inherently different?

HD: An audience is not just sitting there. Hopefully, they are co-experiencing something with you. You are drawing them into an energized space, and you are also feeding off their energy. Something happens in that energized space that affects everyone who enters it. So when somebody comes to you after a show and says, 'You reminded me of when I first heard that song 30 years ago in Stockholm' or something like that, you know you've affected that person's sense of space and time by your actions. So yes, I think the experience of the audience in that sense can be analogous. And again, for the audience the question becomes: 'How can you tell how long or how far you've gone?'

28.3 Kinaesthetic Empathy, or Moving With the Dancers We See

JL: There's a lot of music research on rhythmic entrainment where musicians, dancers, and audience members collectively feel the same beat or rhythm pattern together. And in some ways we can move our bodies in the same way, at least to some extent, tapping our toes or nodding our heads. But it's not the same when

I'm watching dance. One of the marvels is the dancers are doing things I *can't* do, movement-wise. So how is it that we are able to inwardly move along with the dancers?

HD: You're bringing in the relationship between haptics and proprioception into how dancers engage with the audience. In dance we have something called 'kinaesthetic empathy'.[1] Basically that's the ability to sense the movements of the dancer in one's own body even if one cannot move with the same expertise. There is a kind of virtual haptics if you will. You are touched by what you see, what you feel, and what you imagine.

For example, if you do any kind of movement, practice, any kind of full body movement—let's say, for example, you jog, or you run in the morning—and after you jog or you run, you stretch out your body, you stretch out your hamstring or the muscles of your back. What you do in any kind of movement practice is to make yourself aware of your muscular structure, you're aware of how these muscle groups pull on ligaments and tendons, how much it hurts, or what kind of pleasure you get. As you become more involved in your own practice, your awareness grows and you are able to create, in a sense, a virtual body (or, avatar, if you wish) that dances along with the performer. It is through that virtual body you are able to experience kinaesthetic empathy. If the energies are right, you become linked to the performer onstage.

JL: So, this virtual body, is this the substrate for 'metakinesis', the term that the dance critic and theorist John Martin (1933) talked about?

HD: Yes, metakinesis or kinaesthetic empathy, that's the basis of it. You know, for example, that you can reach to the side without looking and know exactly where your cup of coffee is—your awareness is like a measuring device. And even if you knock that cup over, you know, roughly where it is. You also know exactly how to hold it—the fingers grab it. All of these things that we do on a daily basis, it's like we're constantly training this virtual body. Thus, you have a really rigorous practice like dance, it just means that your virtual body, or avatar, may not be as sophisticated in terms of what it can do.

JL: I would suppose that as a choreographer one also has a sense of 'kinaesthetic empathy' when you are working with dancers on a piece. How do you communicate in terms of 'Yes, that's it, that's the timing and movement I want!' or 'No, not quite'?

HD: When I lived in Germany I did a project with a Czech director in Freiburg, and he had a Buddhist monk lead us in tai chi exercises twice a week as a part of our preparation and training. When I was younger, I used to train in Shotokan karate, but practising tai chi in Freiburg was, I think, the first time in many years, that I actually had this kind of deliberate, almost mental, slow-moving training, wherein you go from moving very slowly to get the trajectory of a movement, and then very fast and dynamic. So, in that way we're always working through the material in a dynamic way. When I work with dancers, I give them what I call a controlled or structured improvisation; I give them some material, and then I allow them to play with the material for a while. They're just moving and moving, and when I see something, or a potential for something, I say 'Yes, do that!' or 'Yes, let's explore that'. You're looking for something that catches you, something that is 'true', and then you grab onto it.

When you get to the time of performance, the choreographer knows they have to give up the piece to the dancers, but sometimes we don't want to give it up. We want to control how the piece runs, but at a certain point we have to give it up and let the dancers own it. But since we can never predict where it will go, we want to remain in control as long as possible. But we know we have to give it up. At the same time the dancers are silently saying, 'Just leave it to us . . . trust us'. Afterward there is this huge relief, because we are pleased with what they do, because there is something else that happens that is beyond what we've been seeing in the rehearsal space.

JL: Trust is very important, not just in our fellow musicians and dancers, but also in ourselves. As a musician, I know if I want to play or improvise very rapidly, I cross a temporal threshold where I can no longer control each and every individual motion—my brain can't keep up with them anymore. But the body knows, and I have to trust that my body will perform these things correctly. I just have to think of the entire gesture, or even maybe the initial premise and the goal.

28.4 Time in Music and Time in Dance

HD: What you just said brings me to another way of thinking about time. At a certain point in my choreographic career, I almost entirely stopped choreographing to established musical works and started working mostly with composers on original pieces. My process is so fluid and so experimental that I want to make my own structure. I record all my rehearsals, and on my way home, I drop off these videos at the composer's, because I don't want to be limited by a previous musical structure, a structure that says 'These are the number of beats you have. This is how you need to negotiate those beats. This is the length of the piece'.

When I started working like that, my pieces became much longer; whereas previously a piece might be 15 to 20 minutes long, it became 45 minutes to an hour, according to how we've been working through the choreographic material. Now, I still choreograph to specific pieces of music, if I find a piece of music that I really, really like. And if I have a gig to do, I go back to that old way of dancemaking.

When I am choreographing, I want to see who the dancer is that I'm working with. I want not just their technique—I want to know the identity of that person. And when I start doing that, the length of the piece I am creating changes because I discover new things about the dancers that I can play with. So, the way of exploring time in a rehearsal very often depends on things like, 'Well, what am I looking for?' And if I don't know what I'm looking for that is absolutely fine. I'll find something that will tell me 'This is what I'm looking for'. So it's really curious that I can start without a fixed direction but get to a place or a question that has always intrigued or interested me.

JL: This makes perfect sense to me, because when you say you want to discover who the dancers really are when you are creating dance works, when you are dancing to someone else's music, you have to move with that music, and in a sense, you are moving along with—and in a manner specified by—the musician who creates it. So, if you take the music away, I imagine that while it is a challenge for the dancer(s), it is also liberating, because you do not have to inhabit someone else's movements. On the other hand, perhaps there are pieces of music you encounter, and when you hear them, you immediately want to figure out how to dance to them . . .

HD: Yes, sometimes I can tell with dancers who are really, really, really good, you can see how they play with the music with all the subtleties. That dancer becomes another instrument with the music. The choreographer George Balanchine was perfect at doing that. In many of those performances, I would see the subtlety of a dancer who approached a piece of music in this way, and that in itself is a beauty to look at, especially when you know the music very well.

JL: Right, and I think that's because it's like a musician who has a distinctive personality, as when Glenn Gould plays Bach—you are hearing Bach, and you are also hearing Gould's voice and their identities are crystal clear. It's Gould's ability to inhabit the Bach and still be himself, which means that he knows the Bach so well that his own voice comes through.

HD: There is a beautiful sculpture of a woman that sits at the back of the Plaça de Frederic Marès in Barcelona. I remember watching that statue on two separate occasions; once when the park was open and well kept, and a second time when it was closed and overgrown. The second time the statue seemed like an imprisoned woman. I later decided to choreograph a solo with music by Astor Piazzola and that statue as part of a suite of dances that was based on images I collected from the city of Barcelona.[2] This is an example of a piece of music that's really fixed, and an image that was clearly coming together. Both had these wonderful nuances, and when you are able to find dancers who are capable of playing with all of these nuances you jump at the opportunity.

28.5 The Science of Time and the Practice of Dance

JL: So, to conclude as broadly as we started, what do you think the performing arts can learn from the psychology and neuroscience of time perception, and vice versa?

HD: If psychology is the study of the mind and the how's and why's of human behaviour, and neuroscience the study of the how's and why's of the human nervous system, then perhaps these disciplines can support dance and choreography as the study of behaviours of human bodies as they are motivated by thoughts that allow them to move through all kinds of environments. How, for example, do we learn about the nature of these spaces and our bodies' interactions with other objects or entities in those spaces? Since one of the fundamental assertions I make about human movement is that it is the unfolding of thought that creates a unique relationship to space, time, and consciousness, I believe the disciplines of psychology and the neurosciences can be useful to the dancer/choreographer.

However, this is where we have to be very careful about the difference in these approaches. The assumptions of the dancer and choreographer are often very different from those of the psychologist and the neuroscientist. I am reminded of Michael Shermer's advice about the power that theory has to shape the researcher's observations (Shermer, 1997). Shermer warned against the popular use of scientific theories to explain how the perceptions of an observer can shape what is being observed. He also argued that the context of the person and the belief systems they are embedded in are important considerations as to what can be learned. I believe disciplines and practices turn into belief systems that need to be questioned both in theory and in practice. In this case, the efficacy of any dance or choreographic practice can be questioned by relocating it within other frameworks, in this case within the experiments conducted in psychology and neuroscientific laboratories or using frameworks from physics, chemistry, or the computing sciences, for example. But one also has to keep in mind the environments of the theatre, site-specific performance spaces, and the lived experiences of the dancers or choreographers, and their expressive and communicative intentions. That way, we would move closer to asking more focused questions and getting better results for our experiments about how people think, behave, and respond in the context of dance. If experimental studies reduce dance to simply a form to practise being/becoming good at, or a technique to be analysed for its stylistic content, then key information will be missed.

Notes

1. Kinaesthetic empathy is a term that developed out of the work of critic John Martin (1933, 1939, 1963) and was extended by a host of other writers such as Ann Daly (1992) and Dee Reynolds (2012).
2. https://www.henrydaniel.ca/tango

References

Banes, S. (1993). *Democracy's body: Judson dance theater, 1962–1964*. Duke University Press.
Burt, R. (2006). *Judson dance theater: Performative traces*. Routledge.

Carlson, M. (2018). *Performance: A critical introduction* (3rd ed.). Routledge.

Daly, A. (1992). Dance history and feminist theory: Reconsidering Isadora Duncan and the male Gaze. In L. Senelick (Ed.), *Gender and performance: The presentation of difference in the performing arts* (pp. 239–259). Tufts University/University Press of New England.

Furey, J., & Fortunato, V. (2017). The theory of mindtime. In R. Penrose, D. Chopra, & B. Carter (Eds.), *How consciousness became the universe: Quantum physics, cosmology, neuroscience, parallel universes* (2nd ed., pp. 286–308). Science Publishers.

Goffman, E. (1959). *The presentation of self in everyday life.* Doubleday.

Harding, J. M., & Cindy, R. (2011). *The rise of performance studies: Rethinking Richard Schechner's broad spectrum.* Palgrave Macmillan.

Laroche, J., Himberg, T., & Bachrach, A. (2021). *Making time together: An exploration of participatory time making through collective dance improvisation.* https://hal.archives-ouvertes.fr/hal-03332023/

Martin, J. (1933). *The modern dance.* A. S. Barnes.

Martin, J. (1939). *Introduction to the dance.* Dance Horizons.

Martin, J. (1963). *John Martin's book of the dance.* Tudor Publishing.

Maboungou, Z. (2005). *Heya danse! Poétique, didactique et historique de la danse africaine.* CICIHCA Editions.

Reynolds, D. (2012). *Kinesthetic empathy in creative and cultural practices.* Intellect Books.

Schechner, R. (2020). *Performance studies: An introduction* (4th ed). Routledge.

Shermer, M. (1997). *Why people believe weird things: Pseudoscience, superstition, and other confusions of our time.* W. H. Freeman & Co.

29

Music Is a Unique Artform Because of the Temporal Aspect

Kent Nagano in conversation with Clemens Wöllner

29.1 Preparing to Perform in Time

CLEMENS WÖLLNER (CW): Music has been described as a temporal art *par excellence*, and timing and tempo are central [see Kozak, this volume]. You are known to be highly meticulous in your preparation for performance, particularly with regards to tempi. At the same time, some musicians say that you leave room for temporal changes in the concert during the performance. How do you decide how fast or slow the music should be?

KENT NAGANO (KN): It's important to remember that preparation, rehearsal, and study are absolutely essential for any performance of meaning and quality. It is this never-ending process that allows the artistic depth from which comes the expressive freedom of artistry in a performance. Taking a detour, abbreviating, or omitting this phase will bring the integrity of the performance into question. However, as important as this preparatory process is, it is different from the performance itself. Performance is the moment when true music making is created and communicated with an audience. Nearly all colleagues whom I know would agree that the music itself takes on a life of its own at that performance, and if one does not allow that life to take place, then there will be consequences. Maybe that's what we are referring to: one must allow the freedom of the music to develop at that moment, at that time, and allow the inspiration of that moment to come out of the dialogue between the composer, the interpreter, and the public. There is a conversation taking place in real time, and that is why many performers, including myself, get so nervous before every performance. One can do everything possible to prepare well, but a performance is a performance, and as the dialogue unfolds live, it is not possible to control all of its aspects. Perhaps this is a part of what makes music so universal.

CW: So a performance is always a new situation, you communicate with the audience, and I can imagine that it is a special moment when there is this sense of interconnectedness. Would you say, nevertheless, that there is anything like objective time [see Wittmann, this volume], or in musical terms, a 'best time' like *tempo giusto* [see London, this volume], something that we should strive for or

Kent Nagano in conversation with Clemens Wöllner, *Music Is a Unique Artform Because of the Temporal Aspect*
In: *Performing Time*. Edited by: Clemens Wöllner and Justin London, Oxford University Press. © Oxford University Press 2023.
DOI: 10.1093/oso/9780192896254.003.0030

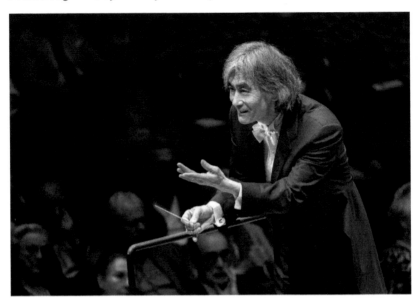

Figure 29.1 Kent Nagano in the Elbphilharmonie concert hall, Hamburg, May 2022. Photo: Marcelo Hernandez.

that would be ideal? Or is it always dependent on the situation, on the musicians, perhaps the audience?

KN: Performance sometimes requires remarkable discipline; because, as an interpreter, as a performer, one must strive to maintain (even though it may sound strange) an element of distance that is necessary, even though one is thoroughly committed and involved emotionally, physically, intellectually, and spiritually [Figure 29.1]. As important as it would be for the performer to be moved, it is the audience who must receive the full possibilities and potential of communication. The content of musical communication is complex, and you've only played and performed well if the audience connects with these emotional, physical, intellectual, and spiritual dimensions. But becoming overly emotional, to limit oneself to purely intellectual communication, to lose oneself physically, brings with it the risk of distraction, which results in compromising the content of what the audience receives. So, while a part of the role of an interpreter is to be profoundly involved, at the same time, one strives to retain an aspect of objectivity, simultaneously, which only an element of distance can provide. This is an extremely difficult balance—sometimes we don't succeed, but it is the ideal.

29.2 Performances Open Up Virtual Realities

CW: We know that for the audience, but also sometimes for performers, music may change our sense of time, our feeling of time passing [see Droit-Volet & Martinelli, this volume; Knowles & Ashley, this volume]. So, for instance, time

seems to run more quickly when we are listening to music we enjoy, but sometimes durations also seem to be longer for complex music. In other words, we feel
that the dimensions of time, and to some extent, space, change when listening
to music [see Wöllner, this volume]. There is also some evidence that time may
change when we're performing [see Bläsing, this volume; Jensenius, this volume],
for example when we're in so-called flow-states. Would you like to say something
about your own experiences in this regard?

KN: Yes, we are entering a period when many people have a marked interest and
fascination with digitally produced virtual reality, and we witness many people
making investments in technology to further the dimensions of this so-called
virtual world—in many ways it is presented as an ideal world. But is it truly? One
only needs to listen to a great performance of Beethoven to be taken into an ideal
world, a parallel world, a virtual world that all would agree is ideal. To this point,
everybody whom I know who has gone to a performance of exceptional quality
has, for a moment, been taken out of the concert hall in which they have been sitting. When this happens, one forgets that there was *Stau* [German: 'traffic jam'],
that they had an argument with their boss, that taxes are due, or that the subway
was on strike—you forget all this *Ärger* [German: 'annoyance'] and irritation.
One will go someplace else for just a moment, and then, eventually you return
from this special ideal world—and where have you been during this time, these
10 minutes, half hour, or even longer? Where has time gone while one has been
gone? They have been in a virtual world.

CW: So music opens a virtual world.

KN: It opens a doorway to a different universe. Everyone who has heard a great performance has had this experience. It happens, organically, fluidly and often.

CW: In other words, we forget the here and now, in a way. And what do you think it is
in the music that leads to these experiences, is it possible to pinpoint it? We know,
of course, that Messiaen stressed the importance of rhythm, being based on different time durations or filled intervals. When you were working with him personally, did you engage in conversations about these aspects, and about timing in
music more generally?

KN: Most fortunately, music is not an exact science. It would be impossible to discuss music only in mathematical terms or only in objective dimensions. And in
this way my work with Messiaen was much more what we might call *Handwerk*
[German: 'craft'] where you learn through conversation, you learn through repetition, you learn through the master observing the student and making comments.
Through this process, one gradually absorbs the aesthetic, content, syntax, style,
and the spirit of what the composer is communicating through his/her art. It is
our responsibility to learn the empirical data, we must know the score perfectly,
memorize the metronome *Zeichen* [German: 'marks'], we must perfectly know
and understand the harmony, how the rhythms function, the modality—but this
is not knowing the music. Information is not enough. As a musician, this is only
the beginning and there needs to be much more for an artistic process to take

place. For me, this very important developmental period with Olivier Messiaen was when I was able to develop sensitivity towards dimensions far beyond the empirical data. But the paradox is that one can only approach this level of artistry if one has already long researched and understood the concrete information and the levels of empirical knowledge and then committed them to memory.

Also, it's important to remember, that in this discussion we are referring to masterpieces when we speak of classical music repertoire. Those masterpieces are the exception. The vast majority of music, while perhaps unique, or inspired, or interesting are not masterpieces. And that implies that much music that we might be exposed to does not have the capacity to move us in the multidimensional ways masterpieces do. Masterworks capture the essence of humanism, the ideals of the *Aufklärung* [German: 'the Enlightenment']. Times change, style and fashion change, *Epoche* [German: 'era'] changes, but fundamental human values remain the same. That is why it is said that music is a 'universal language', a language which 'flies' over entire boundaries, physical and metaphysical: Beethoven lives in San Francisco. He also lives in Tokyo, New York, Beijing, Chicago. Of course, on one level one is speaking metaphorically; however, on the level of *Inhalt* [German: 'content'], Beethoven's music lives, thrives, and inspires universally. It could be said that these ideals of the *Aufklärung*, the ideals of humanism, are what allow the great, exceptional music to exist and travel outside of time. The masterworks are always in fashion—free of trends, mode, popular fads, or era.

cw: I completely agree, as these are some of the fundamental questions that brought me to study and research music myself. I believe, and I would like to hear your thoughts on this, that music can tell us something about fundamental human experiences, such as the one of time passing. In other words, the idea that music is over at the moment when you hear it. But, at the same time, we can hear the past, present, future within the musical moment [see Kozak, this volume; Noble et al., this volume; Wöllner, this volume]. We have memorized what we've just heard, and anticipate what is next. These psychological processes of working and long-term memory as well as prediction of the future are certainly at the core of musical appreciation. On a wider scale, we may connect with other periods in history, with the music our ancestors have heard, something of their time becomes very lively again. So, music is fundamentally related to how we might experience time.

kn: Yes, if we can hear the past through music, which nearly everyone can and does, we hear the past while we are anchored in actuality as well as in the future. In our great repertoire, one has a sense of what the next note, rhythm, or phrase should be or will be. In a way, one is already living there in the future, while one at the same time is also in the present. This existential experiencing, hearing sound only that is in the past, has been long discussed and remarked upon. It has been argued that when we hear the past and recognize it, we sense our identity, from where we came, we are aware of a *Wertesystem* [German: 'a value system']. *Schönheit*—beauty—in itself reflects a *Wertesystem*, as does our sense of timing, dissonance, and resolution. When these factors occur, they at times confirm—a *Bestätigung*—in the concert or idea of who we are. This is part of what makes music such a fascinating artform. It is not saying music is greater or less great than the other artforms, but it is unique because of this temporal aspect.

29.3 Allowing Music and Dance to Breathe

CW: This brings me to another of my questions, and this relates to your work with ballet. We know from many research studies that what we hear may influence what we see, and vice versa [see Doelling et al., this volume; Maes & Leman, this volume]. Music may not only emotionally shape what we see, but may also structure temporal experiences. More specifically, I am familiar with the performances of *Turangalîla* and, more recently, the Beethoven II project you conducted here in Hamburg. How important is it for you, in these collaborations with John Neumeier, to keep the exact timing? Is it more necessary than in concerts or in opera?

KN: Accompanying ballet requires a specialized set of skills. At times, the choreography and its tempo requirements can go against the natural organic rhythm or timing inherent in a work of music. Also, as we have said, when performing music there is an essential element of spontaneity. If one is not skilled, there is a risk of an artificiality in making certain that the tempo, breathing, and phrasing of a performance would be identical in another performance. The specialists of ballet accompaniment are able to maintain musical integrity in spite of the limitations that choreography might impose upon musical constructs. This was an important lesson to learn during my time as a music student while I was employed as a ballet rehearsal pianist, and is largely a reason why I personally do not conduct much ballet in general.

John Neumeier has an unusually deep knowledge of music and creates movement that breathes in ways which are organically sensitive to the musical score. His choreography also has inherent flexibility such that it allows aspects of spontaneity. His aesthetic, to me, is remarkable in that it seems to provide a foundation towards each evening having a unique 'life' of its own. One never feels repetition in a series of performances. Practically speaking, if the musical flow is slightly different than it was the night before, the dancers and choreography interact and are inspired by the music as a living partner. Of course, there will not be a radical interpretive difference between performances, but there will be thousands and thousands of micro variants. John Neumeier is an exceptional artist, he is a great chamber music partner and it has been unusually inspiring to collaborate with him, now twice with discussions of a third time project. In the current ballet, John Neumeier doesn't call the evening a ballet or choreography, he calls it 'Beethoven-Projekt II'. And he didn't call our first collaboration the 'Turangalîla ballet', he called it 'Turangalîla'. In this sense, his thoughts reflect the concept of a total art form which combines music, theatre, and movement. In our work together, I have never sensed an imposition of choreography to a musical soundtrack, where the music is present to serve the choreography—rather one feels no border or separation between the disciplines of music and movement.

CW: He has a very musical eye, I would say.

KN: Yes, a genuine sensitivity to music. From our many conversations, he has shared his fascination with and love of music, as well as his long, deep, and complex relationship with it. Music inspires him and, as mentioned several times, he in turn allows it to live artistically independent. With regard to these particular productions that you mention, we are so very fortunate in Hamburg to have John Neumeier and to have had his deep commitment to our city. To return to my experience as a ballet pianist while I was a student at music school—during this time I not only played ballet class but I was also allowed to participate in choreography rehearsals, which I recall required a certain discipline. A part of learning to collaborate with my colleagues through music, such that they could effectively rehearse their movement, meant developing an understanding that inappropriate interpretive freedom could be distracting. To take a Beethoven symphony and use it as ballet accompaniment is perhaps much less natural in that Beethoven did not conceive of it an accompaniment. Yet with John Neumeier's choreography, we musicians did not sense aesthetic conflict whatsoever.

CW: Although maybe the Seventh is the most danceable one, I would say. I mean it is full of movement, in my ear.

KN: Well, all of the symphonies of Beethoven are full of movement, and are full of historic dance rhythms.

CW: Would you say that the kind of being transported to a different world that you mentioned earlier is different when you *hear* Beethoven's Seventh performed, as opposed to hearing it and seeing dancers moving to it [cf. Bläsing, this volume]? Perhaps, since people are increasingly used to an enormous number of quickly changing visual images every day, seeing something while listening to music may guide and help their imagination, and likely also their attentional span. What would you say, is there something fundamentally different about the experience of only listening, in comparison to listening and seeing a performance?

KN: For me, having a pure audio experience of listening to the Seventh Symphony (or any great repertoire during the concert for that matter) is never an experience involving only what you hear. Attending a concert is a social experience, and on many levels one is interacting with others offering a real texture that is never the same. Often one finds oneself seated next to someone different from the last concert, which affects the collective response to a performance beyond a personal opinion. Collectively we involuntarily sense and sometimes verbally share sensations: 'The ensemble doesn't really seem in form tonight', or 'That was remarkable—the orchestra and conductor were completely engaged in the music'. As an audience, having that audio experience together does not imply that visual aspects are also active. Our auditory reception engages our imagination and provides enormously active visual stimulation in our minds. It is quite a different experience from seeing something concretely represented on the stage. When this happens, one part of our imagination is less active because of concrete visual stimulation. At times, we might find an opera staging distracting to the music because of a concrete visual representation, which counters our own imagined ideal. But if the choreography or staging is great, it can also open up a different world of imagination. In witnessing masterful choreography, one can suddenly be transported to another land, or another culture, or another imaginary space. Many have shared their experience with the Neumeier 'Beethoven-Projekt II' and explained that they suddenly were taken to some fantasy land, a new world, beyond the limits of what they visually perceived. In this way the concrete visual stimulus was an impulse rather than an end result.

CW: I had the same experience. It was really different from just hearing it on a CD or in a concert. The performance was something completely new, of course. For some passages in the music, I heard the music differently than any time before, and I believe the dancers' movements made me aware of these elements. And also, being in a concert and seeing the conductor shaping the music can have a similar impact for an audience, I believe. It could be a bit like a choreography also for the audience, and help them understand and enjoy the music.

KN: Perhaps. It was interesting to speak with the piano and the violin soloists in the Beethoven-Projekt II. They perform very difficult repertoire, but they are also part of the choreography because the dancers are reacting to them and they to the dancers. Both soloists were explaining that, at the beginning, it was very challenging, because they have such close physical contact with the dancers, who were coming up to them and interacting with them as characters. They, of course, must respond in a choreographed way. They explained that it was challenging to have to adapt to that sort of world of performance where, visually, it brought impulses that are not normal to music performers. We usually do have a visual stimulus, but not often in the form of a dancer. They explained that they both learned how to adjust to it, and then use it as an impulse and source of inspiration—that was very interesting.

CW: Yes, it was amazing. I had the feeling that, if I had to play the piano there, I would have gotten quite distracted, so it was fascinating how they kept just playing and performing.

29.4 Being Together in Time

CW: Research in my field has shown that being in synchrony with other people and being at the same time, be it in a musical ensemble, dancing together, or even walking together in time, may lead to social cohesion [see Laroche et al., this volume; Woolhouse, this volume]. This relates to the more humane aspects we have been talking about before. So, would you agree that being in synchrony is key to social connectedness, also in music?

KN: In music we use a word which perhaps could mean the same, but we say 'to be in *ensemble*'—to be together—which, in a way, suggests synchronization. However, it also implies that one has opened up towards and is in a state of awareness of one's colleagues, that you are able to not only be an individual. As a performer, it is essential that one is an individual, but an individual who is also a part of something larger, an ensemble. It is a state that does not necessarily come without practice and is something that can deepen and mature. The *Philharmonisches Staatsorchester Hamburg*, for example: it is astonishing to see that within some of the colleagues who have been in the orchestra for 25, 30, or 40 years and beyond, how great their awareness is of one another. They've known each other so well that they can musically sense how to be in perfect ensemble with each other. In my opinion, ensemble is something that nearly all humans are innately capable of experiencing, but one must develop it.

CW: And it's like reaching a common goal, or being together. It's interesting to hear your thoughts on a musician being an individual and at the same time being one among others and connected. Research has indeed increasingly investigated joint actions in music [see Goebl & Bishop, this volume]. How do musicians reach this sense for each other in an ensemble?

KN: Part of it is just a heightened awareness. In German there's this wonderful word that we don't have in English: *Ahnung* [translatable as 'intuition', 'feel for']. It's just such a wonderful word, because, it's not particularly scientific.

CW: Probably not, and I'm not using it much! It's a very poetic, 19th-century poem word, I would say.

KN: It's what is vital, it's absolutely integral to making good music. Every musician that I know and admire, has developed this to a very acute level.

CW: Fascinating, this certainly relates to empathic skills as well and attention. In comparison, would you say it's perhaps less important simply to be 'on time'?

KN: Well, you can be 'on time' in a number of different ways. It could be defined as being technically or mechanically together in a vertical dimension. But music is much more. Such a definition is far from the art form's existential being, purpose, priority, or goal. Those elements which allow us to express ourselves as humans— *Inhalt* [German: 'content'], emotional expression, direction, line, structure, architecture, or form, harmony—all require a different relationship and understanding of being 'on time'. Experiments have been done by neuroscientists with robotic piano performances, analysing what the difference between mechanical perfection and our human senses are as an ideal. One of them, Dr Daniel Levitin, has published a book on it [see Levitin, 2006, *This is Your Brain On Music*, Penguin]. According to his explanation, that is why a computer that is playing the piano doesn't sound like a human that is playing the piano. You can program everything, but those incremental elements of imperfection are what makes a piece perfect for us as a listener. So, you can play together, but if it's just purely mechanical playing together, that's not music anymore.

CW: Yes, of course, for many genres it's often the deviations from strict metronomic timing, the so-called microtiming, which makes music expressive, interesting, and human. In other words, performing music together in time is definitely much more than simply being together on time in a mechanical way.

KN: To come back to the word I was using, it means to be in *ensemble*, to really be together.

30

Timing, Tempo, and Rhythm

Evidence From the Laboratory and the Concert Stage

Stewart A. Copeland in conversation with Daniel J. Levitin

30.1 Tempo

STEWART A. COPELAND (SAC): As I see it, we have three general topics or zones of inquiry to discuss: groove, that is to say, rhythm; tempo; and the perception of time passing. I don't believe I have anything novel to say about the third one—I probably have the same subjective experience of time passing as you do. If you're busy, it goes by faster. If you're bored, it takes forever. The tempo part I'm really bad at. Here I am, a professional timekeeper, and yet I have a deeply subjective perception of tempo, which changes from moment to moment.

DANIEL J. LEVITIN (DJL): That can help a band or hinder it, depending on whether your bandmates share that perception. It's been reported that there was tension between you and Sting, who had very different conceptions of what it meant to express a song through tempo. Sting preferred the tempo to be rigid, at least from the drums. I assume that's because that predictability would facilitate him being able to place the bass notes and his vocals either slightly ahead of or behind the beat depending on the context and the emotions he wanted to convey. Your view was that tempo should flow and breathe, as you read the room and read the moment. You wanted tempo that was *emotionally accurate*, Sting wanted what you called *algebraically accurate*.

SAC: Sting actually had a very practical consideration, which is he has to be able to sing all the syllables of his beautiful words. And that's the final arbiter for me. I play in a band where we have hit songs that he wrote, and they're damn clever lyrics. I'd like the audience to be able to hear him comfortably do his thing.

Take a song like 'So Lonely', one of the ones that I was the most egregious sinner on, speeding up in the choruses. I wasn't aware I was doing it. But when I set a click to it, I can see how much the tempo goes up and down. We actually tried to play it with a click, but when it came to the choruses, I would speed up to meet my *subjective* feeling of what the tempo is. I'm supposed to be the yardstick—the guy who indicates for the other two (and for everyone else in the room), where the beats are going to land and at what tempo they shall happen. The click stays on

Stewart A. Copeland in conversation with Daniel J. Levitin, *Timing, Tempo, and Rhythm* In: *Performing Time*. Edited by: Clemens Wöllner and Justin London, Oxford University Press. © Oxford University Press 2023. DOI: 10.1093/oso/9780192896254.003.0031 and I'm surprised. With the click going, it felt like the song slowed down in a most disastrous way—like all energy had left the building. Sting didn't hear it that way at all. When we played with the click he said, 'Wow! I'm enjoying this chorus for the first time ever!'

So clearly the very concept of tempo is very subjective.

DJL: Yes, Justin London showed experimentally that the tactus—the place where people *feel* the beat, is not the same as subjective tempo (London, 2011). His paper was actually called 'Tactus ≠ Tempo', and there's an old paper that shows that people with schizophrenia and depression were more likely to experience tempo in a rigid and less adaptable way, compared to people with no psychiatric conditions (Perilli, 1995).

SAC: And many composers only indicate subjective tempo, with markings like *Allegro moderato* or *Largo*, and Wagner gave no tempo markings in his later works:

I supplied my early operas with lavish tempo indications and employed a metronome in order to exclude (so I supposed) any possibility of mistake. The result was that when I had cause to complain of a stupid tempo in, for example, *Tannhäuser*, the defence was invariably made that my metronome mark had been scrupulously observed. This brought home how unsafe it was to apply mathematics to music. I never used the metronome again (Wagner, 1861/1979, p. 58).

I say, yes, absolutely, and that doesn't have as much to do with the *tempo* as to do with the rhythm. The tempo can be very fast, but the rhythm on that fast tempo can be slow. Take heavy metal bands. They play so fast and they've subdivided it so minutely, that actually a larger framework takes over and so it seems, subjectively, slow. Our subjective perception of tempo is bound up with our perception of how much energy is being expended. Look at Justin London's chapter in the current volume:

Musicians know there is more to tempo than just beats per minute, and that simple correlations between BPM [beats per minute] and tempo, as well as between the rate of surface activity and tempo, are problematic ... Taking the complex constellation of auditory and non-auditory cues into account, an energistic account of tempo is developed, with tempo as a summary judgement of energistic cost(s) of musical behaviour, or more precisely, of the effort involved in moving the way the music seems to move. Thus musical tempo is not 'How fast does the music go?' but rather, 'How much energy and effort is required for me to keep up with it? (London, this volume)

DJL: Lots of music musicians play around with tempo and their sense of time. Louis Bellson and Buddy Rich were very precise. You and Art Blakey allow tempo to be governed by the song and what you're feeling in the moment, including reading the room.

SAC: Yes, but . . . there is something to be said for being predictable. The most effective rhythm that gets humans to throw aside all decorum and shake their pudenda at each other in a public place—the thing that makes them do that most profoundly—is a machine. And I suspect that what's going on here is predictability. I sit there on my drums and I watch the audience and when they know something is going to happen and it happens, you can just feel them light up.

DJL: The predictability of tempo is a big part of it, even if it changes—at that point, the performers and the audience have a shared sense of subjective tempo.

SAC: And that's why machines are so ubiquitous in dance music, because it's very easy to know when the next beat is coming. For dancers, provided they're not self-conscious, they see that beat coming down the road and they move in time with it. There's no intellectual activity, it's entirely instinctive. It seems to happen in some machine room in our brain that just triggers all by itself and is like an engine of its own that pushes our pudenda along. The chapter in this book by Doelling makes this point [see Doelling et al., this volume]: 'Rhythms are everywhere in human behaviour . . . rhythms are everywhere in biology.'

The origins of that machine room in our brain, they say, are that rhythm helps us to predict what might happen next, and to facilitate action in the event we need to do something about that impending future.

30.2 Synchronizing and Keeping the Beat

DJL: We know that humans are very good at synchronizing to rhythms (Patel & Iversen, 2014), uniquely so among primates. Dancing and tapping require predictive motor timing in two ways. First, we need to know when the next event is going to occur. Second, we need to anticipate it and send instructions to our limbs some tens of milliseconds in advance so that the actual movement will occur when we want it to.

SAC: Is it known what part of the brain represents the passage of time?

DJL: Yes and no. I'd rephrase the question to start, if I may, because we're tending to think less in terms of *parts* of the brain and more in terms of distributed neural circuits. So, 10 years ago, we would point to a part of the brain and say tempo is *here*. We used to think that the 'machine room in the brain' you invoked was composed of timekeepers in the cerebellum and in the basal ganglia (Grahn, 2012; Levitin, 2009; Wang & Wöllner, 2020). To oversimplify, the machine room/cerebellum keeps track of the timing, and predicts the temporal consequences of events (Avanzino et al., 2015), and the basal ganglia become involved to help coordinate specific movements at specific times (Di Pietro et al., 2004; Grahn & Brett, 2009; Merchant et al., 2008). Those two structures are still believed to be involved, but they might be doing less of the work than we used to think. Rich Ivry, from your alma mater [UC Berkeley] has been studying timing and the cerebellum for more than 30 years. He's come to believe that some of the more interesting cases of timing—such as dance and playing a musical instrument—are not 'done' in the cerebellum, but rather are an emergent property of system dynamics, especially the oscillatory entrainment that falls out of linked neural populations (Breska & Ivry, 2016).

SAC: But surely there are intrinsic properties of neurons themselves that are underlying this?

DJL: Yes. Temporal processing invokes a great many circuits and mechanisms; these underlie both the ability to tell time and generate temporal patterns. Timing does rely on intrinsic and general properties of neurons and neural circuits to solve temporal computations (Paton & Buonomano, 2018). Many circuits have been shown to encode elapsed time in dynamically changing patterns of neural activity and cerebellar neurons, according to lesion and imaging studies, process time in the sub-second range (Grube et al., 2010; Spencer et al., 2003; Teki et al., 2011).

SAC: When we talk about predicting where the beat will be, we're talking about the tactus, the place where people *feel* the rhythm. As a musician or dancer, once you've established it, you can play around with it. You can lay back, or get ahead of it.

DJL: Sinatra famously sang behind the beat. Punk singers would sing ahead of it. What's most interesting to me is when drummers push ahead or lay back. I always feel that Kenny Aronoff, for example, is spot on the beat.

SAC: . . . or slightly pushing ahead with his snare. Yes—that's why they hire him. Or Josh Freese [The Vandals, Guns N' Roses, Nine Inch Nails, Weezer]. Motherfuckers those guys. I don't know how they do it. Then you've got me, speeding up and slowing down with the music . . .

DJL: . . . not deliberately, though, but because it's how you hear it. Like Art Blakey. Drum machines don't do that of course, unless you go all Donald Fagen on them and start editing your recordings of them to make them more human. We tend to think a drum machine has perfect timing. After all, it is a machine. We assume the tempo of the machine is steady, that the time in between each beat is consistent without rushing or dragging. But research has shown that most drum machines and sequencers are not that steady. With errors of up to +/− 12 ms, the mean tempo deviations in these devices can be 3.5% in either direction (Perron, 1994). However, the deviations in these machines seem to go largely unnoticed by most people (including professional drummers).

SAC: For scientists, of course, it's significant, but for the proles on the dance floor, it's closer than Charlie Watts. And Charlie Watts, by the way, is close enough.

30.3 Playing Like a Machine (or Not)

DJL: Even the most professional, seasoned drummers cannot keep time like a drum machine. In a study of professional percussionists, the average discrepancy ranged between 10 and 40 ms or 2–8% of the tempo (Dahl, 2000). So, the best of the ones in that study are about twice as accurate as a drum machine—there's your Kenny Aronoff and Josh Freese—in the worst case, they're twice as variable as a drum machine.

It turns out that these small offsets are pleasing to the listener (Hennig et al., 2011, 2012) and many electronic music programs feature randomizing (or 'humanizing') functions to add imperfections back into the music. The difference though is that human beat variation is not random—that's why Fagen goes in and diddles with it. A professional drummer may shift ahead and behind the beat, but these shifts follow highly precise patterns that last for minutes. Listeners show a strong preference for these long-term correlations in beat fluctuation over the random offsets offered by machines, and those deviations follow a so-called 1/f power distribution (Hennig et al., 2011, 2012). That 1/f shows up not just in the local variations of timing we're talking about here, but in the entire, large-scale temporal coherence of a composition, including a symphony (Levitin et al., 2012). Listeners crave predictability, but also imperfection.

Speaking of Charlie Watts, the Stones always sound to me like a train that is about to jump the rails at any point but you never know where . . .

SAC: Rambling in a cool kind of way . . .

DJL: They never do actually jump the track, but it feels like they're on the verge of it.

SAC: Yes, it's teetering. Audiences love that.

DJL: It sounds like the whole rhythmic structure of the band is about to fall apart at any moment. Where does that come from? Is that due to Charlie?

SAC: That cacophony might have different root causes. It could be that the bass and guitars are swimming wildly in time—it's hard to pull that all apart. You and I are talking about the fundamental rhythm part, but then it's overlaid with a lot of cultural significance: chiefly rebellion and assertive dishevelment, which is what The Rolling Stones are all about. The beat's *here*, but in fact we're kind of, you know, skating on the edge of catastrophe. That's why jam bands thrive. With jam bands, the attraction is the *un*predictability, weirdly, which blows this whole morning's argument about predictability out of the water.

DJL: Yes, but unpredictability in the larger sense—what weird cover song they'll pull out that you've never heard them do before; unpredictable solos and breakdowns. But if you look at Phish, for example, Mike Gordon and Jon Fishman [bass and drums respectively] seem to be locked in to the beat, even as they make space for things to happen. With the Stones it's different. Do you think Charlie is not keeping a steady tempo or is that just an illusion?

SAC: I don't know because music and beat *are* an illusion. I always thought that Charlie's kick drum was on the money forward thrusting, his snare drum was slightly delayed and that tension between the forward thrusting kick and the slightly delayed snare gave it that loosey-goosey feel. It still had the forward propulsion, but that rebellious snare gave it that sexy dishevelment.

Compare that to Buddy Rich. My subjective assessment is there was no tension between the downbeat and the upbeat and the backbeat and the downbeat and anything else. It was all on the money, like a machine. In fact, a lot of people say he was too white for that reason. I don't care. Viscerally, it really transports me once again because of that predictability factor. I like it, but he did all kinds of other things—rhythmic and timbral choices—that were unpredictable. That kept it exciting.

DJL: Bringing us back to Phish.

SAC: And getting back to Art Blakey, he and drummers with that sensibility were playing just in the vicinity of the beat. They were what they like to call 'out'. And their outness was where the sex came from. This concept of the predictability is strong, but the counter predictability introduces a cultural, higher-level aspect of our appreciation of something. It's the tension between what's predictable and we know where it's going to land, spiced with a little danger here because we're skirting on the edge. That's another component probably distantly related in the human psyche. You know the thrill, adventure, danger. Why the hell do humans like danger? Why do we like skiing?

DJL: The adrenaline maybe. One of our authors in this volume argues that the experience of groove is strongest when a rhythm falls within the sweet spot between prediction and surprise.

SAC: Ah see—here I thought I was making stuff up, but of course you eggheads got there decades earlier. Maybe that rebelliousness of the Stones fucking up the rhythm and being dishevelled excites us for that, you know, the tension creates adrenaline.

But I'm just being subjective here about Charlie, Buddy, and Art. You would have to have a computer program to check it—because you and I are going to respond not to whether he's perfect or not, but whether he's *effective* or not, whether it feels good. The computer will tell us, *yeah, it just went up a notch or down a notch right here.*

DJL: Well let's take a look. Here's a computer analysis of Charlie's drum part in *Satisfaction*, using isolated drum tracks so that we're sure we know what we're getting (Figure 30.1). There are lots of ways to do this—you could get real granular and try to figure out the inter-beat interval for every beat, and even for every

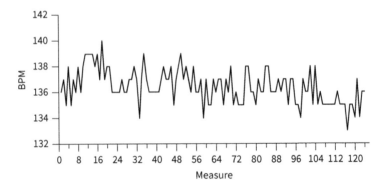

Figure 30.1 Charlie Watts' tempo in 'Satisfaction'.

instrument in each beat. But here, I just calculated the time of the first beat from bar to bar, which yielded a BPM for each bar in 4/4 time.

Here you can see his variability. Those first two bars of the recording are the guitar and bass intro with BPMs of 131.8 and 134.9, not shown here. The graph begins as the drums enter in what I'm going to call bar 1 (even though it's bar 3, this allows us to look at eight-bar phrases on the graph more easily). Charlie comes in a bit faster than the intro at 135.5 and then he's off and running. It would be nice to be able to say 'oh, he always speeds up right before a chorus' or 'coming into a new section' but the graph doesn't show this—he's listening, as it were, to the beat of a different drummer.

Here are some rough statistics (Figure 30.2). The minimum tempo is 133.2 BPM which happens in the outro in bar 119. The maximum is 140.1 BPM and occurs in bar 20, just between the pre-chorus and the chorus; that's a difference of 5.1%. The mean tempo is 136.4 with a standard deviation of 1.28, and a coefficient of variation of 0.94. Sixty-five per cent of his tempos fall within that one standard deviation, and so 65% of the time, he's playing within an astonishing 1.9%.

Charlie is symmetric in his speeding up and slowing down—roughly half the time he's playing faster than the mean (average) and half the time slower. We can visualize this with a histogram of tempos and then trying to fit them a normal distribution (Figure 30.2)

The resulting curve not only *looks* normally distributed, but passes four tests of normality (Kolmogorov–Smirnov, Shapiro–Wilk, D'Agostino–Pearson, and Anderson–Darling).

SAC: So he really *is* accurate, and that train thing you're talking about must come from the way that he speeds up and slows down, and the precise places he does it. Plus the bass and guitars could be skating around, but it's still predictable enough for everybody to have the general idea. We all stomp together. Is there research on how closely all of those stomps land together in time?

DJL: A group out of Yale (Avrunin et al., 2011) presented a paper at the ACM [Association For Computing Machinery] conference showing how people

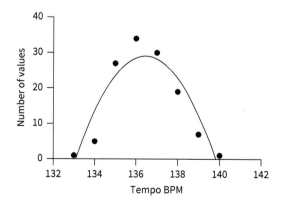

Figure 30.2 Frequency distribution of Charlie Watts' BPM in 'Satisfaction'.

perceive robot dancing. When the robot was really on the beat, they rated it as a better dancer. But interestingly, the ratings of 'most lifelike' came when the robot was only on the beat about half the time.

In my lab, we found in general that the window of simultaneity for audiovisual synchrony is about 40 ms. That means that if you're watching someone dance, their foot can hit the floor 40 ms too early or too late to be truly synchronized with the beat, and your brain will treat it as simultaneous. If *you're* doing the dancing though, the window of simultaneity for audio-tactile synchrony is tighter, at about 25 ms (Levitin et al., 2000). If we're dancing at 120 BPM—the nominal tempo of *Invisible Sun*—one beat occurs every 500 ms. That means our sensitivity of 25 ms is somewhere around a 1/16th note (a 1/20th note to be exact).

30.4 Divvying Up Time

SAC: That brings us to the other part of this conversation, the parcelling of time— how we subdivide beats and rhythms. On one timescale we recognize a 16-bar phrase or 12-bar blues, and we somehow know when we've come around to the end of a 12-bar phrase, and within that we know—or feel—a single bar. We know beats and we even know flourishes within those beats. So, the parcelling of time seems to be something that humans are very into. And that's the part that I do very expertly. And yet the proles on the dance floor—the uninitiated, the unwashed, the untalented, the unblessed—they, too, totally know how to dance to these subdivisions. They know where that downbeat's going to be, and they stomp on it with their big body mass. And then their fingers, their faces, and their necks are doing some other subdivisions of the rhythm that they're executing physically in response to the music. These spontaneous movements are generally synchronized to the beat, but also influenced by other metrical levels (Burger et al., 2014).

DJL: Petri Toiviainen, a great jazz pianist by the way, showed that dancer's movements are not all at the same level of synchrony, depending on the body part (Toiviainen et al., 2010).

SAC: That makes sense. Legs are larger and heavier than arms, you've got different centres of gravity for the limbs and head and torso.

DJL: Arm movements from the body out to the side are at the beat rate or slower, but vertical hand and torso movements occur at the beat rate. Rotation of the torso and swaying of the body from side to side occur at even slower rates. These movement rates may relate to the amount of energy expended to move, and so dancers select slower rates for parts that require more energy (Toiviainen et al., 2010). As you were saying, the length, overall size, and stiffness of a limb also constrain the natural harmonic oscillation rate and variability for movement (Lametti & Ostry, 2010).

Now here's something interesting: head movements tend to be synchronized to low-frequency sounds (e.g. the kick drum or bass guitar in popular music and jazz), whereas hand movements tend to be synchronized to high-frequency sounds (e.g. hi-hat or cymbal). When there is a clear, strong beat in the music, overall body movements tend to be more regular and stable in their timing; when the beat is weaker or less regular, body movements are also less temporally regular (Burger et al., 2014).

SAC: I imagine that professional dancers have finer control over this—they'd have to. We drummers do.

30.5 Evolving Musical Time

SAC: I'm pleased to know that many of the philosophical and theoretical questions about music perception and performance are being addressed empirically. I don't understand all of it, of course, but it seems as though the people in this field are making some interesting observations, through neuroimaging, and psychophysics. I've followed a lot of the evolutionary work and made a film about it for the BBC. As you know, archaeologists discovered a 40,000-year-old flute made from a vulture's femur in a cave in Germany (Conard et al., 2009). That is 30,000 years before the dawn of agriculture—humans didn't know how to plant things or corral animals until around 10,000 BC. We invented musical instruments before we ever got around to what you'd think would be more important, that is, food production.

The archaeologists theorized the purpose of music at that point, or at least a function of it, was to draw people together (Mithen, 2009). Music is very socially cohesive. It relies on predictability to join people together. When we know where the beat's going to be, we can all land on it. It feels good to land on that beat because everyone around us is also landing on that beat. When we all land on that beat together, we feel the power of our tribe. We bond with the larger group around us. That predictability, us all hitting that thing together, is very big. And what's the advantage for us evolutionarily speaking? Well, us 20 bonded *Homo sapiens* can kick those four Neanderthal out of the fruit tree. Human's sense of rhythm and timing makes us more socially successful as a species.

What do you think are the most interesting scientific questions on the horizon?

DJL: A number of them are ones you've raised here. *Why*, and under what circumstances, do we like rhythmic variability versus rhythmic consistency? There's still much to be done on the question of discrimination thresholds—the thresholds of simultaneity and their neural correlates. And to add some precision to the explanations and claims for music's evolutionary origins. Some of the most interesting insights may come from work on neurochemistry. We've got about 100 different neurochemicals in our brains, but only the tools to study about seven of them and so as a consequence, they get more credit than they deserve. Exploring that will be very rewarding.

SAC: I look forward to seeing what all of you come up with. This stuff is fascinating. It's fascinating to understand all that is going on as I sit on my drums and try to keep time for a living.

Acknowledgements

The authors thank Christopher Given Harrison for performing the tempo analysis of the Rolling Stones song mentioned herein, and Lindsay Anne Fleming and Alexandra Bernstein for editorial assistance.

References

Avanzino, L., Lagravinese, G., Bisio, A., Perasso, L., Ruggeri, P., & Bove, M. (2015). Action observation: Mirroring across our spontaneous movement tempo. *Scientific Reports*, 5(1), 1–9.

Avrunin, E., Hart, J., Douglas, A., & Scassellati, B. (2011). Effects related to synchrony and repertoire in perceptions of robot dance. In A. Billard, P. Kahnn, J. A. Adams, & G. Trafton (Eds.), *Proceedings of the 6th International Conference on Human–Robot Interaction* (pp. 93–100). Association For Computing Machinery.

Breska, A., & Ivry, R. B. (2016). Taxonomies of timing: Where does the cerebellum fit in? *Current Opinion in Behavioral Sciences*, 8, 282–288.

Burger, B., Thompson, M. R., Luck, G., Saarikallio, S. H., & Toiviainen, P. (2014). Hunting for the beat in the body: On period and phase locking in music-induced movement. *Frontiers in Human Neuroscience*, 8, 903.

Conard, N. J., Malina, M., & Münzel, S. C. (2009). New flutes document the earliest musical tradition in southwestern Germany. *Nature*, 460(7256), 737–740.

Dahl, S. (2000). The playing of an accent—Preliminary observations from temporal and kinematic analysis of percussionists. *Journal of New Music Research*, 29(3), 225–233.

Di Pietro, M., Laganaro, M., Leemann, B., & Schnider, A. (2004). Receptive amusia: Temporal auditory processing deficit in a professional musician following a left temporo-parietal lesion. *Neuropsychologia*, 42(7), 868–877.

Grahn, J. A. (2012). Neural mechanisms of rhythm perception: Current findings and future perspectives. *Topics in Cognitive Science*, 4(4), 585–606.

Grahn, J. A., & Brett, M. (2009). Impairment of beat-based rhythm discrimination in Parkinson's disease. *Cortex*, 45(1), 54–61.

Grube, M., Cooper, F. E., Chinnery, P. F., & Griffiths, T. D. (2010). Dissociation of duration-based and beat-based auditory timing in cerebellar degeneration. *Proceedings of the National Academy of Sciences of the United States of America*, 107(25), 11597–11601.

Hennig, H., Fleischmann, R., Fredebohm, A., Hagmayer, Y., Nagler, J., Witt, A., Theis, F. J., & Geisel, T. (2011). The nature and perception of fluctuations in human musical rhythms. *PLoS One*, 6(10), e26457.

Hennig, H., Fleischmann, R., & Geisel, T. (2012). Musical rhythms: The science of being slightly off. *Physics Today*, 65(7), 64.

Lametti, D. R., & Ostry, D. J. (2010). Postural constraints on movement variability. *Journal of Neurophysiology*, 104(2), 1061–1067.

Levitin, D. J. (2009). The neural correlates of temporal structure in music. *Music and Medicine*, *1*, 9–13. https://doi.org/10.1177/1943862109338604

Levitin, D. J., Chordia, P., & Menon, V. (2012). Musical rhythm spectra from Bach to Joplin obey a 1/ f power law. *Proceedings of National Academy of Sciences of the United States of America*, *109*(10), 3716–3720. https://doi.org/10.1073/pnas.1113828109

Levitin, D. J., MacLean, K., Mathews, M. V., Chu, L. Y., & Jensen, E. R. (2000). The perception of cross-modal simultaneity. *International Journal of Computing and Anticipatory Systems*, *5*, 323–329.

London, J. (2011). Tactus ≠ tempo: Some dissociations between attentional focus, motor behavior, and tempo judgment. *Empirical Musicology Review*, *6*(1), 43–55.

Merchant, H., Zarco, W., & Prado, L. (2008). Do we have a common mechanism for measuring time in the hundreds of millisecond range? Evidence from multiple-interval timing tasks. *Journal of Neurophysiology*, *99*(2), 939–949.

Mithen, S. (2009). The music instinct: The evolutionary basis of musicality. *Annals of the New York Academy of Sciences*, *1169*(1), 3–12.

Patel, A. D., & Iversen, J. R. (2014). The evolutionary neuroscience of musical beat perception: The Action Simulation for Auditory Prediction (ASAP) hypothesis. *Frontiers in Systems Neuroscience*, *8*, 57. https://doi.org/10.3389/fnsys.2014.00057

Paton, J. J., & Buonomano, D. V. (2018). The neural basis of timing: Distributed mechanisms for diverse functions. *Neuron*, *98*(4), 687–705.

Perilli, G. G. (1995). Subjective tempo in adults with and without psychiatric disorders. *Music Therapy Perspectives*, *13*(2), 104–109.

Perron, M. (1994). *Checking tempo stability of MIDI sequencers* [Paper presentation]. 97th Convention of the Audio Engineering Society, 10–13 November 1994, San Francisco.

Spencer, R. M., Zelaznik, H. N., Diedrichsen, J., & Ivry, R. B. (2003). Disrupted timing of discontinuous but not continuous movements by cerebellar lesions. *Science*, *300*(5624), 1437–1439.

Teki, S., Grube, M., Kumar, S., & Griffiths, T. D. (2011). Distinct neural substrates of duration-based and beat-based auditory timing. *Journal of Neuroscience*, *31*(10), 3805–3812.

Toiviainen, P., Luck, G., & Thompson, M. R. (2010). Embodied meter: Hierarchical eigenmodes in music-induced movement. *Music Perception*, *28*(1), 59–70.

Wagner, R. (1979). On conducting. In *Three Essays* (R. L. Jacobs, Trans.). Eulenburg Books. (Original work published 1861) https://guides.library.yale.edu/c.php?g=525668&p=4810780#s-lg-box-wrap per-18301061

Wang, X., & Wöllner, C. (2020). Time as the ink that music is written with: A review of internal clock models and their explanatory power in audiovisual perception. *Jahrbuch Musikpsychologie*, *29*((e67) 1–22. https://doi.org/10.5964/jbdgm.2019v29.67

Name Index

For the benefit of digital users, indexed terms that span two pages (e.g., 52–53) may, on occasion, appear on only one of those pages.

Note: Figuresare indicated by *f* following the page number

Subject Index

For the benefit of digital users, indexed terms that span two pages (e.g., 52–53) may, on occasion, appear on only one of those pages.

Note: Figures are indicated by *f* following the page number